HIV ESSENTIALS

Seventh Edition

Paul E. Sax, MD
Clinical Director
Division of Infectious Disease and HIV Program
Brigham and Women's Hospital
Professor of Medicine
Harvard Medical School
Boston, MA

Co-Editors

Calvin J. Cohen, MD, MS
Director of Research
Community Research Initiative of New England
Instructor of Medicine
Harvard Medical School
Boston, MA

Daniel R. Kuritzkes, MD
Chief, Division of Infectious Diseases
Director of AIDS Research
Brigham and Women's Hospital
Professor of Medicine
Harvard Medical School
Boston, MA

2014

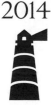

JONES & BARTLETT
LEARNING

World Headquarters
Jones & Bartlett Learning
5 Wall Street
Burlington, MA 01803
978-443-5000
info@jblearning.com
www.jblearning.com

Jones & Bartlett Learning books and products are available through most bookstores and online booksellers. To contact Jones & Bartlett Learning directly, call 800-832-0034, fax 978-443-8000, or visit our website at www.jblearning.com.

Substantial discounts on bulk quantities of Jones & Bartlett Learning publications are available to corporations, professional associations, and other qualified organizations. For details and specific discount information, contact the special sales department at Jones & Bartlett Learning via the above contact information or send an email to specialsales@jblearning.com.

Production Credits

Executive Editor: Nancy Anastasi Duffy
Senior Production Editor: Daniel Stone
Medicine Marketing Manager: Jennifer Sharp
Manufacturing and Inventory Control Supervisor: Amy Bacus

Composition: diacriTech, Chennai, India
Cover Design: Scott Moden
Printing and Binding: Cenveo, Inc.
Cover Printing: Cenveo, Inc.

ISBN-13: 978-1-284-05100-1

6048

Printed in the United States of America
17 18 16 15 14   10 9 8 7 6 5 4 3 2 1

EDITORIAL NOTE

Over the last several years, HIV treatment has improved substantially—so much so that virtually every patient who is able to take antiretroviral therapy can achieve virologic suppression, even those with extensive resistance from prior treatment eras. With the extraordinary success of currently-available regimens, emphasis has shifted in many patients from the sole goal of suppressing viremia to the long term need to prevent and manage non-HIV related complications, in particular cardiovascular disease and malignancies.

The goal of this guide is to provide practitioners actively involved in HIV care with rapid access to practical information useful for patient management. When possible, we have cited US national guidelines from the Department of Health and Human Services and the International AIDS Society–USA; these are available at aidsinfo.nih.gov or www.iasusa.org respectively, and readers are advised to check these sites for the most recent updates. We have also provided recommendations based on our interpretation of clinical trials, cohort studies, case reports, and personal experience.

We continue to dedicate this volume to people living with HIV who have partnered with us to learn how to manage this condition, and to the doctors, nurses, social workers, pharmacists, and other healthcare professionals who focus on HIV as a specialty and continue to teach us how to get better at what we do.

Paul E. Sax, MD
Calvin J. Cohen, MD, MS
Daniel R. Kuritzkes, MD

TABLES AND FIGURES

TABLE OF CONTENTS

TABLE OF CONTENTS (cont'd)

CONTRIBUTORS

Paul E. Sax, MD
Clinical Director, Division of
  Infectious Diseases and HIV Program
Brigham and Women's Hospital
Professor of Medicine
Harvard Medical School
Boston, Massachusetts

Calvin J. Cohen, MD, MS
Director of Research, Community
  Research Initiative of New England
Instructor of Medicine
Harvard Medical School
Boston, Massachusetts

Daniel R. Kuritzkes, MD
Chief, Division of Infectious Diseases
Director of AIDS Research
Brigham and Women's Hospital
Professor of Medicine
Harvard Medical School
Boston, Massachusetts

Burke A. Cunha, MD
Chief, Infectious Disease Division
Winthrop-University Hospital
Mineola, New York
Professor of Medicine
SUNY School of Medicine
Stony Brook, New York

David W. Kubiak, PharmD, BCPS
Infectious Disease Clinical Pharmacist
Brigham and Women's Hospital
Adjunct Clinical Assistant
Professor of Pharmacy
Bouvé College of Health Sciences
School of Pharmacy
Northeastern University
Boston, Massachusetts

ACKNOWLEDGMENTS

To accomplish the task of presenting the data compiled in this reference, a small, dedicated team of professionals was assembled. This team focused their energy and discipline for many months into typing, revising, designing, illustrating, and formatting the many chapters that make up this text. We wish to acknowledge Monica Crowder Kaufman for her important contribution. We would also like to thank the many contributors who graciously contributed their time and energy.

Paul E. Sax, MD
Calvin J. Cohen, MD, MS
Daniel R. Kuritzkes, MD

NOTICE

ABBREVIATIONS FOR ANTIRETROVIRAL AGENTS

3TC	lamivudine	FTC	emtricitabine
ABC	abacavir	IDV	indinavir
ATV	atazanavir	LPV/r	lopinavir/ritonavir
d4T	stavudine	MVC	maraviroc
ddC	zalcitabine	NFV	nelfinavir
ddI	didanosine	NVP	nevirapine
DLV	delavirdine	RAL	raltegravir
DRV	darunavir	RPV	rilpivirine
EFV	efavirenz	RTV	ritonavir
ENF	enfuvirtide	SQV	saquinavir
ETR	etravirine	TDF	tenofovir disoproxil fumarate
EVG	elvitegravir	TPV	tipranavir
EVG/c	elvitegravir/cobicistat	ZDV	zidovudine
FPV	fosamprenavir		

OTHER ABBREVIATIONS

AFB	acid fast bacilli	Enterobacteriaceae:	Citrobacter, Edwardsiella, Enterobacter, E. coli, Klebsiella, Proteus, Providencia, Salmonella, Serratia, Shigella
ALT	alanine transferase		
ANC	absolute neutrophil count		
ARC	AIDS-related complex		
ARDS	adult respiratory distress syndrome	ESR	erythrocyte sedimentation rate
ART	antiretroviral therapy	ESRD	end-stage renal disease
AST	aspartamine transferase	ET	endotracheal
β-lactams	penicillins, cephalosporins, cephamycins (not monobactams or carbapenems)	EVR	early virologic response
		FUO	fever of unknown origin
		GI	gastrointestinal
BAL	bronchoalveolar lavage	gm	gram
BID	twice daily	GU	genitourinary
ICU	intensive care unit	HSV	herpes simplex virus
CD4	CD4 T-cell lymphocyte	HU	hydroxyurea
CIE	counter-immunoelectrophoresis	I & D	incision and drainage
CMV	cytomegalovirus	IFA	immunofluorescent antibody
CNS	central nervous system	IgA	immunoglobulin A
CPK	creatine phosphokinase	IgG	immunoglobulin G
CrCl	creatinine clearance	IgM	immunoglobulin M
CSF	cerebrospinal fluid	IM	intramuscular
CT	computerized tomography	INH	isoniazid
DFA	direct fluorescent antibody	INSTI	integrase strand transfer inhibitor
DIC	disseminated intravascular coagulation		
DNA	deoxyribonucleic acid	IRIS	immune reconstitution inflammatory syndrome
DS	double strength		
e.g.	for example	IV/PO	IV or PO
ELISA	enzyme-linked immunosorbent assay	IV	intravenous
EMB	ethambutol	kg	kilogram
ENT	ear, nose, throat	L	liter

LFT	liver function test	PZA	pyrazinamide
MAC	*Mycobacterium avium* complex	q__d	every__days
mcg	microgram	q__h	every__hours
mcL	microliter	QD	once daily
mg	milligram	qmonth	once a month
mL	milliliter	qweek	once a week
min	minute	RBC	red blood cells
MRI	magnetic resonance imaging	RBV	ribavirin
MRSA	methicillin-resistant *S. aureus*	RNA	ribonucleic acid
MSSA	methicillin-sensitive *S. aureus*	RT-PCR	reverse-transcriptase polymerase chain reaction
NNRTI	non-nucleoside reverse transcriptase inhibitor	RVR	rapid virologic response
NRTI	nucleoside reverse transcriptase inhibitor	SGOT/SGPT	serum transaminases
		SLE	systemic lupus erythematosus
NSAID	nonsteroidal anti-inflammatory drug	sp.	species
OI	opportunistic infection	SQ	subcutaneous
PBS	protected brush specimen	SS	single strength
PCP	*Pneumocystis jirovecii* (carinii) pneumonia	TB	tuberculosis
		TID	three times per day
PCR	polymerase chain reaction	TMP	trimethoprim
PI	protease inhibitor	TMP-SMX	trimethoprim-sulfamethoxazole
PMN	polymorphonuclear leucocytes	VCA	viral capsid antigen
PPD	purified protein derivative	VZV	varicella zoster virus
PO	oral	WBC	white blood cells

Chapter 1
Overview of HIV Infection

OVERVIEW OF HIV INFECTION

Infection with Human Immunodeficiency Virus (HIV-1) leads to a chronic and, without treatment usually fatal infection characterized by progressive immunodeficiency, a long clinical latency period, and opportunistic infections. The hallmark of HIV disease is infection and viral replication within T-lymphocytes expressing the CD4 antigen (helper-inducer lymphocytes), a critical component of normal cell-mediated immunity. Qualitative defects in CD4 responsiveness and progressive depletion in CD4 cell counts increase the risk for opportunistic infections such as *Pneumocystis jirovecii (carinii)* pneumonia, and neoplasms such as lymphoma and Kaposi's sarcoma. HIV infection can also disrupt blood monocyte, tissue macrophage, and B-lymphocyte (humoral immunity) function, predisposing to infection with encapsulated bacteria. Direct attack of CD4-positive cells in the central and peripheral nervous system can cause HIV meningitis, peripheral neuropathy, and dementia.

More than 1 million people in the United States and 30 million people worldwide are infected with HIV. Without treatment, the average time from acquisition of HIV to an AIDS-defining opportunistic infection is about 10 years; survival then averages 1–2 years. There is tremendous individual variability in these time intervals, with some patients progressing from acute HIV infection to death within 1–2 years, and others not manifesting HIV-related immunosuppression for > 20 years after HIV acquisition. Antiretroviral therapy in particular and prophylaxis against opportunistic infections have markedly improved the overall prognosis of HIV disease. The approach to HIV infection is shown in Figure 1.1.

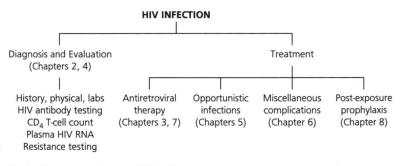

HIV INFECTION

Diagnosis and Evaluation (Chapters 2, 4)

History, physical, labs
HIV antibody testing
CD_4 T-cell count
Plasma HIV RNA
Resistance testing

Treatment

Antiretroviral therapy (Chapters 3, 7)

Opportunistic infections (Chapters 5)

Miscellaneous complications (Chapter 6)

Post-exposure prophylaxis (Chapter 8)

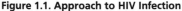

Figure 1.1. Approach to HIV Infection

STAGES OF HIV INFECTION

A. **Viral Transmission.** HIV infection is acquired primarily by sexual intercourse (anal, vaginal, infrequently oral), exposure to contaminated blood (through sharing of needles by injection drug users, less commonly transfusion of contaminated blood products), or maternal-fetal (perinatal) transmission. Sexual practices with the highest risk of transmission include unprotected receptive anal intercourse (especially with mucosal tearing), unprotected receptive vaginal intercourse (especially during menses), and unprotected rectal/vaginal intercourse in the presence of genital ulcers (e.g., primary syphilis, genital herpes, chancroid). Lower risk sexual practices include insertive anal/vaginal intercourse and oral-genital contact. The risk of transmission after a single encounter with an HIV source has been estimated to be 1 in 150 with needle sharing, 1 in 300 with occupational percutaneous exposure, 1 in 300–1000 with receptive anal intercourse, 1 in 500–1250 with receptive vaginal intercourse, 1 in 1000–3000 with insertive vaginal intercourse, and 1 in 3000 with insertive anal intercourse. Transmission risk increases with the number of encounters and when the source of infection has higher HIV RNA plasma levels (Lancet 2001;357:1149–53). Antiretroviral therapy reduces the risk of HIV transmission by more than 90% (N Engl J Med. 2011 Aug 11;365(6):493–505). The mode of transmission does not affect the natural history of HIV disease, though patients with active or past injection drug use may have shortened survival due to comorbid complications (AIDS 2007;21:1185–97).

B. **Acute (Primary) HIV Infection (pp. 4–5).** Acute HIV occurs 1–4 weeks after transmission and is accompanied by a burst of viral replication with a decline in CD4 cell count. Most patients manifest a symptomatic mononucleosis-like syndrome, which is often overlooked. Acute HIV infection is confirmed by demonstrating a high HIV RNA with either a negative HIV antibody test or a reactive ELISA with negative or indeterminate Western blot.

C. **Seroconversion.** Development of a positive HIV antibody test usually occurs within 4 weeks of acute infection, and invariably (with few exceptions) by 6 months.

D. **Asymptomatic HIV Infection.** Asymptomatic HIV lasts a variable amount of time (average 8–10 years) and is accompanied by a gradual decline in CD4 cell counts and a relatively stable HIV RNA level (sometimes referred to as the viral "set point").

E. **Early Symptomatic HIV Infection.** Previously referred to as "AIDS Related Complex (ARC)," findings include thrush or vaginal candidiasis (persistent, frequent, or poorly responsive to treatment), herpes zoster (recurrent episodes or involving multiple dermatomes), oral hairy leukoplakia, peripheral neuropathy, diarrhea, or constitutional symptoms (e.g., low-grade fevers, weight loss).

F. **AIDS is defined** by a CD4 cell count $< 200/mm^3$, a CD4 cell percentage of total lymphocytes $< 14\%$, or one of several AIDS-related opportunistic infections. Common opportunistic infections include *Pneumocystis jirovecii (carinii)* pneumonia, cryptococcal meningitis, recurrent bacterial pneumonia, *Candida esophagitis*, CNS toxoplasmosis, tuberculosis, and non-Hodgkin's lymphoma. Other AIDS indicators in HIV-infected patients include candidiasis of the bronchi, trachea, or lungs; disseminated/extrapulmonary coccidiomycosis, cryptococcosis, or histoplasmosis; chronic (> 1 month) intestinal cryptosporidiosis or isosporiasis; Kaposi's sarcoma; lymphoid interstitial pneumonia/pulmonary lymphoid hyperplasia; disseminated/ extrapulmonary mycobacterial (non-tuberculous) infection; progressive multifocal leukoencephalopathy (PML); recurrent *Salmonella septicemia*; or HIV wasting syndrome.

G. Advanced HIV Disease corresponds with a CD4 cell count < $50/mm^3$. Most AIDS-related deaths occur at this point. Common late stage opportunistic infections are caused by CMV disease (retinitis, colitis) or disseminated *Mycobacterium avium* complex (MAC).

ACUTE (PRIMARY) HIV INFECTION

A. Description. Acute clinical illness associated with primary acquisition of HIV, occurring 1–4 weeks after viral transmission (range: 6 days to 6 weeks). Symptoms develop in 50–90%, but are often mistaken for the flu, mononucleosis, or other nonspecific viral syndrome. More severe symptoms may correlate with a higher viral set point and more rapid HIV disease progression (J AIDS 2007;45:445–8). Even without therapy, most patients recover, reflecting development of a partially effective immune response and depletion of susceptible CD4 cells. Unfortunately, damage to the immune system through depletion of the gut-associated lymphoid tissue occurs rapidly (AIDS 2007;21:1–11) and may not be preventable even with effective ART.

B. Differential Diagnosis includes **EBV, CMV**, viral hepatitis, enteroviral infection, secondary syphilis, toxoplasmosis, HSV with erythema multiforme, drug reaction, Behçet's disease, acute lupus.

C. Signs and Symptoms usually reflect hematogenous dissemination of virus to lymphoreticular and neurologic sites (N Engl J Med 1998;339:33–9):
  - Fever (97%).
  - Pharyngitis (73%). Typically non-exudative (unlike EBV, which is usually exudative).
  - Rash (77%). Maculopapular viral exanthem of the face and trunk is most common, but can involve the extremities, palms and soles.
  - Arthralgia/myalgia (58%).
  - Neurologic symptoms (12%). Headache is most common. Neuropathy, Bell's palsy, and meningoencephalitis are rare, but may predict worse outcome.
  - Oral/genital ulcerations, thrush, nausea, vomiting, diarrhea, weight loss.

D. Laboratory Findings
  1. CBC. Lymphopenia followed by lymphocytosis (common). Atypical lymphocytosis is variable, but usually low level (unlike EBV, where atypical lymphocytosis may be 20–30% or higher). Thrombocytopenia occurs in some.
  2. Elevated Transaminases in some but not all patients.

3. **Depressed CD4 Cell Count.** Can rarely be low enough to induce opportunistic infections, most commonly PCP or mucosal candidiasis.

4. **HIV Antibody.** Usually negative, although persons with prolonged symptoms of acute HIV may have positive antibody tests if diagnosed late during the course of illness.

E. **Confirming the Diagnosis of Acute HIV Infection**
1. **Obtain HIV Antibody** to exclude prior disease.

2. **Order Viral Load Test** (HIV RNA PCR), preferably RT-PCR. HIV RNA confirms acute HIV infection prior to seroconversion when the HIV antibody test is concurrently negative. Most individuals will have very high HIV RNA (> 100,000 copies/mL). Be suspicious of a false-positive test if the HIV RNA is low (< 10,000 copies/mL) (J Infect Dis 2004;190:598–604). For any positive test, it is important to repeat HIV RNA and HIV antibody testing. p24 antigen can also be used to establish the diagnosis, but is less sensitive than HIV RNA PCR.

3. **Order Other Tests/Serologies if HIV RNA Test is Negative.** Order throat cultures for bacterial/viral respiratory pathogens, EBV VCA IgM/IgG, CMV IgM/IgG, HHV-6 IgM/IgG, and hepatitis serologies as appropriate to establish a diagnosis for patient's symptoms.

F. **Management of Acute HIV Infection**
1. **Initiate Antiretroviral Therapy.** Patients with acute HIV infection should be referred to an HIV specialist, who ideally will enroll the patient into a clinical study. Some treatment guidelines now recommend treatment for symptomatic acute HIV, although long term clinical studies comparing treatment with observation have not been conducted. As in chronic infection, once started, treatment should be continued without interruption. Regimens for treatment are similar to those outlined for chronic HIV infection (Table 3.3). Some clinicians elect to start with PI-based treatment given the higher risk of transmitted NNRTI than PI resistance.

2. **Obtain HIV Resistance Genotype** (Chapter 4) because of the possibility of transmission of antiretroviral therapy-resistant virus. Transmitted drug resistance is more easily detectable during acute HIV infection than chronic disease, presumably because some of the transmitted drug mutations revert back to wild-type over time [J Acquir Immune Defic Syndr 2012 Oct 1; 61:258]. A genotype resistance test is preferred; therapy can be started pending results of the test. Again, because transmitted NNRTI resistance completely reduces the activity of initial NNRTI-based therapy, initial treatment with two NRTIs plus a boosted PI is preferred in this setting. If no NNRTI resistance is detected on genotype, therapy may be changed if indicated.

3. **Rationale for Treatment of Acute HIV Infection.** No prospective clinical studies have conclusively documented the benefits of therapy for acute HIV infection, although two randomized and one observational study strongly suggest benefits of early therapy [N Engl J Med 2013; 368:207; N Engl J Med 2013; 368:218; J Infect Dis. 2012 Jan 1;205(1):87.] These benefits include hastening symptom resolution, reducing viral transmission, lowering virologic "set point," reduction of the viral reservoir, and preserving both absolute and virus-specific CD4 responses. Eradication of HIV is not possible with currently available agents (Nat Med 2003;9:727–8), but should HIV cure strategies one day be feasible, it is likely that those treated during acute HIV infection will be the best candidates.

Chapter 2

Diagnosis and Evaluation of HIV Infection

HIV ANTIBODY TESTING

A. Standard HIV Antibody Tests (see also Clin Infect Dis 2007;45:S221–S225 and Journal of Acquired Immune Deficiency Syndromes: 15 December 2010;55:S102–S105.). HIV antibody tests (ELISA, Western blot) and quantitative plasma HIV RNA (HIV viral load) assays are used to diagnose HIV infection (Figure 2.1). Most patients produce antibody to HIV within 6–8 weeks of exposure; 50% will have a positive antibody test by 3–4 weeks, and nearly 100% will have detectable antibody by 6 months. As HIV ELISA testing has become more sensitive, and especially with the use of the combined antigen/antibody assay, patients with recently acquired HIV may have reactive screening tests and negative or indeterminate Western blots. In such situations (positive screening test, negative Western blot), supplemental testing with HIV RNA testing is recommended.

1. ELISA. Usual screening test. All positives should routinely be confirmed with Western blot or other tests, such as an antibody assay that distinguishes between HIV-1 and HIV-2. Fourth-generation screening tests measure both antibody and p24 antigen, shortening the window period between HIV acquisition and a positive screening test.

2. Western Blot. CDC criteria for interpretation:

    a. Positive. At least two of the following bands present: p24, gp41, gp160/120

    b. Negative. No bands present

    c. Indeterminate. HIV band present, but does not meet criteria for positivity

3. Test Performance. Standard method is ELISA screen with Western blot confirmation.

    a. ELISA negative. Western blot is not required (ELISA sensitivity 99.7%, specificity 98.5%). Obtain HIV RNA if acute HIV infection is suspected.

    b. ELISA positive. Laboratories will confirm results with Western blot or an HIV-1/2 differentiation assay. Probability that ELISA and Western blot are both false-positives is extremely low (< 1 per 140,000). Absence of p31 band could be a clue to a false positive Western blot.

    c. Unexpected ELISA/Western blot. Repeat test to exclude clerical/computer error, the most common cause of incorrect results.

4. Indeterminate Western Blot. This occurs in approximately 4–20% of reactive ELISAs, usually due to a single p24 band or weak other bands. HIV-related causes include seroconversion in progress, advanced HIV disease with loss of antibody response, or infection with HIV-2. Non-HIV-related causes include cross-reacting antibody from pregnancy, blood transfusions, organ transplantation, autoantibodies from collagen vascular disease, influenza vaccination, or recipient of HIV vaccine. In low-risk patients, an indeterminate result rarely represents true HIV infection. Since seroconversion-in-progress is generally associated with high HIV RNA levels, the recommended approach is to obtain an HIV RNA test. In addition, most patients with indeterminate Western blots due to seroconversion-in-progress will develop a fully positive HIV test within 1 month.

B. Other HIV Antibody Tests

  1. Home Test Kit (Home Access HIV-1 Test System). This system can be purchased over-the-counter at pharmacies, or ordered by phone or over the Internet (www.homeaccess.com). Users receive a kit that includes a stylet for obtaining a sample of blood from the fingertip, which is then placed on filter paper and mailed to the company for testing. The standard test will return a result within 7 days and costs $44; users can purchase overnight shipping for an additional cost and a more rapid turnaround time. By using a code provided with each kit, users can call and obtain their results anonymously. Phone counseling is available to explain the results, as well as a database of local HIV providers if the test result is positive. The Home Access test employs ELISA testing, which is done in duplicate. All individuals with reactive tests on the system must have results confirmed by standard testing.

  2. OraSure. This office-based test was approved in 1996 and uses a special swab that collects oral mucosal transudate (not saliva) when it is held between the cheek and the gum. This system obtains quantities of antibody that are comparable to or exceed those from serum samples. Once the specimen is collected, it is sent to a central laboratory for ELISA and Western blot testing, which can be performed on the same sample. As a result, the sensitivity and specificity of the test are comparable to standard blood HIV antibody testing (JAMA 1997;277:254).

  3. Rapid HIV Tests (OraQuick ADVANCE Rapid HIV Test; OraQuick In-Home HIV Test; Uni-Gold Recombigen HIV). The OraQuick was approved in 2004 and can be performed on whole blood, plasma, or oral mucosal transudate samples. The UniGold test is limited to blood samples. Results are returned in 10–20 minutes and are comparable in accuracy to a single ELISA test. As a result, *a reactive rapid test must be confirmed with standard ELISA/Western blot serology*. A major advantage of this rapid test includes the ability to give patients a negative result at the time of care; there also is some evidence that individuals given a positive rapid test result are more likely to return for their confirmatory serology results. Since the test can be done at the point of care (no CLIA certification is required), it is particularly useful in the evaluation of source patients of needlestick injuries and for women in labor who did not receive HIV testing during prenatal care. There have been reports of high rates of false positive rapid tests when oral samples are used in low-prevalence settings (Ann Intern Med 2008 Aug 5;149[3]:153–60); as a result, some sites have switched to using blood rapid testing, either with the OraQuick or the Uni-Gold. A version of the mouth swab rapid test from OraQuick was approved for in-home use in 2012; this does not require contact with a health care provider.

C. Selected Other Licensed HIV Diagnostic Tests

  1. p24 Antigen. Approved for diagnosis of acute HIV infection. However, due to low sensitivity of this test, HIV RNA has replaced p24 antigen in clinical practice, and hence this test is rarely ordered.

2. **Nucleic Acid Based Tests.** In the United States, donated blood has been screened with nucleic acid based tests since the late 1990s, shortening the time between infection and detectability of infection to about 12 days. As a result, the rate of acquiring HIV from a blood transfusion is now estimated at one infection per 2 million units transfused (JAMA 2003;289:959). A related test, the Aptima HIV-1 RNA Qualitative Assay, was approved for HIV diagnosis in 2006. Like quantitative HIV RNA tests, this assay can be used to diagnose acute HIV infection before antibodies develop, but results are provided only as positive or negative. Additionally, it can confirm HIV infection in a person with a positive HIV ELISA or rapid test. It is not known whether the rate of false positivity with the Aptima test is lower than the rate with RT-PCR or bDNA.

3. **Combined HIV Antigen/Antibody Combination Assays.** These tests can detect both HIV antibody and p24 antigen. As such, it turns positive before standard ELISA testing, hence shortens the window period between HIV acquisition and detection of antibody. The test can be run on a similar laboratory platform as some HIV antibody tests. The sensitivity of the test for acute HIV compared with HIV RNA testing is somewhat lower as p24 antigen is less likely to be positive than HIV RNA.

QUANTITATIVE PLASMA HIV RNA (HIV VIRAL LOAD ASSAYS)

HIV viral load assays measure the amount of HIV RNA in plasma. The high sensitivity of these assays allows detection of virus in most patients not on antiretroviral therapy. These tests are most commonly used to monitor the response to antiretroviral therapy; they can also be used to diagnose acute HIV infection.

A. Uses of HIV RNA Assay

1. **Confirms Diagnosis of Acute HIV Infection.** A high HIV RNA with a negative or indeterminate HIV antibody test confirms acute HIV infection prior to seroconversion.

2. **Helps in Initial Evaluation of HIV Infection.** Establishes baseline HIV RNA and helps (along with CD4 cell count) determine whether to initiate or defer therapy, as HIV RNA correlates with rate of CD4 decline (Ann Intern Med 1997 Jun 15;126[12]:946–54). Of note, baseline HIV RNA is not as strong a determinant of the indication for therapy as the CD4 cell count.

3. **Monitors Response to Antiviral Therapy.** HIV RNA changes rapidly decline 2–4 weeks after starting or changing effective antiretroviral therapy, with slower decline thereafter. Patients who achieve virologic suppression (less than lower limit of detection of sensitive assays, typically 20-40 cop/mL) have the most durable response to antiviral therapy and the best clinical prognosis. No change in HIV RNA suggests that therapy will be ineffective or the patient is noncompliant.

4. **Estimates Risk for Opportunistic Infection.** For patients with similar CD4 cell counts, the risk of opportunistic infections is higher with higher HIV RNAs. HIV RNA is not formally incorporated into opportunistic infection prevention guidelines.

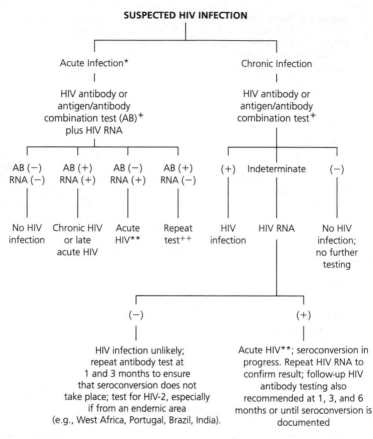

Figure 2.1. Approach to HIV Testing

(–) negative test; (+) positive test

* Occurs 1–4 weeks after viral transmission. Most patients manifest a viral syndrome (fever, pharyngitis ± rash/arthralgias), which is often mistaken for mononucleosis or the flu and therefore overlooked

** HIV RNA in acute HIV infection should be very high (usually > 100,000 copies/mL)

\+ All positive ELISA tests must be confirmed by a different second test; most commonly this is a Western blot, but some sites might use an HIV differentiation assay that distinguishes HIV-1 from HIV-2

++ May be "HIV controller" (controls virus without requiring medications) or laboratory error

B. Assays and Interpretation

1. **Tests, Sensitivities, and Dynamic Range.** Several assays are used, each with advantages and disadvantages; most US sites use RT-PCR (Roche or Abbott) which has replaced the older (and less accurate) bDNA assay. Any assay can be used to diagnose acute HIV infection and guide/monitor therapy, but the same test should be used to follow patients longitudinally.

   a. **RT-PCR Amplicor** (Roche): Sensitivity = 400 copies/mL; dynamic range = 400–750,000 copies/mL. Assay discontinued, no longer in wide use.

   b. **RT-PCR Ultrasensitive 1.5** (Roche): Sensitivity = 50 copies/mL; dynamic range = 50–75,000 copies/mL. Assay discontinued, no longer in wide use.

   c. **bDNA Versant 3.0** (Bayer): Sensitivity = 75 copies/mL; dynamic range = 75–500,000 copies/mL

   d. **Nucleic acid sequence-based amplification** (NASBA), NucliSens HIV-1 QT (bioMerieux). Sensitivity = 10 copies/mL; dynamic range = 176–3.5 million copies/mL (depends on volume)

   e. **Real Time HIV-1 assay** (Abbott): PCR-based assay. Sensitivity = 40 copies/mL; dynamic range = 40–10 million copies/mL

   f. **COBAS AmpliPrep/COBAS TagMan HIV-1 test** (Roche): Sensitivity = 20 copies/mL; dynamic range = 20–10 million copies/mL

2. **Correlation Between HIV RNA and CD4 Cell Count.** HIV RNA assays correlate inversely with CD4 cell counts, but do so imperfectly (e.g., some patients with high CD4 counts have relatively high HIV RNA levels, and vice versa.) For any given CD4, higher HIV RNA levels correlate with more rapid CD4 decline. In response to antiretroviral therapy, changes in HIV RNA generally precede changes in CD4 cell count.

3. **Significant Change in HIV RNA Assay.** This is defined by at least a 2-fold (0.3 log) change in viral RNA (accounts for normal variation in clinically stable patients), or a 3-fold (0.5 log) change in response to new antiretroviral therapy (accounts for intralaboratory and patient variability). For example, if a HIV RNA result = 50,000 copies/mL, then the range of possible actual values = 25,000–100,000 copies/mL, and the value needed to demonstrate antiretroviral activity is ≤ 17,000 copies/mL.

C. Indications for HIV RNA Testing. This test is indicated for the diagnosis of acute HIV infection and for initial evaluation of newly diagnosed HIV. It is the single most important monitoring test for HIV treatment efficacy; it should be performed 2–8 weeks after starting a new antiretroviral regimen. If HIV RNA is detectable at 2–8 weeks, repeat every 4–8 weeks until suppression to <200 copies/mL, then every 3–6 months. Clinically stable patients with long term virologic suppression may reduce the frequency of HIV RNA testing to 1–2 times yearly.

INITIAL ASSESSMENT OF HIV-INFECTED PATIENTS

A. **Clinical Evaluation.** The history and physical examination should focus on diagnoses associated with HIV infection. Compared to patients without HIV, the severity, frequency, and duration of these conditions are usually increased in HIV disease.

1. **Dermatologic:** Severe herpes simplex (oral/anogenital); herpes zoster (especially recurrent, cranial nerve, or disseminated); molluscum contagiosum; staphylococcal abscesses; tinea nail infections; Kaposi's sarcoma (from HHV-8 infection); petechiae (from ITP); seborrheic dermatitis; new or worsening psoriasis; eosinophilic pustular folliculitis; severe cutaneous drug eruptions (especially sulfonamides)

2. **Oropharyngeal:** Oral candidiasis; oral hairy leukoplakia (from EBV); Kaposi's sarcoma (most commonly on palate or gums); gingivitis/periodontitis; warts; aphthous ulcers (especially esophageal/perianal)

3. **Constitutional symptoms:** Fatigue, fevers, chronic diarrhea, weight loss

4. **Lymphatic:** Persistent, generalized lymphadenopathy

5. **Others:** Active TB (especially extrapulmonary); non-Hodgkin's lymphoma (especially CNS); unexplained leukopenia, anemia, thrombocytopenia (especially ITP); myopathy; miscellaneous neurologic conditions (cranial/peripheral neuropathies, Guillain-Barre syndrome, mononeuritis multiplex, aseptic meningitis, cognitive impairment)

B. **Baseline Laboratory Testing (Table 2.1)** (See also Clin Infect Disease Clin Infect Dis. 2013 Nov 13.).

Table 2.1. Baseline Laboratory Testing for HIV-Infected Patients*

Test	Rationale
Repeat HIV serology (ELISA/confirmatory Western blot)	Indicated for patients unable to document a prior positive test, and for "low risk" individuals with a positive test (to detect computer/clerical error). Repeat serology is now less important since HIV RNA testing provides an additional means of confirming HIV infection. Also useful in ruling out cases of suspected factitious HIV
CBC with differential, platelets	Detects cytopenias (e.g., ITP) seen in HIV. Needed to calculate CD4 cell count
Chemistry panel ("SMA 20")	Detects renal dysfunction and electrolyte/LFT/glucose abnormalities, which may accompany HIV and associated infections (e.g., HIV nephropathy, HCV)
Fasting lipid profile	Since HIV and many antiretroviral agents influence lipid levels, a lipid profile before treatment provides a useful baseline
CD4 cell count	Determines the urgency of antiretroviral therapy and need for opportunistic infection (OI) prophylaxis. Best test for defining risk of OI's and prognosis

Table 2.1. Baseline Laboratory Testing for HIV-Infected Patients* (cont'd)

Test	Rationale
HIV RNA assay ("viral load")	Provides a marker for the pace of HIV disease progression. Determines response to antiretroviral therapy
HIV resistance genotype	Identifies patients infected with a resistant virus (some resistance now detected in approximately 15% of newly diagnosed patients in the US)
Tuberculin skin test (standard 5 TU of PPD) or interferon gamma release assay (IGRA)	Detects latent TB infection and targets patients for preventive therapy. Anergy skin tests are not recommended due to poor predictive value. HIV is the most powerful co-factor for the development of active TB
PAP smear	Risk of cervical cancer is nearly twice as high in HIV-positive women vs. uninfected controls; some advocate anal pap smears for gay men
Toxoplasmosis serology (IgG)	Identifies patients at risk for subsequent cerebral/systemic toxoplasmosis and the need for prophylaxis. Those with negative tests should be counseled on how to avoid infection
Syphilis serology (VDRL or RPR)	Identifies co-infection with syphilis, which is epidemiologically-linked to HIV. Disease may have accelerated course in HIV patients
Hepatitis C serology (anti-HCV)	Identifies HCV infection and usually chronic carriage. If positive, follow with HCV genotype and HCV viral load assay. If patient is antibody-negative but at high-risk for hepatitis, order HCV RNA to exclude a false-negative result
Hepatitis B serologies (HBsAb, HBcAb, HBsAg)	Identifies patients who are immune to hepatitis B (HBsAb) or chronic carriers (HBsAg). If all three are negative, hepatitis B vaccine is indicated
Hepatitis A serology (anti-HAV)	Identifies candidates for hepatitis A vaccine; if anti-HAV positive, already immune
G6PD screen	Identifies patients at risk for dapsone or primaquine-associated hemolysis
CMV serology (IgG)	Identifies patients who should receive CMV-negative or leukocyte-depleted blood if transfused
VZV serology (IgG)	Identifies patients at risk for varicella (chickenpox), and those who should avoid contact with active varicella or herpes zoster patients. Serology-negative patients exposed to chickenpox should receive varicella-zoster immune globulin (VZIG); some advocate varicella vaccine if CD4 > 350/mm³
Chest x-ray	Sometimes ordered as a baseline test for future comparisons. May detect healed granulomatous diseases/other processes. Indicated in all tuberculin skin test positive patients
HLA-B*5701	Needed if therapy with abacavir is planned. Patients negative for HLA-B*5701 have almost no risk of severe hypersensitivity reaction to abacavir

*   See also Clin Infect Dis 2009;49:651–681

Table 2.2. Laboratory Monitoring Schedule for Patients Prior to and After Initiation of Antiretroviral Therapy (Updated February 12, 2013)

	Entry into care	Follow-up before ART	ART initiation or modification[1]	2–8 weeks post-ART initiation or modification	Every 3–6 months	Every 6 months	Every 12 months	Treatment failure	Clinically indicated
HIV serology	√ If diagnosis has not been confirmed								
CD4 count	√	every 3–6 months	√		√	In clinically stable patients with suppressed viral load, CD4 count can be monitored every 6–12 months (see text)		√	√
Viral load	√	every 3–6 months	√	√[2]	√[3]			√	√
Resistance testing	√		√[4]					√	√
HLA-B*5701 testing			√ if considering ABC						

Tropism testing		✓ if considering a CCR5 antagonist				✓ if considering a CCR5 antagonist or for failure of CCR5 antagonist-based regimen	✓
Hepatitis B serology[5]	✓	✓ may repeat if HBsAg (−) and HBsAb (−) at baseline					✓
Hepatitis C serology, with confirmation of positive results	✓	✓				✓	✓
Basic chemistry[6]	✓	every 6–12 months	✓	✓	✓		✓

Table 2.2. Laboratory Monitoring Schedule for Patients Prior to and After Initiation of Antiretroviral Therapy (Updated February 12, 2013) (cont'd)

	Entry into care	Follow-up before ART	ART initiation or modification[1]	2–8 weeks post-ART initiation or modification	Every 3–6 months	Every 6 months	Every 12 months	Treatment failure	Clinically indicated
ALT, AST, T. bilirubin	√	every 6–12 months	√	√	√				√
CBC with differential	√	every 3–6 months	√	√ if on ZDV	√				√
Fasting lipid profile	√	if normal, annually	√	consider 4–8 weeks after starting new ART		√ if abnormal at last measurement	√ if normal at last measurement		√
Fasting glucose or hemoglobin A1C	√	if normal, annually	√		√ if abnormal at last measurement	√ if normal at last measurement			√

Urinalysis[7]	✓			✓	✓ if on TDF[8]	✓	✓
Pregnancy test		✓ if starting EFV					✓

[1] This table pertains to laboratory tests done to select an ARV regimen and monitor for treatment responses or ART toxicities. Please refer to the HIV Primary Care guidelines for guidance on other laboratory tests generally recommended for primary health care maintenance of HIV patients [1].

[2] ART may be modified for treatment failure, adverse effects, or regimen simplification.

[3] If HIV RNA is detectable at 2–8 weeks, repeat every 4–8 weeks until suppression to <200 copies/mL, then every 3–6 months.

[4] Viral load typically is measured every 3 to 4 months in patients on ART. However, for adherent patients with suppressed viral load and stable immunologic status for more than 2 to 3 years, monitoring at 6 month intervals may be considered.

[5] For ART-naïve patients, if resistance testing was performed at entry into care, repeat testing is recommended in this case. For virologically suppressed patients who are switching therapy for toxicity or convenience, viral amplification will not be possible and therefore resistance testing should not be performed. Results from prior resistance testing can be used to help in the construction of a new regimen.

[6] If HBsAg is positive at baseline or prior to initiation of ART, TDF + (FTC or 3TC) should be used as part of ARV regimen to treat both HBV and HIV infections. If HBsAg, and HBsAb, and anti-HBc are negative at baseline, hepatitis B vaccine series should be administered.

[7] Serum Na, K, HCO₃, Cl, BUN, creatinine, glucose (preferably fasting); some experts suggest monitoring phosphorus while on TDF; determination of renal function should include estimation of creatinine clearance using Cockcroft-Gault equation or estimation of glomerular filtration rate based on MDRD equation.

[8] For patients with renal disease, consult "Guidelines for the Management of Chronic Kidney Disease in HIV-Infected Patients: Recommendations of the HIV Medicine Association of the Infectious Diseases Society of America" [2].

[9] More frequent monitoring may be indicated for patients with evidence of kidney disease (e.g. proteinuria, decreased glomerular dysfunction) or increased risk of renal insufficiency (e.g. patients with diabetes, hypertension).

Acronyms: 3TC = lamivudine, ABC = abacavir, ALT = alanine aminotransferase, ART = antiretroviral therapy, AST = aspartate aminotransferase, CBC = complete blood count, EFV = efavirenz, FTC = emtricitabine, HBsAb = hepatitis B surface antibody, HBsAg = hepatitis B surface antigen, HBV = hepatitis B virus, MDRD = modification of diet in renal disease (equation), TDF = tenofovir, ZDV = zidovudine

Reproduced from: Guidelines for the Use of Antiretroviral Agents for HIV-1-infected Adults and Adolescents: Recommendations of the Panel on Clinical Practices for Treatment of HIV Infection; aidsinfo.nih.gov.

Table 2.3. Use of CD4 Cell Count for Interpretation of Patient Signs and Symptoms in HIV Infection

CD4 (cells/mm³)	Associated Conditions
> 500	Most illnesses are similar to those in HIV-negative patients. Some increased risk of bacterial infections (pneumococcal pneumonia, sinusitis), herpes zoster, tuberculosis, skin conditions
200–500*	Bacterial infections (especially pneumococcal pneumonia, sinusitis), cutaneous Kaposi's sarcoma, vaginal candidiasis, ITP
50–200*	Thrush, oral hairy leukoplakia, classic HIV-associated opportunistic infections (e.g., *P. jirovecii [carinii]* pneumonia, cryptococcal meningitis, toxoplasmosis). For patients receiving prophylaxis, most opportunistic infection do not occur until CD4 cell counts < 100/mm³ (Ann Intern Med 1996;124:633–42)
< 50*	"Final common pathway" opportunistic infections (disseminated *M. avium* complex, CMV retinitis), HIV-associated wasting, neurologic disease (neuropathy, encephalopathy)

*　Patients remain at risk for all processes noted in earlier stages

C.　CD4 Cell Count (Lymphocyte Subset Analysis)

　　1.　Overview. Acute HIV infection is characterized by a decline in CD4 cell count, followed by a gradual rise associated with clinical recovery. Chronic HIV infection shows progressive declines (~ 50–80 cells/year, but with wide interpatient variability) in CD4 cell count without treatment, followed by more rapid decline 1–2 years prior to opportunistic infection (AIDS-defining diagnosis). Cell counts remain stable over 5–10 years in 5% of patients, while others may show rapid declines (> 300 cells/year). Since variability exists within individual patients and between laboratories, it is useful to repeat any value that is clinically unexpected.

　　2.　Uses of CD4 Cell Count

　　　　a.　Gives context of degree of immunosuppression for interpretation of symptoms/signs (Table 2.3)

　　　　b.　Used to guide therapy. Although HIV treatment is now recommended in the United States regardless of CD4 cell count, the urgency of starting therapy is much greater with counts < 200. In other parts of the world, therapy is generally not started in asymptomatic patients until the CD4 is < 350. For prophylaxis against PCP, toxoplasmosis, and MAC/CMV infection, CD4 cell counts of 200/mm³, < 100/mm³, and < 50/mm³ are used as threshold levels, respectively

　　　　c.　Provides estimate of risk of opportunistic infection or death. CD4 cell counts < 50/mm³ are associated with a markedly increased risk of death (median survival 1 year without treatment), although some patients with low counts survive > 3 years even without antiretroviral therapy. Prognosis is heavily influenced by HIV RNA, presence/history of opportunistic infections or neoplasms, performance status, and the immunologic response to antiretroviral therapy.

Chapter 3

Treatment of HIV Infection

INITIATION OF ANTIRETROVIRAL THERAPY (Table 3.2)

Combination antiretroviral therapy has led to dramatic reductions in HIV-related morbidity and mortality for patients with severe immunosuppression (CD4 < 200 cells/mm³) or a prior AIDS-defining illness [N Engl J Med 1997 Sep 11;337(11):725–33]. Treatment of asymptomatic patients is now recommended across the spectrum of HIV disease, as there is increasing evidence that such therapy is associated with a reduced risk of both HIV-related and non-HIV related complications, and furthermore reduces the risk of HIV transmission. Potential benefits of starting antiretroviral therapy with relatively high CD4 cell counts include reduction in HIV RNA, prevention of immunodeficiency, delayed time to onset of AIDS, reduced non-AIDS morbidity (cardiovascular, hepatic, neoplastic), decreased risk of drug toxicity, viral transmission, and selecting resistant virus. A cohort study published in 2009 found that deferral of ART until after the CD4 cell count fell to < 500 cells/mm³ was associated with nearly a two-fold increased risk of death [N Engl J Med 2009; 360:1815–1826]; a second study suggested that improved outcome was seen when treatment was started before the CD4 reached 350, but not at higher levels [Lancet 2009; DOI: 10.1016/S0140–6736(09)60612–7]. A multinational randomized clinical trial for asymptomatic patients with CD4 cell counts between 350 and 550 found that immediate ART had two major benefits: 1) a 96% reduction in HIV transmission to uninfected partners and; 2) a significant reduction in HIV-related clinical events, mostly tuberculosis. (N Engl J Med. 2011 Aug 11;365(6):493–505.) Potential risks of early antiretroviral therapy include reduced quality of life (from side effects/inconvenience), earlier development of drug resistance (with consequent transmission of resistant virus), limitation in future antiretroviral choices, unknown long-term toxicity of antiretroviral drugs, and the cost of therapy.

The primary goals of therapy are prolonged suppression of viral replication to undetectable levels (HIV RNA < 20–75 copies/mL depending on assay), restoration/preservation of immune function, and improved clinical outcome. Once initiated, antiretroviral therapy should be continued indefinitely, as intermittent treatment has been associated with increased risk of HIV-related and non-HIV-related complications (N Engl J Med 2006 Nov 30;355[22]:2283–96). Deferral of antiretroviral therapy may be considered in select patients who are not ready or willing to start treatment, in particular those with relatively preserved CD4 cell counts (>350 cells/mm³). In these untreated individuals, regular clinical and laboratory monitoring is essential.

Table 3.1. Antiretroviral Agents Used for HIV Infection

Drug (abbreviation; trade name, manufacturer)	Formulations	Usual Adult Dosing§
NUCLEOSIDE (AND NUCLEOTIDE) REVERSE TRANSCRIPTASE INHIBITORS (NRTIs)		
Abacavir sulfate (ABC; Ziagen, GlaxoSmithKline; also available generically)	300-mg tablets; 20-mg/mL oral solution	300 mg BID or 600 mg QD
Abacavir sulfate/lamivudine (Epzicom, GlaxoSmithKline)	600/300-mg tablet	One 600/300-mg tablet QD

Table 3.1. Antiretroviral Agents Used for HIV Infection (cont'd)

Drug (abbreviation; trade name, manufacturer)	Formulations	Usual Adult Dosing§
NUCLEOSIDE (AND NUCLEOTIDE) REVERSE TRANSCRIPTASE INHIBITORS (NRTIs) (cont'd)		
Abacavir sulfate/lamivudine/zidovudine (Trizivir, GlaxoSmithKline)	300/150/300-mg tablet	One 300/150/300-mg tablet BID
Didanosine (ddI; Videx/Videx EC, Bristol-Myers Squibb; Oncology/Immunology; also available generically)	125-, 200-, 250-, 400-mg delayed-release enteric-coated capsules; 100-, 167-, 250-mg powder	Capsule: < 60 kg: 250 mg QD ≥ 60 kg: 400 mg QD 250 mg QD with tenofovir (best avoided) Powder: < 60 kg: 167 mg BID ≥ 60 kg: 250 mg BID probably Administration: Take on empty stomach at least 30 minutes before or 2 hours after meal
Emtricitabine (FTC; Emtriva, Gilead Sciences)	200-mg capsule	200 mg QD
Lamivudine (3TC; Epivir, GlaxoSmithKline)	150-, 300-mg tablets; 10-mg/mL oral solution	150 mg BID or 300 mg QD
Lamivudine/zidovudine (Combivir, GlaxoSmithKline; also available generically)	150/300-mg tablet	One 150/300-mg tablet BID
Stavudine (d4T; Zerit, Bristol-Myers Squibb Virology)	15-, 20-, 30-, 40-mg capsules; 1-mg/mL oral solution	< 60 kg: 30 mg BID ≥ 60 kg: 40 mg BID
Tenofovir disoproxil fumarate (TDF; Viread, Gilead Sciences)	300-mg tablet	One 300-mg tablet QD
Tenofovir disoproxil fumarate/emtricitabine (Truvada, Gilead Sciences)	300/200-mg tablet	One 300/200-mg tablet QD
Zidovudine (ZDV; Retrovir, GlaxoSmithKline; also available generically)	100-mg capsule; 300-mg tablet; 10-mg/5 mL oral solution; 10-mg/mL IV solution	200 mg TID or 300 mg BID (or with 3TC as Combivir or with abacavir and 3TC as Trizivir) 5–6 mg/kg daily

Table 3.1. Antiretroviral Agents Used for HIV Infection (cont'd)

Drug (abbreviation; trade name, manufacturer)	Formulations	Usual Adult Dosing§
NON-NUCLEOSIDE REVERSE TRANSCRIPTASE INHIBITORS (NNRTIs)*		
Delavirdine mesylate (DLV; Rescriptor, Agouron)‡	100-, 200-mg tablets	400 mg TID (100-mg tablets can be dispersed in water; 200-mg tablet should be taken intact). Separate dosing from ddI or antacids by 1 hour, with or without food
Efavirenz (EFV; Sustiva, Bristol-Myers Squibb Oncology/ Immunology; outside USA known as Stocrin)‡	50-, 100-, 200-mg capsules; 600-mg tablet	600 mg QD; best taken prior to bed to reduce incidence of CNS side effects
Etravirine (ETR; Intelence, Janssen Therapeutics)	100-mg tablets; 200-mg tablets	Two 100-mg tablets twice daily after a meal or one 200-mg tablet twice daily after a meal
Nevirapine (NVP; Viramune, Boehringer Ingelheim; also available generically)‡	200-mg tablet; 50-mg/ 5 mL oral suspension (pediatric)	200 mg QD × 2 weeks, then 200 mg BID
Nevirapine Extended Release (NVP XR, Viramune XR, Boehringer Ingelheim)	400 mg tablet	200 mg immediate release QD x 14 days then 400 mg XR QD thereafter
Rilpivirine (RVP, Edurant, Janssen Therapeutics)	25-mg tablet	1 tablet daily with a meal
COMBINATION NRTI/NNRTI		
Efavirenz/emtricitabine/ tenofovir (Atripla, Bristol-Myers Squibb & Gilead)	One 600/200/300-mg tablet daily on an empty stomach, generally given before bed	One 600/200/300-mg tablet daily
Tenofovir/emtricitabine/rilpivirine (Complera, Gilead and Janssen)	300/200/25 mg tablet	One tablet daily with a meal
PROTEASE INHIBITORS (PIs)†		
Atazanavir sulfate (ATV; Reyataz, Bristol-Myers Squibb Virology)‡	100-, 150-, 200-, 300-mg capsules	400 mg QD, or 300 mg QD in combination with ritonavir 100 mg QD. For treatment-experienced patients, or when used with tenofovir or efavirenz or nevirapine use: 300 mg in combination with 100 mg of ritonavir. Take with food

Table 3.1. Antiretroviral Agents Used for HIV Infection (cont'd)

Drug (abbreviation; trade name, manufacturer)	Formulations	Usual Adult Dosing[§]
PROTEASE INHIBITORS (PIs)[†] (cont'd)		
Darunavir (DRV; Prezista, Janssen Therapeutics)	400-, 600-mg, 800 mg tablets	600 mg BID with ritonavir 100 mg BID (treatment experienced); 800 mg QD with ritonavir 100 mg QD (treatment naïve)
Fosamprenavir (FPV; Lexiva, GlaxoSmithKline)[‡]	700-mg tablet	PI-naïve patients: 1400 mg BID, or 700 mg BID in combination with ritonavir 100 mg BID, or 1400 mg QD in combination with ritonavir 200 mg QD or 100 mg QD. PI-experienced patients: 700 mg BID in combination with ritonavir 100 mg BID
Indinavir sulfate (IDV; Crixivan, Merck)[‡]	200-, 333-, 400-mg capsules	800 mg TID, or 800 mg BID in combination with ritonavir 100 mg or 200 mg BID Administration: Unboosted: Take 1 hour before or 2 hours after meals; may take with skim milk/low-fat meal Boosted: Take with or without food. Separate dosing from ddI by 1 hour
Lopinavir/ritonavir (LPV/r; Kaletra, Abbott)[‡]	200/50 mg tablet; 80/20-mg/mL oral solution	Two tablets (400/100 mg) BID; 5 mL oral solution BID. Four tablets (800/200 mg) QD an option for treatment-naïve patients With EFV or NVP: 3 tablets (600/150 mg) BID or 6.7 mL BID
Nelfinavir mesylate (NFV; Viracept, Agouron/Pfizer)	250-, 625-mg tablets; 50-mg/gm oral powder	750 mg TID or 1250 mg BID. Take with food
Ritonavir (RTV; Norvir, Abbott)[‡]	100-mg tablet or capsule; 600 mg/7.5 mL solution; 80 mg/mL oral solution	600 mg BID as sole PI; 100–400 mg daily in 1–2 divided doses as pharmacokinetic booster for other PIs Administration: Take with food or up to 2 hours after a meal to improve tolerability

Table 3.1. Antiretroviral Agents Used for HIV Infection (cont'd)

Drug (abbreviation; trade name, manufacturer)	Formulations	Usual Adult Dosing§
PROTEASE INHIBITORS (PIs)† (cont'd)		
Saquinavir (SQV; Invirase, Roche)‡	200-, 500-mg hard-gel capsules	1000 mg BID in combination with ritonavir 100 mg BID. Take with food
Tipranavir (TPV; Aptivus, Boehringer Ingelheim)‡	250-mg soft-gel capsule	500 mg BID in combination with ritonavir 200 mg BID. Take with food
FUSION INHIBITORS		
Enfuvirtide (T-20; Fuzeon, Roche)‡	Injectable (lyophilized powder). Each single-use vial contains 108 mg of enfuvirtide to be reconstituted with 1.1 mL of sterile water for injection for delivery of approximately 90 mg/mL	90 mg BID IV. Administered subcutaneously into upper arm, anterior thigh, or abdomen
CCR5 ANTAGONIST		
Maraviroc (MVC; Selzentry, Pfizer)	150-, 300-mg tablets	150 mg, 300 mg or 600 BID depending on concomitant drugs (see p. 205 for details); may be taken with or without food
INTEGRASE INHIBITORS		
Raltegravir (RAL; Isentress, Merck)	400-mg tablet	One 400-mg tablet BID with or without food
		1. Dolutegravir (DTG; Tivicay); ViiV) 2. 25 mg tablet 3. No integrase inhibitor resistance: One 25 mg QD; with integrase inhibitor resistance: One 25 mg tablet twice BID

Table 3.1. Antiretroviral Agents Used for HIV Infection (cont'd)

COMBINATION NRTI/INTEGRASE INHIBITOR		
Tenofovir/emtricitabine/ elvitegravir/cobicistat (TDF/FTC/ EVG/c; Stribild, Gilead Sciences)	300 mg/200 mg/150 mg/ 150 mg tablet	One tablet daily with food.

*   Nevirapine and efavirenz are cytochrome p450 CYP3A4 inducers; delavirdine is an inhibitor; etravirine has mixed effects. Consult package insert for full drug interaction profile.

†   All protease inhibitors are hepatically metabolized by the cytochrome p450 system; they also are specific inhibitors of CYP3A4 and have induction effects on other enzymes. Consult package insert for full drug-drug interaction profile.

‡   Consult package insert for full drug interaction profile.

§   See Chapter 9 for dosing adjustments in renal or hepatic insufficiency. Unless otherwise stated, medication may be taken with or without food.

SELECTION OF AN OPTIMAL INITIAL ANTIRETROVIRAL REGIMEN (Tables 3.2–3.3)

Selection of the optimal initial antiretroviral regimen must take into consideration antiviral potency, tolerability, and safety. In the DHHS and IAS-USA Guidelines (Tables 3.3 and 3.4), all recommended regimens consist of three active agents: an NRTI pair (containing 3TC or FTC as one of the drugs) plus either an NNRTI or a ritonavir-boosted PI. As such, choosing a specific regimen therefore can be reduced to four major decisions (see Table 3.2).

Table 3.2. Major Decisions in Selecting the Initial Antiretroviral Regimen*

Decision	Comment
What is the optimal NRTI to pair with 3TC or FTC?	Because of the availability of once-daily, fixed-dose formulations and a low risk of lipoatrophy, clinicians should choose between either TDF (co-formulated with FTC as Truvada) or ABC (co-formulated with 3TC as Epzicom). ABC therapy should be preceded by testing for HLA-B*5701 to reduce the risk of ABC hypersensitivity. Some studies have suggested that ABC treatment is associated with an increased risk of myocardial infarction (Lancet 2008 Apr 26;371[9622]: 1417–26; AIDS 2008 Sep 12;22[14]:F17–24). Furthermore, ABC/3TC had a higher rate of virologic failure compared with TDF/FTC in patients with a baseline HIV RNA greater than 100,000 copies per mL (N Engl J Med. 2009 Dec 3;361[23]:2230–40). Based on these data, the DHHS guidelines list TDF/FTC as the preferred NRTI pair. The IAS-USA Guidelines list both as recommended, provided the HIV RNA is < 100,000 cop/mL; TDF/FTC is recommended if the HIV RNA is > 100,000 cop/mL.

Table 3.2. Major Decisions in Selecting the Initial Antiretroviral Regimen* (cont'd)

Decision	Comment
Should the third drug be an NNRTI or a PI or an integrase inhibitor?	NNRTI-based regimens—in particular those EFV—are in general simpler to take than PI-based treatments. EFV-based regimens have also demonstrated superior antiviral activity in prospective clinical trials (N Engl J Med 2008 May 15;358[20]:2095–106), although interestingly, immunologic response was better with the boosted PI. While PI-based regimens have a somewhat higher pill burden and more drug-drug interactions, they confer a lower risk of resistance in the case of virologic failure. The integrase strand transfer inhibitors (INSTI) raltegravir and elvitegravir (with cobicistat as a PK booster) demonstrated comparable efficacy to EFV in prospective clinical trials, with fewer drug-related adverse effects (Lancet 2009 Sep 5;37[9692]:796–806, Lancet 30 June 2012;379 (9835):2439–2448). In prospective randomized trials, dolutegravir was superior to EFV and DRV/r, non-inferior to RAL (NEJM 2013;369;1807–19; Lancet 2013; 381 (9868): 735–43).
If an NNRTI-based regimen is chosen, which agent should be used?	In general, EFV is the preferred NNRTI due to comparable or superior antiviral activity to all comparators in prospective clinical trials. It is also available as a single-tablet triple regimen combined with TDF and FTC. However, EFV should be avoided in women of childbearing potential who may wish to become pregnant and may be difficult to tolerate for patients with psychiatric disease. In these contexts, Rilpivirine is also available as a single-pill regimen with TDF and FTC. Comparative clinical trials with EFV showed that RPV was better tolerated (less rash and CNS side effects), but with a higher risk of virologic failure, especially in patients with viral loads > 100,000 cop/mL (Lancet 2011; 378:229–37). NVP can lead to severe hypersensitivity (risk of which is diminished if CD4 is < 250 in women, 400 in men), requires dose escalation, and appears to be less effective than EFV; as a result, it is rarely selected for initial therapy today in the United States.
If a PI-based regimen is chosen, which PI should be used?	Comparative clinical trials have suggested more favorable tolerability and efficacy with ATV + RTV and DRV + RTV over LPV/r (Lancet 2008;372:646–55 and AIDS 2008;22:1389–97), and treatment guidelines hence list ATV + RTV and DRV + RTV as preferred.

Table 3.2. Major Decisions in Selecting the Initial Antiretroviral Regimen* (cont'd)

Decision	Comment
Should a single-tablet regimen be used?	Some data suggest that adherence and clinical outcomes are improved with regimens that consist of one tablet daily compared with those that are multiple pills (AIDS. 2010 Nov 27;24(18):2835–40. PLoS One. 2012;7(2):e31591). There are three combination tablets approved for initial therapy of HIV: TDF/FTC/EFV, TDF/FTC/RPV, and TDF/FTC/EVG/c. All three had excellent rates of virologic suppression in prospective clinical trials. While TDF/FTC/EFV has been available the longest, it may not be suitable for some patients with psychiatric disease or in women of childbearing potential. TDF/FTC/RPV should be avoided in patients with HIV RNA > 100,000 cop/mL, and TDF/FTC/EVG/c should not be given to patients with estimated GFR < 70 ml/min.

* All recommended regimens consist of three active agents: an NRTI pair (containing 3TC or FTC as one of the drugs) plus either an NNRTI or a PI. Information on adverse drug reactions and drug-drug interactions highlight important differences between available agents. Combinations not listed as "Preferred" or "Alternative" regimens in Table 3.3 should in general be avoided.

Table 3.3. DHHS Guidelines: Preferred and Alternative Antiretroviral Regimens for Antiretroviral Therapy-Naïve Patients (Last updated October 31, 2013)
Selection of a regimen should be individualized based on virologic efficacy, toxicity, pill burden, dosing frequency, drug-drug interaction potential, resistance testing results, and comorbid conditions. The regimens in each category are listed in alphabetical order. Adapted from: Panel on Clinical Practices for Treatment of HIV Infection, Guidelines for the use of Antiretroviral Agents in HIV-Infected Adults and Adolescents, Department of Health and Human Services, October 31, 2013.

A combination antiretroviral therapy (ART) regimen generally consists of two NRTIs plus one active drug from one of the following classes: NNRTI, PI (generally boosted with RTV), INSTI, or a CCR5 antagonist. Selection of a regimen should be individualized on the basis of virologic efficacy, toxicity, pill burden, dosing frequency, drug-drug interaction potential, and the patient's resistance testing results and comorbid conditions. Rating of Recommendations: A = Strong; B = Moderate; C = Optional Rating of Evidence: I = data from randomized controlled trials; II = data from well-designed nonrandomized trials or observational cohort studies with long-term clinical outcomes; III = expert opinion

Preferred Regimens (Regimens with optimal and durable efficacy, favorable tolerability and toxicity profile, and ease of use)
The preferred regimens for non-pregnant patients are arranged by chronological order of FDA approval of components other than nucleosides and, thus, by duration of clinical experience.

Table 3.3. DHHS Guidelines: Preferred and Alternative Antiretroviral Regimens for Antiretroviral Therapy-Naïve Patients (Last updated October 31, 2013) (cont'd)

Preferred Regimens (Regimens with optimal and durable efficacy, favorable tolerability and toxicity profile, and ease of use)

NNRTI-Based Regimen • EFV/TDF/FTCª **(AI)**	**Comments** • **EFV** is teratogenic in non-human primates. A regimen that does not include EFV should be strongly considered in women who are planning to become pregnant or who are sexually active and not using effective contraception.
PI-Based Regimens *(in alphabetical order)* • ATV/r + TDF/FTCª **(AI)** • DRV/r (once daily) + TDF/FTCª **(AI)** **INSTI-Based Regimen** • RAL + TDF/FTCª **(AI)** • EVG/COBI/TDF/FTC **(AI)** • DTG + ABC/3TC in patients who are HLA-B*5701 negative **(AI)** • DTG + TDF/FTC **(AI)**	• **TDF** should be used with caution in patients with renal insufficiency. • **ATV/r** should not be used in patients who require >20 mg omeprazole equivalent per day. • **EVG/COBI/TDF/FTC** should not be started in patients with estimated creatinine clearance (CrCl) < 70 mL/min, and should be changed to an alternative ARV regimen if CrCl falls below 50 mL/min on therapy • **COBI** is a potent CYP 3A inhibitor. It can increase the concentration of other drugs metabolized by this pathway. • **EVG/COBI/TDF/FTC** should not be used with other antiretroviral drugs or with nephrotoxic drugs

Alternative Regimens (Regimens that are effective and tolerable but have potential disadvantages compared with preferred regimens. An alternative regimen may be the preferred regimen for some patients.)

NNRTI-Based Regimens *(in alphabetical order)* • EFV + ABC/3TCª **(BI)** • RPV/TDF/FTCª **(BI)** • RPV + ABC/3TCª **(BIII)** **PI-Based Regimens** *(in alphabetical order)* • ATV/r + ABC/3TCª **(BI)** • DRV/r + ABC/3TCª **(BII)** • FPV/r (once or twice daily) + ABC/3TCª or TDF/FTCª **(BI)** • LPV/r (once or twice daily) + ABC/3TCª or TDF/FTCª **(BI)**	**Comments** • RPV is not recommended in patients with pretreatment HIV RNA >100,000 copies/mL. • Higher rate of virologic failures reported in patients with pre-ART CD4 count <200 cells/mm³. • Use of PPIs with **RPV** is contraindicated. • **ABC** should not be used in patients who test positive for HLA-B*5701. • Use **ABC** with caution in patients with known high risk of CVD or with pretreatment HIV RNA >100,000 copies/mL. • **Once-daily LPV/r** is not recommended for use in pregnant women.

Table 3.3. DHHS Guidelines: Preferred and Alternative Antiretroviral Regimens for Antiretroviral Therapy-Naïve Patients (Last updated October 31, 2013) (cont'd)

Alternative Regimens (Regimens that are effective and tolerable but have potential disadvantages compared with preferred regimens. An alternative regimen may be the preferred regimen for some patients.) (cont'd)	
INSTI-Based Regimen • RAL + ABC/3TC[a] **(BIII)**	

[a]3TC may substitute for FTC or vice versa.

The following combinations in the recommended list above are available as coformulated fixed-dose combinations: ABC/3TC, EFV/TDF/FTC, EVG/COBI/TDF/FTC, LPV/r, RPV/TDF/FTC, TDF/FTC, and ZDV/3TC.

Key to Abbreviations: 3TC = lamivudine, ABC = abacavir, ART = antiretroviral therapy, ARV = antiretroviral, ATV/r = atazanavir/ritonavir, COBI = cobicistat, CrCl = creatinine clearance, CVD = cardiovascular disease, DRV/r = darunavir/ritonavir, DTV = dolutegravir, EFV = efavirenz, EVG = elvitegravir, FDA = Food and Drug Administration, FPV/r = fosamprenavir/ritonavir, FTC = emtricitabine, INSTI = integrase strand transfer inhibitor, LPV/r = lopinavir/ritonavir, NNRTI = non-nucleoside reverse transcriptase inhibitor, NRTI = nucleos(t)ide reverse transcriptase inhibitor, PI = protease inhibitor, PPI = proton pump inhibitor, RAL = raltegravir, RPV = rilpivirine, RTV = ritonavir, TDF = tenofovir, ZDV = zidovudine

Reproduced from: Panel on Clinical Practices for Treatment of HIV Infection. Guidelines for the use of Antiretroviral Agents in HIV-infected Adults and Adolescents. Department of Health and Human Services. October 31, 2013.

Table 3.4. 2012 IAS-USA Guidelines: Recommended and Alternative Initial Antiretroviral Regimens, Including Strength of Recommendations and Quality of Evidence[a]

	Recommended Regimens	Alternative Regimens[b]	Comments
NNRTI plus NRTIs	Efavirenz/tenofovir/ emtricitabine (AIa) Efavirenz plus abacavir/lamivudine[c,d] (AIa) in HLA-B*5701– negative patients with baseline plasma HIV-1 RNA<100000 copies/mL	Nevirapine plus tenofovir/ emtricitabine or abacavir/ lamivudine (BIa) Rilpivirine/ tenofovir/emtricitabine (or rilpivirine plus abacavir/ lamivudine) (BIa)	Severe hepatotoxicity and rash with nevirapine are more common in initial therapy when CD4 cell count is >250/μL in women and >400/μL in men.
PI/r plus NRTIs[c]	Darunavir/r plus tenofovir/ emtricitabine (AIa) Atazanavir/r plus tenofovir/	Darunavir/r plus abacavir/ lamivudine (BIII) Lopinavir/r[d] plus tenofovir/	Other alternative PIs include fosamprenavir/r

Table 3.4. 2012 IAS-USA Guidelines: Recommended and Alternative Initial Antiretroviral Regimens, Including Strength of Recommendations and Quality of Evidence[a] (cont'd)

	Recommended Regimens	Alternative Regimens[b]	Comments
	emtricitabine (AIa) Atazanavir/r plus abacavir/lamivudine (AIa) in patients with plasma HIV-1 RNA<100000 copies/mL	emtricitabine(BIa)(or abacavir/lamivudine) (BIa)	and saquinavir/r but indications to use these options for initial treatment are rare.
InSTI plus NRTIs[c]	Raltegravir plus tenofovir/emtricitabine (AIa)	Raltegravir plus abacavir/lamivudine (BIIa) Elvitegravir/cobicistat/tenofovir/emtricitabine (BIb)	Raltegravir is given twice daily

Abbreviations: InSTI, integrase strand transfer inhibitor; NRTI, nucleos(t)ide reverse transcriptase inhibitor; NNRTI, nonnucleoside reverse transcriptase inhibitor; PI, protease inhibitor; /r, ritonavir-boosted.

[a] Ratings of the strength of the recommendations and quality of evidence are described in the eBox. Fixed-dose combinations are recommended when available and appropriate. Current fixed-dose combinations available are efavirenz/tenofovir/emtricitabine; tenofovir/emtricitabine; abacavir/lamivudine; rilpivirine/tenofovir/emtricitabine; lopinavir/ritonavir; zidovudine/lamivudine; and, if approved, elvitegravir/cobicistat/tenofovir/emtricitabine.

[b] Zidovudine/lamivudine is an alternative NRTI component of NNRTI-,PI /r-, and raltegravir-based regimens, but the toxicity profile of zidovudine reduces its utility.

[c] HLA-B*5701screening is recommended before abacavir administration to reduce the risk of hypersensitivity reaction.

[d] Avoiding the use of abacavir or lopinavir/ritonavir might be considered for patients with or at high risk of cardiovascular disease.

Reproduced from *JAMA*. 2012;308(4):387–402.

Table 3.5. Advantages and Disadvantages of Antiretroviral Components Recommended as Initial Antiretroviral Therapy (Last updated February 12, 2013)

ARV Class	ARV Agent(s)	Advantages	Disadvantages
NNRTIs (in alphabetical order)		**NNRTI Class Advantages:** • Long half-lives	**NNRTI Class Disadvantages:** • Greater risk of resistance at the time of treatment failure with NNRTIs than with PIs • Potential for cross resistance • Skin rash • Potential for CYP450 drug interactions • Transmitted resistance more common with NNRTIs than with PIs

Table 3.5. Advantages and Disadvantages of Antiretroviral Components Recommended as Initial Antiretroviral Therapy (cont'd)

ARV Class	ARV Agent(s)	Advantages	Disadvantages
	EFV	• Virologic responses non-inferior or superior to all comparators to date • Once-daily dosing • Coformulated with TDF/FTC	• Neuropsychiatric side effects • Teratogenic in nonhuman primates. Several cases of neural tube defect in infants born to women who were exposed to EFV in the first trimester of pregnancy reported. • Dyslipidemia
	NVP	• No food effect • Fewer lipid effects than EFV • Once-daily dosing with extended-release tablet formulation	• Higher incidence of rash, including rare but serious HSRs (SJS or TEN), than with other NNRTIs • Higher incidence of hepatotoxicity, including serious and even fatal cases of hepatic necrosis, than with other NNRTIs • Contraindicated in patients with moderate or severe (Child-Pugh B or C) hepatic impairment • ART-naive patients with high pre-treatment CD4 counts (>250 cells/mm^3 for females, >400 cells/mm^3 for males) are at higher risk of symptomatic hepatic events. NVP is not recommended in these patients unless benefit clearly outweighs risk. • Early virologic failure of NVP + TDF + (FTC or 3TC) in small clinical trials
	RPV	• Once-daily dosing • Coformulated with TDF/FTC • Smaller pill size than co-formulated TDF/FTC/EFV or TDF/FTC/EVG/COBI	• Not recommended for use in patients with pre-ART HIV RNA >100,000 copies/mL because the rate of virologic failures is higher in these patients • Higher rate of virologic failures observed in patients with pre-ART CD4 count < 200 cells/mm^3 • More NNRTI, TDF-, and 3TC-associated mutations at virological failure than with regimen containing EFV + two NRTIs • Meal requirement • Absorption depends on lower gastric pH.

Table 3.5. Advantages and Disadvantages of Antiretroviral Components Recommended as Initial Antiretroviral Therapy (cont'd)

ARV Class	ARV Agent(s)	Advantages	Disadvantages
		• Compared with EFV: – Fewer discontinuations for CNS adverse effects – Fewer lipid effects – Fewer rashes – Smaller pill size	• Contraindicated with PPIs • RPV-associated depression reported • Use RPV with caution when coadministered with a drug having a known risk of torsades de pointes.
PIs (in alphabetical order)		**PI Class Advantages:** • Higher genetic barrier to resistance than NNRTIs and RAL • PI resistance uncommon with failure (boosted PIs)	**PI Class Disadvantages:** • Metabolic complications such as dyslipidemia, insulin resistance, hepatotoxicity • GI adverse effects • CYP3A4 inhibitors and substrates: potential for drug interactions (more pronounced with RTV-based regimens)
	ATV (unboosted)	• Fewer adverse effects on lipids than other PIs • Once-daily dosing • Low pill burden • Good GI tolerability • Signature mutation (I50L) not associated with broad PI cross resistance	• Indirect hyperbilirubinemia sometimes leading to jaundice or scleral icterus • PR interval prolongation: generally inconsequential unless ATV combined with another drug with similar effect • Unboosted ATV should not be coadministered with TDF, EFV, or NVP (See ATV/r.) • Nephrolithiasis, cholelithiasis • Skin rash • Food requirement • Absorption depends on food and low gastric pH
	ATV/r	• RTV boosting: higher trough ATV concentration and greater antiviral effect	• More adverse effects on lipids than unboosted ATV • More hyperbilirubinemia and jaundice than unboosted ATV • Food requirement

Table 3.5. Advantages and Disadvantages of Antiretroviral Components Recommended as Initial Antiretroviral Therapy (cont'd)

ARV Class	ARV Agent(s)	Advantages	Disadvantages
		• Once-daily dosing • Low pill burden	• Absorption depends on food and low gastric pH. • RTV boosting required with TDF and EFV. With EFV, use ATV 400 mg and RTV 100 mg once daily (PI-naive patients only). • Should not be coadministered with NVP • Nephrolithiasis, cholelithiasis
	DRV/r	• Once-daily dosing • Potent virologic efficacy	• Skin rash • Food requirement
	FPV/r	• Twice-daily dosing resulted in efficacy comparable to LPV/r • Once-daily dosing possible with RTV 100 mg or 200 mg daily • No food effect	• Skin rash • Hyperlipidemia • Once-daily dosing results in lower APV concentrations than twice-daily dosing • For FPV/r 1400/200 mg: requires 200 mg of RTV • Fewer data on FPV/r 1400/100 mg dose than on DRV/r and ATV/r
	LPV/r	• Coformulated • No food requirement • Greater CD4 count increase than with EFV-based regimens	• Requires 200 mg per day of RTV • Lower drug exposure in pregnant women—may need dose increase in third trimester • Once-daily dosing not recommended in pregnant women • Once-daily dosing results in lower trough concentration than twice-daily dosing • Possible higher risk of MI associated with cumulative use of LPV/r • PR and QT interval prolongation have been reported. Use with caution in patients at risk of cardiac conduction abnormalities or receiving other drugs with similar effect.

Table 3.5. Advantages and Disadvantages of Antiretroviral Components Recommended as Initial Antiretroviral Therapy (cont'd)

ARV Class	ARV Agent(s)	Advantages	Disadvantages
	SQV/r	• Similar efficacy but less hyperlipidemia than with LPV/r	• Highest pill burden (6 pills per day) among available PI regimens • Requires 200 mg of RTV • Food requirement • PR and/or QT interval prolongations in a healthy volunteer study • Pretreatment ECG recommended • SQV/r is not recommended for patients with any of the following conditions: (1) congenital or acquired QT prolongation; (2) pretreatment ECG >450 msec; (3) on concomitant therapy with other drugs that prolong QT interval; (4) complete AV block without implanted pacemakers; (5) risk of complete AV block.
INSTI (in alphabetical order)	EVG	• Co-formulation with cobicistat (COBI)/TDF/FTC • Once daily dosing • Non-inferior to EFV/TDF/FTC and ATV/r + TDF/FTC	• COBI – potent CYP3A4 inhibitor – significant interactions with CYP3A substrates • COBI inhibits active tubular secretion of creatinine and can decrease CrCL without affecting renal glomerular function • Has potential for new onset or worsening of renal impairment • Only recommended for patients with baseline CrCl > 70 mL/min; therapy should be discontinued if CrCl decreased to < 50mL/min • Food requirement
	RAL	• Virologic response noninferior to EFVsuperior at 4–5 years	• Twice-daily dosing • Lower genetic barrier to resistance than with boosted PI-based regimens

Table 3.5. Advantages and Disadvantages of Antiretroviral Components Recommended as Initial Antiretroviral Therapy (cont'd)

ARV Class	ARV Agent(s)	Advantages	Disadvantages
		• Fewer drug-related adverse events and lipid changes than EFV • No food effect • Fewer drug-drug interactions than EVG/COBI,/TDF/FTC, PI-, NNRTI, or MVC	• Increase in creatine kinase, myopathy, and rhabdomyolysis have been reported • Rare cases of severe hypersensitivity reactions (including SJS and TEN) have been reported.
CCR5 Antagonist	MVC	• Virologic response noninferior to EFV in post hoc analysis of MERIT study (See text.) • Fewer adverse effects than EFV	• Requires viral tropism testing prior to initiation of therapy, which results in additional cost and possible delay in initiation of therapy • More MVC-treated than EFV-treated patients discontinued therapy due to lack of efficacy in MERIT study • Less long-term experience in ART-naive patients than with boosted PI- or NNRTI-based regimens • Limited experience with dual-NRTIs other than ZDV/3TC • Twice-daily dosing • CYP 3A4 substrate; dosing depends on presence or absence of concomitant CYP3A4 inducer(s) or inhibitor(s)
Dual-NRTI pairs (in alphabetical order)	ABC/3TC	• Virologic response noninferior to ZDV/3TC • Better CD4 count responses than with ZDV/3TC • Once-daily dosing • Coformulation • No food effect • No cumulative TAM-mediated resistance	• Potential for ABC HSR in patients with HLA-B*5701 • Inferior virologic responses in patients with baseline HIV RNA >100,000 copies/mL when compared with TDF/FTC in ACTG 5202 study; but not in the HEAT study. • Some observational cohort studies show increased potential for cardiovascular events, especially in patients with cardiovascular risk factors

Table 3.5. Advantages and Disadvantages of Antiretroviral Components Recommended as Initial Antiretroviral Therapy (cont'd)

ARV Class	ARV Agent(s)	Advantages	Disadvantages
	TDF/FTC	• Better virologic responses than with ABC/3TC in patients with baseline viral load >100,000 copies/mL in ACTG 5202 study; however, this was not seen in the HEAT study. • Active against HBV; recommended dual-NRTI for HIV/HBV coinfection • Once-daily dosing • No food effect • Coformulated (TDF/FTC, EFV/TDF/FTC, EVG/COBI/TDF/FTC, and RPV/TDF/FTC) • No cumulative TAM-mediated resistance	• Potential for renal impairment, including proximal tubulopathy and acute or chronic renal insufficiency • Early virologic failure of NVP + TDF + (FTC or 3TC) in small clinical trials • Potential for decrease in BMD
	ZDV/3TC	• Coformulated (ZDV/3TC and ZDV/3TC/ABC) • No food effect (although better tolerated with food) • Preferred dual NRTI in pregnant women	• Bone marrow suppression, especially anemia and neutropenia • GI intolerance, headache • Mitochondrial toxicity, including lipoatrophy, lactic acidosis, hepatic steatosis • Compared with TDF/FTC, inferior in combination with EFV • Less CD4 increase compared with ABC/3TC • Twice-daily dosing

Table 3.5. Advantages and Disadvantages of Antiretroviral Components Recommended as Initial Antiretroviral Therapy (cont'd)

Key to Abbreviations: 3TC = lamivudine, ABC = abacavir, APV = amprenavir, ART = antiretroviral therapy, ARV = antiretroviral, ATV = atazanavir, ATV/r = atazanavir/ritonavir, AV = atrioventricular, BMD = bone mineral density, CNS = central nervous system, COBI = cobicistat, CrCl = creatinine clearance, CYP = cytochrome P, d4T = stavudine, ddI = didanosine, DRV/r = darunavir/ritonavir, ECG = electrocardiogram, EFV = efavirenz, EVG = elvitegravir, FPV = fosamprenavir, FPV/r = fosamprenavir/ritonavir, FTC = emtricitabine, GI = gastrointestinal, HBV = hepatitis B virus, HSR = hypersensitivity reaction, INSTI = integrase strand transfer inhibitor, LPV/r = lopinavir/ritonavir, MI = myocardial infarction, msec = milliseconds, MVC = maraviroc, NNRTI = non-nucleoside reverse transcriptase inhibitor, NRTI = nucleoside reverse transcriptase inhibitor, NVP = nevirapine, PI = protease inhibitor, PPI = proton pump inhibitor, RAL = raltegravir, RPV = rilpivirine, RTV = ritonavir, SJS = Stevens-Johnson syndrome, SQV/r = saquinavir/ritonavir, TAM = thymidine analogue mutation, TDF = tenofovir, TEN = toxic epidermal necrosis, ZDV = zidovudine

METABOLIC AND MORPHOLOGIC COMPLICATIONS OF THERAPY

The metabolic and morphologic changes that occur with HIV therapy are sometimes grouped under the term "lipodystrophy syndrome." Key features include *subcutaneous lipoatrophy*, which is most evident in the face, limbs, and buttocks; and *regional fat accumulation*, which may occur in the posterior or anterior portions of the neck and in the midsection, as a manifestation of visceral adiposity. Patients may have predominantly lipoatrophy, fat accumulation, or both. Lipoatrophy has become less common since the principal causative agents stavudine and zidovudine are rarely used today. These morphologic changes are often accompanied by metabolic derangements, including lipid dysregulation (increased triglycerides and total cholesterol; reduced HDL cholesterol) and insulin resistance. The etiology of the lipodystrophy syndrome is poorly understood, and there are clearly both host and treatment factors.

A. Lipoatrophy

1. **Overview.** The most important host risk factor is the stage of HIV disease, as patients with more advanced HIV-related immunosuppression are at greatest risk. Among treatment-related factors, the leading hypothesis is that NRTI-induced mitochondrial toxicity induces fat cell apoptosis, and NRTIs with the highest *in vitro* inhibition of the mitochondrial enzyme polymerase gamma pose the greatest risk. Based on this hypothesis, a hierarchy of treatment-associated risk for lipoatrophy would be as follows: *highest risk* for dideoxynucleosides (stavudine, didanosine, and zalcitabine); *intermediate risk* for zidovudine; and *lowest risk* for tenofovir, abacavir, lamivudine, and emtricitabine. While one study showed a greater degree of mild lipoatrophy with efavirenz versus lopinavir/r treatment, (AIDS 2009;23:1109–18) in general the NNRTI class of medications has not been implicated in this process.

2. **Treatment.** Treatment strategies for lipoatrophy consist of drug substitutions, insulin-sensitizing agents, and plastic surgery. Substituting tenofovir or abacavir for stavudine or zidovudine leads to a gradual increase in limb fat that is often accompanied by a subjective improvement in facial appearance (AIDS 2006;20:2043–50). Such improvements occur slowly after antiretroviral switches and may not be evident to the patient for several months or at all. The tenofovir substitution strategy may also improve lipid abnormalities. Substituting an NNRTI for the PI-component of the regimen has had no consistent effect on morphologic changes (AIDS 2005;19:917–25). Although there was initial optimism that insulin-sensitizing agents would help reverse lipoatrophy, the bulk of prospective data do not support a role for this approach, and such drugs are not recommended in the absence of established medical indications (e.g., hyperglycemia). Finally, cosmetic surgery for facial lipoatrophy can often dramatically improve appearance. The most common

approach is injection of biologically inert substances such as polylactic acid (Sculptra). Patient satisfaction after polylactic acid injections is extremely high, and thus far the procedure appears safe. The major drawbacks to this treatment approach include the lack of long-term efficacy and safety data, relatively high cost, and lack of effect on lipoatrophy of the arms and legs. Patients should be informed that most insurance policies and state-funded programs will not cover the cost of polylactic acid injections.

B. Fat Accumulation

   1. Overview. Fat accumulation can be highly disfiguring; when fat accumulation is in the form of visceral adiposity, it is associated with increased cardiovascular risk. The neck, upper body, and intra-abdominal (visceral) sites are most often involved. (Neck fat accumulation in the posterior compartment is often referred to as a buffalo hump.) Despite the similarity to Cushing's syndrome, serum cortisol levels are not elevated. While fat accumulation syndrome is anecdotally linked to PI-based therapy, cases have occurred in the absence of PIs as well; one prospective study found that patients treated with atazanavir/r based regimens had greater fat accumulation that those receiving efavirenz (Clin Infect Dis 2011; 53(2):185–196).

   2. Treatment. No treatment modification has consistently led to improvement. Exercise may reduce central fat accumulation, and weight loss may reduce neck fat, but improvements are generally modest. Recombinant growth hormone reduces central fat accumulation, but treatment is expensive and associated with a risk of other side effects, including glucose intolerance and carpal tunnel syndrome. The injectable growth hormone releasing factor tesamorelin appears safe and modestly effective for this indication (J Clin Endocrinol Metab. 2010 Jun 16); it is approved for this indication at a dose of 2 mg once daily. The beneficial effects of tesamorelin in reducing visceral adiposity wane quickly when the medication is stopped; as such, the optimal duration of therapy is unknown, and some patients continue it indefinitely. Liposuction of neck fat accumulation is the most rapidly effective technique, but recurrences are possible. Insurance coverage for neck liposuction can sometimes be deemed medically necessary if the fat accumulation leads to medical problems such as neck pain or sleep apnea.

C. Prevention of Lipodystrophy. Since morphologic changes are only slowly reversible and may be permanent in some patients, the best strategy is to choose treatments that are least likely to induce these abnormalities. Of currently preferred NRTI combinations, tenofovir/emtricitabine and abacavir/lamivudine induce less fat atrophy than zidovudine/lamivudine (Table 3.6). In addition, providers should consider a proactive switching strategy for patients receiving long-term zidovudine/lamivudine. Regimens containing stavudine should be avoided unless there are no alternatives.

Table 3.6. Treatment and Prevention of Body Habitus Changes Associated with Antiretroviral Therapy

Treatment	• Substitute tenofovir or abacavir for thymidine analogue • Polylactic acid injections for facial lipoatrophy • Weight loss and exercise for fat accumulation • Liposuction for dorsocervical fat accumulation • Tesamorelin for central fat accumulation
Prevention	• Start therapy before advanced HIV disease • Select initial NRTI backbones less likely to induce lipoatrophy (i.e., emtricitabine/tenofovir or abacavir/lamivudine) • Consider proactive switch to tenofovir DF or abacavir for patients still on thymidine analogues (ZDV or d4T)

D. **Lipid Abnormalities.** Multiple abnormalities in lipid metabolism were reported in HIV-infected patients before the availability of combination antiretroviral therapy, including increased levels of very low-density lipoprotein (VLDL) cholesterol and triglycerides and decreased levels of high-density lipoprotein (HDL) cholesterol, low-density lipoprotein (LDL) cholesterol, and apolipoprotein B (JAMA 2003;289:2978–82). However, soon after the introduction of PIs, a dramatic increase in triglyceride levels and, to a lesser extent, total cholesterol levels were evident in PI-treated patients.

1. **Antiretroviral Therapy and Dyslipidemia.** The PIs are all associated to varying degrees with clinically significant dyslipidemia. Among recommended boosted PIs, atazanavir and darunavir appear to have the lowest risk of hyperlipidemia, possibly because they use only 100 mg/day of ritonavir. Other components of the antiretroviral regimen may also induce lipid disturbances: d4T, ZDV, and ABC are all more likely to raise lipids than tenofovir, and efavirenz increases lipids, especially triglycerides, more than nevirapine, etravirine, and rilpivirine. Raltegravir, maraviroc, elvitegravir/c, and dolutegravir increase lipids less than efavirenz. Treatment of HIV may have the favorable effect of raising HDL cholesterol, particularly with nevirapine and efavirenz.

2. **Treatment of Dyslipidemia.** Various approaches can be taken to treat PI-associated dyslipidemia. As for HIV-negative patients, the first step consists of therapeutic lifestyle changes, including dietary counseling, reduction in alcohol intake, smoking cessation, and increased aerobic exercise. Unfortunately, lifestyle changes alone are often insufficient to reverse lipid abnormalities in patients with HIV. The two most widely used pharmacological strategies are substitution of the potentially offending antiretroviral agent with an alternative antiretroviral and use of lipid-modifying drug therapy. In patients who are virologically suppressed and have no or little presumed antiretroviral resistance, the former strategy is generally safe but may not lower lipids into the desirable range (AIDS 2005;19:1051–8). When switching antiretroviral drugs it is important to weigh the risks of new treatment-related toxicities and virologic relapse against the risks of potential drug interactions and new treatment-related toxicities from lipid-lowering agents. Table 3.7 cites some potential switch strategies; if there is more than one possible offending agent, the changes should be made sequentially

to ensure that the initial change is well tolerated. The use of lipid-lowering agents in HIV-infected patients is notable for a relative lack of efficacy and a high risk of drug interactions, particularly between the statins and PIs. Nonetheless, lipid abnormalities should be aggressively treated just as in HIV-negative patients, especially when other cardiac risk factors are present.

Elevations in LDL cholesterol will usually require statin therapy. Most of the statins, with the exception of pravastatin, fluvastatin, pitavastatin, and rosuvastatin, are metabolized by the cytochrome P450 enzyme system via the 3A4 isoform (CYP3A4). Most PIs and cobicistat inhibit CYP3A4, potentially leading to elevated statin levels increasing the risk of statin-related toxicity, including rhabdomyolysis (Clin Infect Dis 2002;35:e111–2). We generally prefer atorvastatin as the initial statin of choice, so long as the starting dose is low and the patient is closely monitored for hepatic/ muscle toxicity. Not all statin-ART drug-drug interactions are mediated through CYP3A4: rosuvastatin levels may increase significantly when given with lopinavir/r through unclear mechanisms, and darunavir appears to increase pravastatin levels. The optimal management of HIV-related hypertriglyceridemia is unclear; for levels greater than 500 mg/dL, aggressive dietary modification and use of fibrates should be implemented to reduce the risk of pancreatitis.

Table 3.7. Drug-Induced Dyslipidemia and Switch Therapy

Cause	Switch To	Comments
Protease inhibitors (PIs): ritonavir, indinavir, saquinavir, nelfinavir, lopinavir/r, tipranavir, fosamprenavir	Atazanavir or atazanavir/ ritonavir or darunavir/ ritonavir or rilpivirine or raltegravir or dolutegravir	Need to use boosted atazanavir if patient is also on tenofovir. Do not use unboosted atazanavir if there is any history of PI resistance or PI-related treatment failure; do not use rilpivirine if there is any history of NRTI resistance. If patient is on a proton pump inhibitor, atazanavir and rilpivirine should in general be avoided.
d4T or ZDV	Tenofovir	Use with caution in patients with impaired renal function; if necessary, reduce dose per package insert guidelines
Efavirenz	Nevirapine or Rilpivirine or Etravirine	Avoid NVP women with CD4 > 250/mm^3 or men with CD4 > 400/mm^3 due to increased risk of hepatotoxicity

ANTIRETROVIRAL THERAPY ADVERSE EFFECTS

Although the tolerability and safety of antiretroviral therapy has improved substantially, adverse events have been reported with all the available agents. In addition, subjective side effects remain one of the most common causes of medication non-compliance and treatment failure. Certain drugs — such as d4T, ddl, and indinavir — are now rarely used in developed countries due to their relatively poor adverse event profile, but may still be used in resource-limited settings that do not have access to the newest agents. In addition, recently-approved compounds necessarily have less comprehensive data on side effects that are either particularly rare or might not occur except after prolonged exposure.

Clinicians should be particularly alert to potential side effects that may occur in patients who already have underlying disease processes, or who are taking concomitant medications with overlapping toxicities. For example, individuals co-infected with hepatitis B and C generally have higher rates of hepatotoxicity; those with psychiatric disease are more prone to the adverse CNS effects of efavirenz; and patients with pre-existing renal disease may be more likely to experience tenofovir nephrotoxicity. Table 3.8 was adapted from DHHS Guidelines for the Use of Antiretroviral Agents in HIV-1-Infected Adults and Adolescents, last updated February –, 2013.

Table 3.8. Antiretroviral Therapy-Associated Common and/or Severe Adverse Effects (Last updated February 12, 2013)

Adverse Effects	NRTIs	NNRTIs	PIs	INSTI	EI
Bleeding events			**All PIs:** ↑ spontaneous bleeding, hematuria in hemophilia **TPV:** Reports of intracranial hemorrhage. Risks include CNS lesions; trauma; surgery; hypertension; alcohol abuse; coagulopathy, anti-coagulant, or anti-platelet agents including vitamin E		
Bone marrow suppression	**ZDV:** Anemia, neutropenia				
Cardiovascular disease (CVD)	**ABC** and **ddI:** Associated with myocardial infarction (MI) in some but not all cohort studies. Risk greatest among those with traditional CVD risk factors.		**PIs:** Associated with MI and stroke in some cohort studies. Risk greatest among those with traditional CVD risk factors. Limited data on newer PIs (ATV, DRV, TPV). **SQV/r, ATV + RTV,** and **LPV/r:** PR interval prolongation. Risks include structural heart disease, conduction system abnormalities, cardiomyopathy, ischemic heart disease, and coadministration with		

Table 3.8. Antiretroviral Therapy-Associated Common and/or Severe Adverse Effects (Last updated February 12, 2013; last reviewed February 12, 2013) (cont'd)

Adverse Effects	NRTIs	NNRTIs	PIs	INSTI	EI
			drugs that prolong PR interval. **SQV/r:** QT interval prolongation in a healthy volunteer study. Risks include underlying heart conditions, pre-existing prolonged QT or arrhythmia, or use with other QT-prolonging drugs. ECG prior to SQV initiation is recommended and should be considered during therapy.		
Central nervous system (CNS) effects	**d4T:** Associated with rapidly progressive ascending neuromuscular weakness resembling Guillain-Barré syndrome (rare)	**EFV:** Somnolence, insomnia, abnormal dreams, dizziness, impaired concentration, depression, psychosis, suicidal ideation. Most symptoms subside or diminish after 2–4 weeks. Bedtime dosing may reduce symptoms. Risks include history of psychiatric illness, concomitant use of agents with neuropsychiatric effects, and ↑ plasma EFV concentrations due to genetic factors or absorption (i.e., with food).		**RAL:** Depression (uncommon)	

Cholelithiasis			**ATV:** • History of kidney stones increases risk and patients may present with cholelithiasis and kidney stones concurrently • Typically presents as abdominal pain • Reported complications include cholecystitis, pancreatitis, choledocholithiasis, and cholangitis • Median time to onset is 42 months (range 1–90 months)
Diabetes mellitus (DM)/insulin resistance	ZDV, **d4T**, and **ddI**		• Reported for some **PIs** (**IDV, LPV/r**), but not all PIs studied • **ATV +/– RTV** not found to alter insulin sensitivity
Dyslipidemia	**d4T > ZDV > ABC:** • ↑ LDL and TG	**EFV** • ↑ TG • ↑ LDL • ↑ HDL	↑ LDL, ↑ TG, ↑ HDL: **all RTV-boosted PIs** TG: **LPV/r = FPV/r** and **LPV/r > DRV + RTV and ATV + RTV**

Table 3.8. Antiretroviral Therapy-Associated Common and/or Severe Adverse Effects (Last updated February 12, 2013; last reviewed February 12, 2013) (cont'd)

Adverse Effects	NRTIs	NNRTIs	PIs	INSTI	EI
Gastrointestinal (GI)	Nausea and vomiting: **ddI** and **ZDV** > other **NRTIs** Pancreatitis: **ddI**		GI intolerance (diarrhea, nausea, vomiting) Diarrhea: common with **NFV**. **LPV/r** > **DRV + RTV** and **ATV + RTV**	Nausea and diarrhea: EVG/COBI/TDF/FTC	
Hepatic effects	Reported for most **NRTIs** **ddI**: prolonged exposure linked to noncirrhotic portal hypertension, some cases with esophageal varicees Steatosis: most commonly seen with **ZDV, d4T,** or **ddI** Flares: hepatitis B virus (HBV)-coinfected patients may develop severe hepatic flare when **TDF, 3TC,** and **FTC** are withdrawn or when HBV resistance develops.	**NVP > other NNRTIs** **NVP:** • Severe hepatic toxicity with **NVP** is often associated with skin rash or symptoms of hypersensitivity. • For ARV-naïve patients, risk is greater for women with pre-**NVP** CD4 count >250 cells/mm³ and men with pre-**NVP** CD4 count >400 cells/mm³. Risk is higher for women.	**All PIs:** Drug-induced hepatitis and hepatic decompensation (and rare cases of fatalities) have been reported with all PIs to varying degrees. **TPV/r** has a higher frequency of hepatic events than other PIs. **IDV, ATV:** jaundice due to indirect hyperbilirubinemia		

			TPV/r: Contraindicated in patients with moderate to severe hepatic insufficiency (Child-Pugh classification B or C)	
		• 2-week dose escalation of **NVP** reduces risk of rash and possibly hepatotoxicity if related to hypersensitivity. • Given high risk in those with competent immune systems, **NVP** should never be used for post-exposure prophylaxis in HIV-uninfected individuals. • **NVP** is contraindicated in patients with Child-Pugh classification B or C.	**NVP:** • Hypersensitivity syndrome of hepatic toxicity and rash that may be accompanied by fever, general malaise, fatigue, myalgias, arthralgias, blisters, oral lesions, conjunctivitis, facial edema, eosinophilia,	
Hypersensitivity reaction (HSR) (excluding rash alone or Stevens Johnson syndrome [SJS])		**ABC:** • HLA-B*5701 screening prior to initiation of **ABC.** Should not be started if HLA-B*5701 is positive. • Symptoms of HSR include (in descending frequency): fever, skin rash, malaise, nausea, headache, myalgia, chills,		

Table 3.8. Antiretroviral Therapy-Associated Common and/or Severe Adverse Effects Last updated February 12, 2013; last reviewed February 12, 2013 (cont'd)

Adverse Effects	NRTIs	NNRTIs	PIs	INSTI	EI
	diarrhea, vomiting, abdominal pain, dyspnea, arthralgia, respiratory symptoms • Worsen with continuation of **ABC** • Median onset 9 days; ~ 90% of reactions within first 6 weeks • Onset of rechallenge reactions is within hours of rechallenge dose	granulocytopenia, lymphadenopathy, or renal dysfunction. • For ARV-naïve patients, risk is greater for women with pre-**NVP** CD4 count >250 cells/mm^3 and men with pre-**NVP** CD4 count >400 cells/mm^3. Risk is higher for women. • 2-week dose escalation of **NVP** reduces risk.			
Lactic acidosis	**NRTIs**, especially **d4T, ZDV**, and **ddI** • Insidious onset with GI prodrome, weight loss, and fatigue. May be rapidly progressive, with tachycardia, tachypnea, jaundice, muscular weakness, mental status changes, respiratory distress, pancreatitis, and organ failure.				

	• Mortality up to 50% in some case series, especially in patients with serum lactate >10 mmol/L • Increased risk: female sex, obesity Laboratory findings: • ↑ lactate (often >5 mmol/L), anion gap, AST, ALT, PT, bilirubin • ↑ amylase and lipase in patients with pancreatitis • ↓ arterial pH, serum bicarbonate, serum albumin	
Lipodystrophy	Lipoatrophy: **Thymidine analogs (d4T > ZDV)** May be more likely when combined with **EFV** vs. **boosted PI**.	Lipohypertrophy: Trunk fat increase observed with **EFV**, **PI**, and **RAL**-containing regimens; however, causal relationship has not been established.
Myopathy/ elevated CPK	**ZDV:** myopathy	**RAL:** ↑ CPK. muscle weakness and rhabdomyolysis

Table 3.8. Antiretroviral Therapy-Associated Common and/or Severe Adverse Effects Last updated February 12, 2013; last reviewed February 12, 2013 (cont'd)

Adverse Effects	NRTIs	NNRTIs	PIs	INSTI	EI
Nephrotoxicity/urolithiasis	**TDF:** ↑ serum creatinine, proteinuria, hypophosphatemia, urinary phosphate wasting, glycosuria, hypokalemia, non-anion gap metabolic acidosis Concurrent use of **PI** may increase risk.		**IDV:** ↑ serum creatinine, pyuria; hydronephrosis or renal atrophy **IDV, ATV:** Stone, crystal formation; adequate hydration may reduce risk.	**EVG/COBI/TDF/FTC:** • COBI can cause non-pathologic decrease in CrCl. • May increase risk of TDF-related neph-rotoxicity	
Osteopenia/osteoporosis	**TDF:** Associated with greater loss of bone mineral density (BMD) compared with **ZDV**, **d4T**, and **ABC**.	Decreases in BMD observed in studies of regimens containing different **NRTIs** combined with either **NNRTIs** or **PIs**.			
Peripheral neuropathy	Peripheral neuropathy (pain and/or paresthesias, lower extremities > upper extremities): **d4T > ddI** and **ddC** (can be irreversible) **d4T:** Associated with rapidly progressive ascending neuromuscular weakness resembling Guillain-Barré syndrome (rare)				

Rash		All NNRTIs	ATV, DRV, FPV	MVC
Stevens-Johnson syndrome (SJS)/ toxic epidermal necrosis (TEN)	ddl, ZDV: Reported cases	NVP > DLV, EFV, ETR For NVP risks include: • Female sex • Black, Asian, Hispanic race/ethnicity	FPV, DRV, IDV, LPV/r, ATV: Reported cases	

Key to Abbreviations: 3TC = lamivudine, ABC = abacavir, ALT = alanine aminotransferase, ARV = antiretroviral, AST = aspartate aminotransferase, ATV = atazanavir, ATV/r = atazanavir + ritonavir, BMD = bone mineral density, CrCl = creatinine clearance, CNS = central nervous system, COBI = cobicistat, CPK = creatine phosphokinase, CVD = cardiovascular disease, d4T = stavudine, ddC = zalcitabine, ddl = didanosine, DLV = delavirdine, DM = diabetes mellitus, DRV = darunavir, DRV/r = darunavir + ritonavir, ECG = electrocardiogram, EFV = efavirenz, EI = entry inhibitor, ETR = etravirine, EVG = elvitegravir, FPV = fosamprenavir, FPV/r = fosamprenavir + ritonavir, FTC = emtricitabine, GI = gastrointestinal, HBV = hepatitis B virus, HDL = high-density lipoprotein, HSR = hypersensitivity reaction, IDV = indinavir, INSTI = integrase strand transfer inhibitor, LDL = low-density lipoprotein, LPV/r = lopinavir + ritonavir, MI = myocardial infarction, MVC = maraviroc, NFV = nelfinavir, NNRTI = non-nucleoside reverse transcriptase inhibitor, NRTI = nucleoside reverse transcriptase inhibitor, NVP = nevirapine, PI = protease inhibitor, PT = prothrombin time, RAL = raltegravir, RPV = rilpivirine, RTV = ritonavir, SJS = Stevens-Johnson syndrome, SQV = saquinavir, SQV/r = saquinavir + ritonavir, TDF = tenofovir disoproxil fumarate, TEN = toxic epidermal necrosis, TG = triglyceride, TPV = tipranavir, TPV/r = tipranavir + ritonavir, ZDV = zidovudine

Reproduced from: Guidelines for the Use of Antiretroviral Agents for HIV-1-infected Adults and Adolescents: Recommendations of the Panel on Clinical Practices for Treatment of HIV Infection; aidsinfo.nih.gov.

REFERENCES AND SUGGESTED READINGS

AACE Diabetes Mellitus Clinical Practice Guidelines Task Force. American Association of Clinical Endocrinologists medical guidelines for clinical practice for the management of diabetes mellitus. *Endocr Pract*, 2007. 13 (Suppl 1):1–68.

American Diabetes Association. Clinical Practice Recommendations 2008. *Diabetes Care*, 2008. 31 (Suppl 1): S1–104.

Ann Intern Med, 2009. Mar 3;150(5):301–13.

Baylor MS, Johann-Liang R. Hepatotoxicity associated with nevirapine use. *J Acquir Immune Defic Syndr*, 2004. 35(5):538–9.

Bersoff-Matcha SJ, Miller WC, Aberg JA, et al. Sex differences in nevirapine rash. *Clin Infect Dis*, 2001. 32(1):124–9.

Bolhaar MG, Karstaedt AS. A high incidence of lactic acidosis and symptomatic hyperlactatemia in women receiving highly active antiretroviral therapy in Soweto, South Africa. *Clin Infect Dis*, 2007. 45(2):254–60.

Cazanave C, Dupon M, Lavignolle-Aurillac V, et al. Reduced bone mineral density in HIV-infected patients: prevalence and associated factors. *AIDS*, 2008. 22(3): 395–402.

D:A:D Study Group, Sabin CA, Worm SW, et al. Use of nucleoside reverse transcriptase inhibitors and risk of myocardial infarction in HIV-infected patients enrolled in the D:A:D study: a multi-cohort collaboration. *Lancet*, 2008. 371(9622):1417–26.

Dear Health Care Provider letter. Important safety information: intracranial hemorrhage in patients receiving Aptivus[a] (tipranavir) capsules. Boehringer Ingelheim Pharmaceuticals, Inc. June 30, 2006.

denBrinker M, Wit FW, Wertheim-van Dillen PM, et al. Hepatitis B and C virus co-infection and the risk for hepatotoxicity of highly active antiretroviral therapy in HIV-1 infection. *AIDS*, 2000. 14(18):2895–902.

De Wit S, Sabin CA, Weber R, et al. Incidence and risk factors for new-onset diabetes in HIV-infected patients: the Data Collection on Adverse Events of Anti-HIV Drugs (D:A:D) study. *Diabetes Care*, 2008. 31(6):1224–9.

Dieterich DT, Robinson PA, Love J, Stern JO. Drug-induced liver injury associated with the use of nonnucleoside reverse-transcriptase inhibitors. *Clin Infect Dis*, 2004. 38 (Suppl 2):S80–9.

Dube MP, Stein JH, Aberg JA, et al. Guidelines for the evaluation and management of dyslipidemia in human immunodeficiency virus (HIV)-infected adults receiving antiretroviral therapy: recommendations of the HIV Medical Association of the Infectious Disease Society of America and the Adult AIDS Clinical Trials Group. *Clin Infect Dis*, 2003. 37(5):613–27.

European AIDS Clinical Society. Prevention and Management of Non-Infectious Co-Morbidities in HIV. November 1, 2009; http://www.europeanaidsclinicalsociety.org/guidelinespdf/2_Non_Infectious_Co_Morbidities_in_HIV.pdf.

Fagot JP, Mockenhaupt M, Bouwes-Bavinck J-N, for the EuroSCAR study group. Nevirapine and the risk of Stevens-Johnson syndrome or toxic epidermal necrolysis. *AIDS*, 2001. 15(14):1843–8.

Falcó V, Rodríguez D, Ribera E, et al. Severe nucleoside-associated lactic acidosis in human immunodeficiency virus-infected patients: report of 12 cases and review of the literature. *Clin Infect Dis*, 2002. 34(6):838–46.

Fisac C, Fumero E, Crespo et al. Metabolic benefits 24 months after replacing a protease inhibitor with abacavir, efavirenz or nevirapine. *AIDS*, 2005. 19: 917–25.

Fleischer R, Boxwell D, Sherman KE. Nucleoside analogues and mitochondrial toxicity. *Clin Infect Dis*. 2004; 38(8):e79–80.

Geddes R, Knight S, Moosa MY, et al. A high incidence of nucleoside reverse transcriptase inhibitor (NRTI)-induced lactic acidosis in HIV-infected patients in a South African context. *S Afr Med J*, 2006. 96(8):722–4.

Guyader D, Poinsignon Y, Cano Y, Saout L. Fatal lactic acidosis in a HIV-positive patient treated with interferon and ribavirin for chronic hepatitis C. *J Hepatol*. 2002;37(2):289–291.

Hare CB, Vu MP, Grunfeld C, Lampiris HW. Simvastatin-nelfinavir interaction implicated in rhabdomyolysis and death. *Clin Infect Dis*, 2002. 35:e111–2.

Hammer SM, et al. A controlled trial of two nucleoside analogues plus indinavir in persons with human immunodeficiency virus infection and CD4 cell counts of 200 per cubic millimeter or less. *N Engl J Med*, 1997 Sep 11. 337(11):725–33.

Haubrich RH, Riddler SA, DiRienzo AG, Komarow L, Powderly WG, et al. AIDS Clinical Trials Group

(ACTG) A5142 Study Team. *AIDS*, 2009 Jun 1. 23(9):1109–18.

HIV Neuromuscular Syndrome Study Group. HIV-associated neuromuscular weakness syndrome. *AIDS*, 2004. 18(10):1403–12.

J Clin Endocrinol Metab, 2010 Jun 16.

Keiser O, Fellay J, Opravil M, et al. Adverse events to antiretrovirals in the Swiss HIV Cohort Study: effect on mortality and treatment modification. *Antivir Ther*, 2007. 12(8):1157–64.

Kitihata MM, et al. NA-ACCORD. *N Engl J Med*, 2009. 360:1815–26. *Lancet*, 2008. 372:646–55.

Lafeuillade A, Hittinger G, Chadapaud S. Increased mitochondrial toxicity with ribavirin in HIV/HCV coinfection. *Lancet*, 2001. 357(9252):280–1.

Mallal S, Phillips E, Carosi G, et al. HLA-B*5701 screening for hypersensitivity to abacavir. *N Engl J Med*, 2008. 358(6):568–79.

Molina J-M, Andrade-Villanueva J, Echevarria J, et al. Conference on Retroviruses and Opportunistic Infections; February 3–6, 2008. Boston, MA. Abstract 37.

Molina J-M, Andrade-Villanueva J, Echevarria J, et al. Efficacy and safety of once daily atazanavir/ritonavir compared to twice-daily lopinavir/ritonavir, each in combination with tenofovir and emtricitabine in ARV-naïve HIV-1-infected subjects: The CASTLE Study, 48-week results. Lancet, 2008 Aug 23. 372(9639): 604–6.

Moyle GJ, Sabin CA, Cartledge J, et al. A randomized comparative trial of tenofovir DF or abacavir as replacement for a thymidine analogue in persons with lipoatrophy. *AIDS*, 2006. 20:2043–50.

National Heart, Lung and Blood Institute. Third Report of the Expert Panel on Detection, Evaluation, and Treatment of High Blood Cholesterol in Adults (Adult Treatment Panel III). Available at http://www.nhlbi.nih.gov/guidelines/cholesterol/index.htm.

National Osteoporosis Foundation. Clinician's Guide to Prevention and Treatment of Osteoporosis. Available at http://www.nof.org/professionals/Clinicians_Guide.htm.

O'Brien ME, Clark RA, Besch CL, et al. Patterns and correlates of discontinuation of the initial HAART regimen in an urban outpatient cohort. *J Acquir Immune Defic Syndr*, 2003. 34(4):407–14.

Ortiz R, Dejesus E, Khanlou H, et al. Efficacy and safety of once-daily darunavir/ritonavir versus lopinavir/ritonavir in treatment-naive HIV-1-infected patients at week 48. *AIDS*, 2008. 22:1389–97.

Pozniak AL, Gallant JE, DeJesus E, et al. Tenofovir disoproxil fumarate, emtricitabine, and efavirenz versus fixed-dose zidovudine/lamivudine and efavirenz in antiretroviral-naïve patients: virologic, immunologic, and morphologic changes–a 96-week analysis. *J Acquir Immune Defic Syndr*, 2006. 43(5):535–40.

Qaseem A, Snow V, Shekelle P, et al. Screening for osteoporosis in men: a clinical practice guideline from the American College of Physicians. *Ann Intern Med*, 2008. 148(9):680–4.

Raffi F, Rachlis A, Stellbrink HJ, et al. Once-daily dolutegravir versus raltegravir in antiretroviral-naïve adults with HIV-1 infection: 48 week results from the randomised, double-blind, non-inferiority SPRING-2 Study Group. *Lancet* 2013;381 (9868):735–43.

Riddler SA, Smit E, Cole SR, et al. Impact of HIV infection and HAART on serum lipids in men. *JAMA*, 2003. 289:2978–82.

Rodriguez-Novoa S, Barreiro P, Rendón A, et al. Influence of 516G>T polymorphisms at the gene encoding the CYP450-2B6 isoenzyme on efavirenz plasma concentrations in HIV-infected subjects. *Clin Infect Dis*, 2005. 40(9):1358–61.

Saag M, Balu R, Phillips E, et al. High sensitivity of human leukocyte antigen-b*5701 as a marker for immunologically confirmed abacavir hypersensitivity in white and black patients. *Clin Infect Dis*, 2008. 46(7):1111–8.

Saves M, Raffi F, Clevenbergh P, et al. and the APROCO Study Group. Hepatitis B or hepatitis C virus infection is a risk factor for severe hepatic cytolysis after initiation of a protease inhibitor-containing antiretroviral regimen in human immunodeficiency virus-infected patients. Antimicrob Agents Chemother, 2000. 44(12). 3451–5.

Schambelan M, Benson CA, Carr A, et al. Management of metabolic complications associated with antiretroviral therapy for HIV-1 infection: recommendations of an International AIDS Society-USA panel. *J Acquir Immune Defic Syndr*. 2002;31(3):257–275.

SMART Study Group; El-Sadr WM, Lundgren JD, Neaton JD, et al. CD4+ count-guided interruption of antiretroviral treatment. *N Engl J Med*, 2006. 355(22): 2283–96.

Smith KY, Patel P, Fine D, Bellos N, Sloan L, Lackey P, Kumar PN, Sutherland-Phillips DH, Vavro C, Yau L, Wannamaker P, Shaefer MS; HEAT Study Team. *AIDS*, 2009 Jul 31. 23(12):1547–56.

Smith KY, Weinberg WG, Dejesus E, et al. Fosamprenavir or atazanavir once daily boosted with ritonavir 100 mg, plus tenofovir/emtricitabine, for the initial treatment of HIV infection: 48-week results of ALERT. *AIDS Res Ther*, 2008. 5(1):5.

Sulkowski MS, Thomas DL, Chaisson RE, Moore RD. Hepatotoxicity associated with antiretroviral therapy in adults infected with human immunodeficiency virus and the role of hepatitis C or B virus infection. *JAMA*, 2000. 283(1):74–80.

Thompson, MA, Aberg, JA, Cahn, P, et al. Antiretroviral treatment of adult HIV infection: 2010 recommendations of the International AIDS Society USA Panel. *JAMA*, 2010. 304(3):321–33.

Tien PC, Schneider MF, Cole SR, et al. Antiretroviral therapy exposure and incidence of diabetes mellitus in the Women's Interagency HIV Study. *AIDS*, 2007. 21(13):1739–45.

Van Leth F, Phanuphak P, Ruxrungtham K, et al. Comparison of first-line antiretroviral therapy with regimens including nevirapine, efavirenz, or both drugs, plus stavudine and lamivudine: a randomised open-label trial, the 2NN Study. *Lancet*, 2004. 363(9417):1253–63.

Walmsley S, Antela A, Clumeck N, et al. Dolutegravir plus abacavir-lamivudine for the treatment of HIV-1 infection. *N Engl J Med* 2013; 369:1807–18.

When to start consortium timing of initiation of antiretroviral therapy in AIDS-free HIV-1-infected patients: a collaborative analysis of 18 HIV cohort studies. *Lancet*, 2009. 373:1352–63.

Wohl DA, McComsey G, Tebas P, et al. Current concepts in the diagnosis and management of metabolic complications of HIV infection and its therapy. *Clin Infect Dis.* 2006;43(5):645–653.

Chapter 4

Treatment Failure and Resistance Testing

ANTIRETROVIRAL TREATMENT FAILURE (Table 4.1)

Antiretroviral treatment failure can be defined in various ways. These include **virologic failure** (inability to achieve virologic suppression, or occurrence of virologic rebound), **immunologic failure** (progressive CD4 decline), and **clinical failure** (HIV disease progression). Causes of treatment failure include inadequate adherence, preexisting drug resistance, regimen complexity, side effects, and suboptimal pharmacokinetics. All of these factors can lead to persistent viral replication and evolution of drug resistance.

Regimens for treatment-experienced patients with virologic failure need to be individualized, with the help of resistance testing. Such testing can identify drugs that are likely to be active in patients with prior treatment failures, although other factors, such as regimen tolerability, drug-drug interactions, and achievable plasma concentrations are also important. Choosing an individualized antiretroviral regimen, optimally containing at least two fully active agents, is critical in maximizing the chances for virologic suppression.

Poor medication adherence is the most common cause of treatment failure (J Infect Dis 2005;191:339–347). With poor adherence, subinhibitory drug levels occur, allowing ongoing viral replication and potentially the emergence of resistant virus. Such resistant variants are likely preexisting mutants that have escaped drug control or host immune failure. The level of adherence required to prevent treatment failure varies depending on the regimen used. In the early protease inhibitor (PI) era, there was a sharp increase in failure rates when adherence fell below 95% (Ann Intern Med 2000;133:21–30). More recent analyses suggest that lower levels of adherence are required when using NNRTI, boosted PI, and integrase-based, likely due to the longer plasma half-life of these classes of drugs compared with PIs (Clin Infect Dis 2006;43:939–41) and the higher barrier to resistance of boosted vs. non-boosted PIs (J Infect Dis 2005 Jun 15;191[12]:2046–52).

For patients with virologic failure due to noncompliance, the first step is to establish how much of the combination regimen is being taken. Pharmacy refill frequency has been shown to be a generally reliable proxy for adherence, often better than patient self-report [J Infect Dis 2006 Oct 15;194(8):1108–14]. Often a patient will have stopped an entire regimen simultaneously either due to poor tolerability or psychosocial issues. In this context, virologic failure usually occurs *without* the development of antiretroviral drug resistance, as viremia occurs in the absence of selective pressure of the antivirals. Starting a new regimen (one with the goal of fewer side effects) or restarting the same regimen with a renewed emphasis on the importance of adherence may result in treatment virologic suppression.

A. Types of Treatment Failure

1. **Virologic Failure** is most strictly defined as the inability to achieve or maintain virologic suppression. The HIV RNA level should be < 200 copies/mL after 24 weeks or < 50 copies/mL by 48 weeks after starting therapy; most patients have achieved these benchmarks by 24 weeks except in those with very high baseline HIV RNA. Virologic rebound is seen when there is repeated detection of

HIV RNA at levels > 200 cop/mL after virologic suppression in either treatment-naïve or treatment-experienced patients.

2. **Immunologic Failure** was previously defined as a failure to increase the CD4 cell count by 25–50 cells/mm^3 above baseline during the first year of therapy, or as a decrease in CD4 cell count to below baseline count while on therapy. However, it is now recognized that a minority of patients experience little to no CD4 increase despite virologic suppression. There is no consensus on the definition of immunologic failure in these cases, nor is there a proven treatment strategy to improve immunologic response if the HIV RNA is suppressed.

3. **Clinical Failure** is the occurrence or recurrence of HIV-related events after at least 3 months on potent antiretroviral therapy, excluding events related to an immune reconstitution inflammatory syndrome (IRIS, see definition below in section D). Once IRIS-related clinical events are excluded, clinical failure is exceedingly rare among patients adherent to antiretrovirals—clinicians should strongly suspect medication non-compliance when it occurs.

4. **Usual Sequence of Treatment Failure.** Virologic failure usually occurs first, followed by immunologic failure, and finally by clinical progression (J Infect Dis 2000;181: 946–953). These events may be separated by months or years and may not occur in this order in all patients.

B. **Goals After Virologic Failure.** When patients have detectable HIV RNA on treatment, clinicians should attempt to identify the cause of their lack of response and set a treatment goal of achieving full virologic suppression. The availability of drugs from older classes with enhanced activity against resistant virus and newer agents from novel classes make this an attainable goal for virtually every treatment-experienced patient (Clin Infect Dis 2009; 49:1441–9). In addition to improving clinical and immunologic outcomes, this strategy will also prevent the selection of additional resistance mutations (Ann Intern Med 2000;133:471–473; J Acquir Immune Defic Syndr 2005;40:34–40). Provided that medication adherence issues and regimen tolerability have been addressed, the regimen should be changed sooner than later.

In rare cases, achieving an undetectable HIV RNA level in patients with an extensive prior treatment history may not be possible. The main goals in these patients should be partial suppression of HIV RNA below the pretreatment baseline level, which in turn leads to the preservation of immune function and the prevention of clinical progression. A likely explanation for this phenomenon is that continued antiretroviral therapy in the face of resistance selects for less fit virus, ultimately leading to less immediate immunologic damage (J Infect Dis 2000;181:946–953; AIDS 2004;18:1539–1548). It is well documented that such patients on treatment have a slower CD4 cell decline than those not on therapy who have wild-type virus (Lancet 2004;364:51–62). Consequently, even with extensive drug resistance and virologic rebound, antiviral therapy should be continued, since stopping therapy is associated with higher rates of disease progression (J Infect Dis 2002;186:189–197; N Engl J Med 2003;349:837–846).

C. Antiretroviral Regimens After Virologic Failure

  1. Timing of Switch. The likelihood of achieving an undetectable HIV RNA level after virologic failure is greater when treatment is changed prior to the accumulation of multiple resistance mutations. Two additional important factors influencing the outcome of subsequent treatment are the level of virologic rebound and degree of CD4 decline (J Acquir Immune Defic Syndr 1999:22:132–138; HIV Clin Trials 2005;6:281–290). For example, in the TORO studies of enfuvirtide plus an optimized background regimen versus an optimized background regimen alone, study participants with a CD4 cell count > 100/mm^3 and/or an HIV RNA level < 100,000 copies/mL were significantly more likely to respond to therapy with or without enfuvirtide (HIV Clin Trials 2005;6:281–290). An additional predictor is having a greater number of active drugs in the optimized background regimen.

  2. Delayed Switch Strategy. Patients with extensive drug resistance may be clinically stable, with relatively preserved CD4 cell counts. If 2 fully active drugs are not available, deferring a switch to preserve active drug classes reduces the risk of selecting further resistance with sequential monotherapy. This delayed switch strategy is most defensible when the CD4 cell count is in a clinically safe range (> 200/mm^3) and the patient is amenable and adherent to a strategy of regular clinical and laboratory monitoring. The risk of this approach is the selection of additional resistance mutations, which may compromise future options; a delayed switch was associated with worse clinical outcomes (AIDS 2008 Oct 18;22[16]:2097–106). Delayed switching of failing regimens should generally be avoided given the availability since 2008 of several agents with activity against resistant viruses. If delayed switching is unavoidable, however, due to patient refusal to change therapy or other issues, providers should ensure that the regimen is less likely to select for additional resistance mutations (see "Holding" Regimens, below).

  3. "Holding" Regimens. For patients who cannot switch therapy (adherence or financial barriers, no availability of at least 2 active agents), it is reasonable to continue a regimen chosen to maintain clinical stability—sometimes referred to as a "holding" regimen. In the face of incomplete viral suppression, holding regimens should have the following components: (1) at least 2 NRTIs, one of them 3TC or FTC; and (2) a boosted PI based on tolerability. The NRTIs seem particularly important in maintaining a low HIV RNA level in patients with incomplete viral suppression (J Infect Dis 2005;192: 1537–44). There is no evidence that NNRTIs continue to exert antiviral or other benefit after resistance develops, and continuing them may select for further NNRTI mutations, limiting subsequent response to new agents in this drug class, such as etravirine; similarly, integrase inhibitors should also generally be stopped since some (but not all) strains resistant to raltegravir and elvitegravir are susceptible to dolutegravir.

4. **Blips.** It is important to emphasize that transient, low-level detectable HIV RNA levels—sometimes called "blips"—are often not indicative of virologic failure. In one study, 10 patients with virologic suppression (HIV RNA < 50 copies/mL) underwent intensive analysis with 36 visits over approximately 3 months (JAMA 2005;293:817–829). Of more than 700 viral load measurements, 26 samples showed transient low-level viremia. However, blips did not predict subsequent treatment failure or indicate underlying resistance. As a result, clinicians should not act based on single viral load measurements above the limit of detection but should confirm these results before changing treatment. In contrast, patients with persistent low-level viremia (> 200 and < 1000 HIV RNA copies/mL) have exhibited increases in immune activation and a higher risk of viral resistance evolution and subsequent virologic failure (AIDS 2004;18:981–989). There is an increased frequency of detecting low-level HIV RNA (20–200 cop/mL) with the newer more sensitive HIV RNA assays [J Acquir Immune Defic Syndr 2009 Feb 25]. While some studies indicate an increased risk of eventual virologic failure in those who have HIV RNA repeatedly detected between 20–200 cop/mL, the optimal strategy for managing these patients is not known. For now our practice is not to switch treatments in patients who have newly detectable HIV RNA < 200 cop/mL on this newer assay especially if not confirmed with a second value.

D. **Immunologic and Clinical Failure.** Most cases of immunologic and clinical failure are seen after virologic rebound, in particular in patients who have completely stopped antiretroviral therapy. However, patients who have virologic suppression will rarely experience a limited CD4 response, or even a decline. Factors variably associated with poor immunologic response include older age, hepatitis C virus coinfection, cirrhosis, use of NNRTI- rather than PI-based therapy, use of zidovudine (which can reduce total white blood cell count), and the combination of tenofovir plus didanosine (J Infect Dis 2006;193:259–268; Clin Infect Dis 2005;41:901–905). These cases of poor CD4 response, even with virologic suppression, likely have a prominent host component, and therefore are usually not related to any specific antiretroviral strategy (Ahuja et al, Nat Med 2008;14[4]:413–420). The management of patients with poor CD4 response despite virologic suppression is not well established, and no particular strategy has been proven to improve the CD4 cell count. Our practice is to modify the antiretroviral regimen only if there is a specific component known to reduce CD4 response (e.g., tenofovir + ddI, or ZDV-induced leukopenia). Importantly, the clinical prognosis for patients with virologic responses even without substantial CD4 increases is superior to those with comparable CD4 cell counts who do not have suppression of viremia (Ann Intern Med 2000;133:401–410). Actual clinical progression to AIDS-related complications in the face of virologic suppression is rare, and often a manifestation of the immune reconstitution inflammatory syndrome (IRIS) rather than actual HIV disease progression. Such cases represent an enhanced immune response to a preexisting opportunistic process and not the acquisition of a new infection (Clin Infect Dis 2006;42:418–427). In cases of IRIS, the current antiretroviral therapy should be continued, with treatment of the underlying process and, if necessary, adjunctive anti-inflammatory therapy with corticosteroids to treat the symptoms of IRIS.

Table 4.1. Management of Antiretroviral Treatment Failure

Type of Failure	Recommended Approach	Comments
Virologic failure *Limited or intermediate prior treatment*	Assess for adherence and regimen tolerability. Obtain genotype resistance test. Select new regimen based on resistance test results and tolerability	Usually associated with limited or no detectable resistance. If no resistance is found, consider re-testing for resistance 2–4 weeks after resuming antivirals. Stop NNRTIs if resistance is detected. Likelihood of virologic suppression is high if adherence is good
Extensive prior treatment	Assess for adherence and regimen tolerability. Obtain resistance test—consider phenotype, "virtual phenotype," or phenotype-genotype combination if level of resistance is likely to be high, especially to the protease inhibitor drug class. Obtain viral tropism assay to assess possible use of CCR5 antagonist. Select new regimen using at least 2 new active agents; if 2 new active agents not available, continue a "holding" regimen	In patients with resistance to NRTIs, NNRTIs, and PIs, the new regimen should generally contain: (1) at least one and if possible two drugs from a new drug class (integrase inhibitor, CCR5 antagonist, or fusion inhibitor); (2) a boosted PI with activity against resistant viruses (darunavir generally preferred over tipranavir). For patients with documented PI resistance, the superiority of darunavir over other PIs has been demonstrated in several studies [Lancet 2007 Apr 7;369 (9568):1169–78; Lancet 2007 Jul 7;370 (9581):49–58]. The only exception would be those viruses with documented resistance to darunavir but preserved susceptibility to tipranavir. A holding regimen should generally contain 3TC or FTC plus a boosted PI; NNRTIs and integrase inhibitors should never be used.
Low-level HIV RNA (20–200 copies)	Assess for adherence, drug-drug interactions, intercurrent illness, recent immunizations. Consider repeat test in 3–4 weeks	For low-level viremia followed by undetectable HIV RNA ("blip"), no treatment change is necessary. If HIV RNA is then detectable on repeat testing at > 200 copies/mL, obtain resistance test as described above, and treat accordingly. For repeated values between 20–200 cop/mL, the optimal management strategy is unknown; our practice currently is not to modify treatment.

Table 4.1. Management of Antiretroviral Treatment Failure (cont'd)

Type of Failure	Recommended Approach	Comments
Immunologic failure *Detectable HIV RNA*	Assess for adherence and tolerability. If non-adherent, resume treatment after barriers to adherence are addressed. If adherent, obtain resistance testing and alter therapy as described above.	If HIV RNA is back to pre-treatment baseline, non-adherence is the most likely explanation.
Suppressed HIV RNA	Investigate for modifiable conditions that may be associated with impaired CD4 response (chronic HCV, treatment with ZDV, TDF + ddI). If no modifiable conditions found, continue current regimen.	Prognosis for patients with suppressed HIV RNA and immunologic failure better than for those with comparable CD4 cell counts and detectable viremia.
Clinical failure *Detectable HIV RNA*	Treat OI with appropriate anti-infective therapy. Assess for antiretroviral adherence and tolerability. Send resistance test and choose new regimen based on results of test and other treatment options.	OIs (IRIS excluded) most commonly occur in those not on antiretroviral therapy due to poor compliance and/or regimen tolerability.
Suppressed HIV RNA	Continue current antiretrovirals. Treat OI with appropriate anti-infective therapy. If symptoms persist and IRIS is likely, use adjunctive corticosteroids.	IRIS most likely when baseline CD4 cell count is low (< 200/mm³); onset usually weeks to months after starting a potent regimen. IRIS been reported with virtually all OIs. True clinical progression with suppressed HIV RNA is unusual; IRIS should not be considered a sign of antiretroviral treatment failure.

IRIS = immune reconstitution inflammatory syndrome, OI = opportunistic infection

---

PRINCIPLES OF RESISTANCE TESTING

HIV drug resistance most commonly occurs as a result of non-suppressive antiretroviral regimens. Less commonly, resistance occurs as a result of transmission of a resistant strain. The prevalence of drug resistance among patients with sustained viral replication while taking antiretroviral therapy is high. In a random sample of HIV-infected American adults, NRTI resistance was found in 71% of samples, PI resistance in 41%, NNRTI resistance in 25%, and triple-class resistance in 13% (AIDS 2004;18:1393–1401). Studies have demonstrated that the presence of resistance before starting a new antiretroviral regimen increases the likelihood that the regimen will fail, and that patients whose treatment is chosen with information from resistance testing have better short-term virologic outcomes than control subjects without use of resistance tests.

Resistance testing is a highly complex diagnostic strategy that for maximal effect requires both a thorough review of the patient treatment history and an understanding of the strengths and limitations of the resistance assays. Both genotypic and phenotypic criteria for resistance are under continuous evaluation and evolution. It is therefore important to consult with updated guidelines, such as those published by the International AIDS Society. (https://www.iasusa.org/tam/article/update-drug-resistance-mutations-hiv-1-march-2013; see Appendix 1)

In a patient's resistance testing history, the occurrence of a given mutation implies that this resistance will persist even when the selective pressure for this mutation is removed and the mutation is no longer detectable by conventional resistance testing. For example, the occurrence of the M184V mutation selected by 3TC or FTC therapy may no longer appear on resistance tests after these drugs have been stopped. However, viruses that still harbor this mutation are "archived" and will re-emerge with resumption of these agents. Although there are literally hundreds of genotypic mutations described, certain mutations or patterns of mutations are more common or important than others. These are discussed below.

The correlation between the presence of resistance and response to a given combination of drugs is not always absolute. For example, even when viruses harbor several primary PI resistance mutations, ritonavir-boosted PIs may retain significant antiviral effect since achievable drug levels exceed levels required for inhibition of these strains; additionally, certain agents (notably darunavir, etravirine, and tipranavir) were specifically developed due to their retained activity against many viruses with resistance to other drugs within the same class. Among the NRTIs, it is well established that 3TC (and presumably FTC) continue to reduce HIV RNA even after development of substantial in vitro resistance to these drugs [Clin Infect Dis 2005 Jul 15;41(2):236–42]. As a result of these and other factors, continuing antiretroviral therapy even after widespread antiviral drug resistance leads to a better virologic, immunologic, and clinical outcome.

TYPES OF RESISTANCE TESTING

Two types of resistance testing can be ordered: genotypic and phenotypic. Genotype tests describe mutations known to be associated with resistance to specific drugs. Phenotype tests measure the ability of individual drugs to inhibit a recombinant virus that is derived from the patient's isolate. Advantages and disadvantages of the two types of resistance tests are described in Table 4.2.

Table 4.2. Genotype vs. Phenotype Resistance Testing

Method	Advantages	Disadvantages
Genotype testing	• Rapid turnaround (1–2 weeks) • Less expensive than phenotyping • Detection of mutations may precede phenotypic resistance • Widely available from multiple commercial and academic labs • More sensitive than phenotype for detecting mixtures of resistant and wild-type virus, especially for patients not on treatment • Two FDA-approved genotype assays (TRUGENE, ViroSeq)	• Indirect measure of resistance • Relevance of some mutations is unclear • Unable to detect minority variants (< 20–25% of viral sample) • Complex mutational patterns may be difficult to interpret • Interpretation of results variable depending on the laboratory
Phenotype testing	• Provides direct and quantitative measure of resistance • Methodology can be applied to any antiretroviral agent, including new drugs, for which genotypic correlates of resistance are unclear • Can assess interactions among mutations • Accurate with non-B HIV subtypes • May offer an estimate of the ability of resistant viruses to grow compared with wild-type strains ("replication capacity")	• Susceptibility cut-offs not standardized between assays • Clinical cut-offs not defined for some agents • Unable to detect minority variants (< 20–25% of viral sample) • Complex technology with longer turnaround (3–4 weeks) • More expensive than genotyping • Availability limited to two laboratories in USA (Monogram and Virco)

A.   Genotype Testing. In most settings where resistance testing is indicated, genotype testing is preferred over phenotype testing, as a larger number of studies having validated the predictive value of genotype testing to help enhance treatment response. Genotype testing is also more easily standardized from lab-to-lab, less expensive, and has faster turnaround time. Standard genotype resistance tests offer results for NRTIs, NNRTIs, and PIs; testing for genotypic resistance to integrase inhibitors must be ordered separately.

B.   Phenotype Testing. Phenotype testing, usually in conjunction with a genotype test, may be of particular value in the following clinical scenarios: (1) occurrence of certain viral strains that make sequencing difficult for the laboratory; (2) highly complex or contradictory genotype results, especially in multiple PI-resistant cases; and (3) when used in conjunction with therapeutic drug monitoring of protease inhibitors (rarely done in the

United States currently). Phenotype testing is especially useful when deciding whether to use tipranavir or darunavir, as these are the most active agents against highly PI-resistant strains. In such a setting, predicting tipranavir or darunavir activity based on genotype testing is often difficult; in contrast, clinical cutoffs are provided by phenotype testing that detail whether these drugs are fully active, partially active, or inactive virologically.

C. Other Options for Resistance Testing. One of the companies that performs phenotype testing (Monogram) offers a combined phenotype/genotype test, called a "Phenosense GT." This test provides the most complete representation of resistance status, with a direct correlation between detected mutations and in vitro susceptibility. The combined test has the highest cost among commercially available assays. Another company (Virco) used to offer a test sometimes referred to as a "virtual" phenotype. Called "VircoType HIV," this test used standard genotype results to predict drug susceptibility based on associations of detected mutations with existing phenotypes in a database. The company stopped offering this test in December, 2013.

D. Co-Receptor Tropism Assay. HIV enters the CD4 cell using both the CD4 receptor and either a CCR5 receptor (R5-tropic viruses) or a CXCR4 receptor (X4-tropic viruses). R5-tropic viruses are commonly transmitted and predominate in early infection. Over time, there is a shift in virus population to those that use both receptors (dual tropic) or to a mixture of R5 and X4 viruses. The CCR5 antagonist drug maraviroc is only active against R5-tropic viruses. As a result, when considering use of this agent, a co-receptor tropism assay should be ordered. It is reasonable to consider repeating this test for patients who experience virologic failure on maraviroc.

One available tropism assay currently is a modification of the Monogram phenotype; results return in 3–4 weeks, and indicate whether the viral population is R5-tropic, of dual or mixed tropism (D/M), or X4-tropic. The report also provides a summary statement about whether CCR5 antagonist drugs will be active. A second version of this assay is available for patients who have virologic suppression; it is potentially useful for those who may need to switch to a maraviroc-containing regimen due to toxicity, but no prior tropism test is available. Importantly, there has not yet been clinical validation of this second assay. Finally, a genotypic tropism assay is also available from Quest Laboratories. It provides similar information to the phenotypic assay, with results returning in 1–2 weeks and at much lower cost than the phenotype.

INDICATIONS FOR AND APPROACH TO RESISTANCE TESTING

Since the introduction of resistance testing in the late 1990s, indications for resistance testing have expanded significantly (Table 4.3), and resistance testing is now indicated in virtually every setting where a patient starts or changes therapy and has detectable virus on HIV RNA testing. A suggested approach to HIV drug resistance testing is shown in Figure 4.1.

Table 4.3. Summary of Clinical Situations in Which Resistance Testing is Recommended

Clinical Setting	Comments
Before initiation of therapy Primary (acute and early) infection	Resistance testing is recommended. If treatment is started before results of resistance testing return, initial therapy may be altered based on resistance test results
First evaluation of chronic HIV-1 infection	Resistance testing is recommended, including for patients for whom therapy is delayed, because plasma wild-type isolates may replace drug-resistant virus with time in the absence of treatment
Treatment initiation for chronic HIV-1 infection	Resistance testing is recommended because of a rising prevalence of baseline HIV-1 drug resistance in untreated patients with chronic infection, unless preexisting data or stored samples for testing are available
In antiretroviral-treated patients with virologic failure	Resistance testing is recommended. The decision to change therapy should integrate treatment history, new and prior resistance results (if available), and evaluation of adherence and possible drug interactions
In pregnancy[a]	Resistance testing is recommended before initiation of therapy to effectively treat the mother and prevent mother to child transmission
Other considerations and general recommendations	Post-exposure prophylaxis should consider treatment history and resistance data from the source, when available. A sudden increase in HIV-1 plasma RNA may reflect superinfection, possibly with drug-resistant virus. Plasma samples to be tested for drug resistance should contain at least 500 HIV-1 RNA copies/mL to ensure successful PCR amplification required for all sequencing approaches. It is preferable that the blood sample for resistance testing be obtained while the patient is receiving the failing regimen, if possible Resistance testing should be performed by laboratories that have appropriate operator training, certification, and periodic proficiency assurance. Genotypic and phenotypic test results should be interpreted by individuals knowledgeable in antiretroviral therapy and drug resistance patterns. Inhibitory quotient testing is not recommended for clinical decision making.

[a] If resistance test results are available from before the pregnancy, clinical judgment should guide whether retesting for resistance is necessary.

Reproduced from: Clin Infect Dis 2008;47(2):266–285—Antiretroviral Drug Resistance Testing in Adult HIV-1 Infection: 2008 Recommendations of an International AIDS Society–USA Panel.

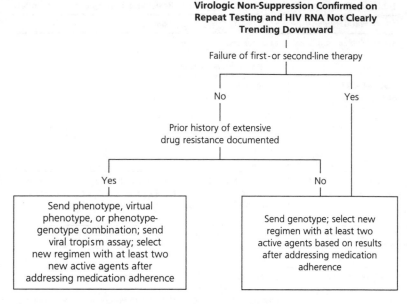

Figure 4.1. Approach to HIV Drug Resistance Testing

IMPORTANT GENOTYPIC RESISTANCE PATTERNS
(SEE ALSO APPENDIX 1: DRUG RESISTANCE MUTATIONS IN HIV-1, P. 231)

A. Nucleoside Reverse Transcriptase Inhibitors (NRTI's)
1. 3TC/FTC: M184V

- M184V emerges rapidly (days-weeks) in non-suppressive treatment regimens. This leads to a large reproducible increase in resistance of the virus to 3TC and FTC. On its own, M184V reduces the susceptibility of viruses to abacavir and ddI; however, these drugs do retain clinically significant antiviral activity even with M184V. Some studies (e.g. NEJM 2006;43:535–40) have indicated that the incidence of M184V on treatment failure is lower in patients treated with FTC than 3TC, possibly due to FTC's longer half-life and greater potency.

- Despite this resistance, significant antiviral activity of 3TC/FTC-containing regimens is often maintained for a prolonged period of time. Common explanations include: (1) M184V increases viral susceptibility to certain other NRTI's, notably ZDV, d4T, and tenofovir; (2) viruses with M184V have a lower replication capacity in vitro than wild-type viruses; and (3) 3TC/FTC exert an antiviral effect despite the presence of high-level phenotypic resistance.

- The combination of rapid development of resistance to 3TC/FTC, the potential benefits of the M184V mutation otherwise, and the excellent tolerability of these drugs leads to a clinical dilemma: should the drug be continued even in the face of resistance? Our practice is typically to continue the 3TC/FTC in patients who otherwise have extensive resistance and may benefit from the reduced viral fitness imparted by the M184V mutation. Supportive data for this approach is derived from studies in which patients receiving 3TC and having M184V experienced significant increases in HIV RNA after 3TC was discontinued (Clin Infect Dis 2005;41:236–42; AIDS 2006;20:795–803).

2. ZDV/d4T: Thymidine-Associated Mutations (TAMs)

- The thymidine-associated mutations are M41L, D67N, K70R, L210W, T215Y, and K219Q.
- TAMs emerge slowly and sequentially with ZDV and d4T-containing regimens. As ZDV and d4T are combined with 3TC or FTC for initial therapy, the M184V mutation generally evolves before the occurrence of TAMs.
- As with other non-suppressive regimens, in general the longer a patient is on an ZDV or d4T-containing regimen with a detectable HIV RNA, the greater the number of TAMs the patient will accumulate.
- The degree of resistance to ZDV and d4T as well as other NRTI's correlates with the total number of TAMs. Only 1 or 2 TAMs may reduce susceptibility to ZDV or d4T, whereas 3 or more TAMs are required to reduced susceptibility (and virologic response) to ABC, ddI, and TDF. (Note that M184V plus only 1 TAM will reduce viral susceptibility to ABC.)
- Often patients will evolve along one of two different TAM pathways: (1) M41L, L210W, T215Y: this occurs more commonly and is associated with broader resistance, including all other NRTI's as well as TDF; or (2) D67N, K70R, and K219Q: this induces a lower-level of resistance, and TDF treatment retains significant activity.

3. Tenofovir: K65R

- K65R reduces in vitro susceptibility to tenofovir, 3TC, ddI, and abacavir. In patients with prior ZDV or d4T treatment and associated TAMs, selection of K65R rarely occurs.
- As with the TAMs described above, in a typical combination regimen using TDF, 3TC or FTC, and EFV, the first mutations to appear are M184V (selected by 3TC and FTC) and NNRTI-associated mutations. In patients with continued non-suppressive therapy, K65R may also develop.
- The consequence of M184V and K65R is broad NRTI resistance (analogous to multiple TAMs). Viruses harboring the K65R mutation remain susceptible to ZDV, and are sometimes "hypersusceptible," indicating that ZDV is more active vs. K65R mutants than against wild-type virus.
- Rates of K65R development are substantially higher in HIV subtype C than B. Subtype C is more common in Africa, B in North America and Western Europe.
- As with M184V, in vitro data suggest that K65R reduces replication capacity, and that both together reduce replication capacity more than either one alone.

- K65R also may develop in treatment-naïve patients placed on abacavir, ddI, or d4T-containing initial regimens. More commonly, however, d4T will select for TAMs, and ddI and abacavir for L74V.

4. Abacavir, ddI: L74V

- Virologic failure of initial therapy with abacavir or ddI (plus 3TC or FTC) most commonly selects initially for the M184V mutation, followed by L74V.
- L74V reduces susceptibility to ABC and ddI; ZDV remains fully active. The data on TDF activity are conflicting.

5. Multinucleoside Resistance Patterns: Q151M and T69ins

- Before the triple-therapy era, Q151M and T69 insertion mutation pattern (T69ins) developed in patients who were on prolonged ZDV/ddI or d4T/ddI-containing regimens with virologic failure.
- The occurrence of these mutational patterns is rare today.
- Q151M reduces susceptibility to all NRTI's except tenofovir.
- If the T69ins is accompanied by 1 or more TAMs, all NRTI's (including TDF) show reduced susceptibility.

B. Non-Nucleoside Reverse Transcriptase Inhibitors (NNRTI's). Unsuccessful treatment with NNRTI's leads rapidly to selection of NNRTI-associated resistance mutations. These mutations generally share two important properties: (1) a nearly complete loss of antiviral activity (contrast 3TC or FTC resistance); and (2) a high degree of cross-resistance between nevirapine, delavirdine, and efavirenz. As a result, sequencing of these older NNRTI's after resistance develops is not possible. The most common resistance mutation selected by efavirenz is K103N, and nevirapine often selects for Y181C, except when given with ZDV. Less common mutational patterns seen with NNRTI's are L100I, V106A/M, Y181C/I, Y188L, G190S/A, and M230L.

Etravirine was the first NNRTI with documented clinical activity against some NNRTI-resistant viruses. In the DUET studies, treatment-experienced patients with documented NNRTI resistance received either etravirine or placebo; they also received an optimized background regimen containing at least DRV + RTV, plus other agents selected by the investigators. At 24 weeks, viral load and CD4 cell count data significantly favored etravirine over placebo (Lancet 2007;370:39–48). In this study, response to etravirine was diminished only when patients had at least three of the following mutations (which are also included in the IAS–USA set): V90I, A98G, L100I, K101E/P, V106I, V179D/F, Y181C/I/V, and G190A/S. Importantly, baseline presence of the K103N mutation—the most common mutation seen in patients with treatment failure on efavirenz—does not reduce response to etravirine.

The newest NNRTI rilpivirine most commonly selects for the resistance mutation E138K. This mutation reduces susceptibility to all other NNRTIs, including etravirine. Subsequent treatment strategies for patients with the E138K mutation would therefore include at least 2 active agents outside the NNRTI drug class.

C. Protease Inhibitors (PI's)

1. Nelfinavir: D30N

- Virologic failure on a nelfinavir-containing regimen is most commonly associated with the D30N mutation, sometimes with N88D. While conferring high-level resistance to NFV, other PI's retain activity against these viruses.

- Clinical studies have confirmed that second PI's—especially when "boosted" with ritonavir–can be used to salvage virologic failures with D30N mutations. A potential disadvantage of this strategy is that 3TC and sometimes other NRTI-based mutations are often present as well.
- A minority of treatment failures with nelfinavir will select for the L90M mutation, which is associated with broader resistance to PI's than D30N. The L90M pathway is more common in non-subtype B viruses, which are considerably more prevalent outside of the United States and Western Europe.

2. Atazanavir: I50L

- In patients without prior PI treatment, unboosted atazanavir selects for the I50L mutation, usually after selection of 3TC or other NRTI resistance. As with D30N and nelfinavir, I50L reduces susceptibility to ATV but not to other PI's.
- On phenotype testing, viruses with I50L alone often demonstrate hypersusceptibility to other PI's—that is, non-ATV PI's appear to be more active against these viruses than against wild-type strains. The clinical significance of this phenomenon is unknown, as there are no controlled studies evaluating sequencing of PI's after ATV failure.
- PI-experienced patients treated with ATV rarely select for I50L, and more typical PI-mutations emerge.
- The resistance pattern selected by boosted ATV in treatment-naive patients is thus far unknown. One study showed no PI resistance mutations or virologic rebound on boosted ATV, analogous to other boosted PI's (presented at 13th CROY, Denver, CO, 2006 Abst. 107LB).

3. Fosamprenavir: I50V

- Use of unboosted FPV may select for the I50V mutation, generally occurring (as with NFV and ATV) along with some degree of NRTI resistance.
- I50V reduces susceptibility to lopinavir, ritonavir, and darunavir; other PI's retain activity, at least as measured by phenotype testing.
- Sequencing of PI's after development of I50V or other patterns of FPV failure has not been studied in controlled trials.
- Since unboosted fosamprenavir may select for mutations that confer cross resistance to darunavir (the most important PI in treatment-experienced patients), it generally should be avoided.

4. General protease inhibitor resistance mutations: L10F/I/R/V, V32I, M46I/L, I54V/M/L, V82A/F/T/S, I84V/A/C, and L90M

- The presence of an increasing number of mutations from the above list generally confers broad PI resistance to all FDA-approved PI's.
- With < 4 mutations from the above list, ritonavir-boosted atazanavir and lopinavir had similar virologic activity; with 4 or more such mutations, lopinavir was more active (AIDS 2006;20:847–53).
- When choosing a new regimen for patients with any PI resistance, phenotype testing is generally preferred; use of a "virtual phenotype" would be an acceptable option if phenotype is unavailable. Tipranavir and darunavir are currently

the PI's with the greatest activity against PI-resistant viruses and darunavir is generally preferred due to favorable tolerability, safety, and fewer drug-drug interactions.

- The darunavir-related resistance mutations are V11I, V32I, L33F, I47V, I50V, I54L/M, T74P, L76V, I84V, L89V. If patients have none of these mutations, they may be treated with once-daily darunavir/ritonavir (800/100 mg daily; AIDS 2011;25:929–39). If they have one or more of these mutations and still retain full or partial susceptibility to darunavir based on phenotype testing, they should receive twice daily darunavir/ritonavir (600/100 mg twice daily).

D. Integrase Inhibitor Resistance As with other antiretroviral drug classes treatment failure with raltegravir or elvitegravir may select for mutations that confer resistance to these agents. Because the use of integrace inhibitors both in clinical trials and clinical practice occurred after a more complete understanding of optimal antiretroviral strategies, which employed multiple active agents, resistance to these agents is relatively rare.

The resistance pattern for raltegravir generally involves a major mutation at one of Q148H/K/R, N155H, or Y143R/H/C, with addition of one or more minor mutations that decrease susceptibility further. The most common inital mutation with elvitegravir failure is E92Q. Cross-resistance between raltegravir and elvitegravir can be assumed; that is, no significant antiviral effect can be expected by switching from one drug to the other once resistance has developed. By contrast, the integrase inhibitor dolutegravir retains activity against many raltegravir and elvitegravir resistant viruses. Dolutegravir is least likely to be active against viruses with mutations at position 148 along with other mutations.

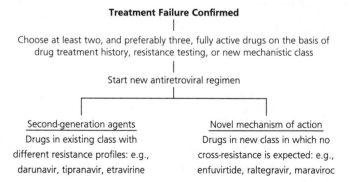

Treatment Failure Confirmed
|
Choose at least two, and preferably three, fully active drugs on the basis of drug treatment history, resistance testing, or new mechanistic class
|
Start new antiretroviral regimen
|

Second-generation agents	Novel mechanism of action
Drugs in existing class with different resistance profiles: e.g., darunavir, tipranavir, etravirine	Drugs in new class in which no cross-resistance is expected: e.g., enfuvirtide, raltegravir, maraviroc

Figure 4.2. Approach to Patients with Virologic Failure and Multiclass Resistance

Reproduced from: Department of Health and Human Services Panel on Antiretroviral Guidelines for Adults and Adolescents. Aidsinfo.nih.gov

Chapter 5

Prophylaxis and Treatment of Opportunistic Infections

PROPHYLAXIS OF OPPORTUNISTIC INFECTIONS

Patients with HIV disease are at risk for infectious complications not otherwise seen in immunocompetent patients. Such opportunistic infections occur in proportion to the severity of immune system dysfunction (reflected by CD4 cell count depletion). While community acquired infections (e.g., pneumococcal pneumonia) can occur at any CD4 cell count, the "classic" HIV-related opportunistic infections (PCP, toxoplasmosis, cryptococcus, disseminated *M. avium* complex, CMV) generally do not occur until CD4 cell counts are dramatically reduced. Specifically, it is rare to encounter PCP in HIV patients with CD4 > 200/mm^3, and CMV and disseminated MAC typically occur at median CD4 < 50/mm^3. Furthermore, for patients receiving suppressive antiretroviral therapy, opportunistic infections occur very infrequently, regardless of the CD4 cell count. Indications for prophylaxis and specific prophylaxis regimens are summarized in Table 5.1 and detailed in Table 5.2. The US Public Health Service/Infectious Diseases Society of America guidelines for the prevention and treatment of opportunistic infections in persons infected with HIV can be found at aidsinfo.nih.gov, and were last updated June 17, 2013 (see http://aidsinfo.nih.gov/guidelines/html/4/adult-and-adolescent-oi-prevention-and-treatment-guidelines/318/introduction).

Table 5.1. Overview of Prophylaxis of Selected Opportunistic Infections (see Table 5.2 for details)

Infection	Indication for Prophylaxis	Intervention
PCP	CD4 < 200/mm^3	TMP-SMX
TB *(M. tuberculosis)*	PPD > 5 mm (current or past) or contact with active case	INH
Toxoplasma	IgG Ab (+) and CD4 < 100/mm^3	TMP-SMX
MAC	CD4 < 50/mm^3	Azithromycin
S. pneumoniae	CD4 > 200/mm^3	Pneumococcal polysaccharide and conjugate vaccines
Hepatitis B	Susceptible patients	Hepatitis B vaccine
Hepatitis A	Susceptible patients	Hepatitis A vaccine
Influenza	All patients	Annual flu vaccine
VZV	CD4 > 200/mm^3, VZV antibody negative	Varicella vaccine

Ab = antibody; HA = Hepatitis A; HCV = Hepatitis C virus; VZIG = varicella-zoster immune globulin; VZV = varicella-zoster virus; other abbreviations (p. ix)

Table 5.2 Prophylaxis to Prevent First Episode of Opportunistic Disease

Pathogen	Indication	First choice	Alternative
Pneumocystis pneumonia (PCP)	CD4+ count < 200 cells/µL or oropharyngeal candidiasis CD4+ < 14% or history of AIDS-defining illness CD4+ count > 200 but < 250 cells/µL if monitoring CD4+ count every 1–3 months is not possible Note: Patients who are receiving pyrimethamine/sulfadiazine for treatment or suppression of toxoplasmosis do not require additional PCP prophylaxis	Trimethoprim-sulfamethoxazole (TMP-SMX), 1 DS PO daily; or 1 SS daily	TMP-SMX 1 DS PO tiw; **or** Dapsone 100 mg PO daily or 50 mg PO bid; **or** Dapsone 50 mg PO daily + pyrimethamine 50 mg PO weekly + leucovorin 25 mg PO weekly; **or** Dapsone 200 mg PO weekly + pyrimethamine 75 mg PO weekly + leucovorin 25 mg PO weekly; **or** Aerosolized pentamidine 300 mg via Respigard II™ nebulizer every month; **or** Atovaquone 1,500 mg PO daily; **or** Atovaquone 1,500 mg PO daily + pyrimethamine 25 mg PO daily + leucovorin 10 mg PO daily
Toxoplasma gondii encephalitis	Toxoplasma IgG – positive patients with CD4+ count < 100 cells/µL	TMP-SMX, 1 DS PO daily	TMP-SMX 1 DS PO tiw; **or** TMP-SMX 1 SS PO daily;

Table 5.2 Prophylaxis to Prevent First Episode of Opportunistic Disease (cont'd)

Pathogen	Indication	First choice	Alternative
			or Dapsone 50 mg PO daily + pyrimethamine 50 mg PO weekly + leucovorin 25 mg PO weekly; **or** Dapsone 200 mg PO weekly + pyrimethamine 75 mg PO weekly + leucovorin 25 mg PO weekly; **or** Atovaquone 1,500 mg PO daily + pyrimethamine 25 mg PO daily + leucovorin 10 mg PO daily
	Seronegative patients receiving PCP prophylaxis not active against toxoplasmosis should have toxoplasma serology retested if CD4+ count decline to < 100 cells/μL Prophylaxis should be initiated if seroconversion occurred		
Mycobacterium tuberculosis infection (TB) (Treatment of latent TB infection or LTBI)	(+) diagnostic test for LTBI, no evidence of active TB, and no prior history of treatment for active or latent TB; **or** Close contact with a person with infectious TB, with no evidence of active TB, regardless of screening test results	Isoniazid (INH) 300 mg PO daily or 900 mg PO/DOT biw for 9 months–both plus pyridoxine 25 mg PO daily; **or** For persons exposed to drug-resistant TB, selection of drugs after consultation with public health authorities	Rifampin (RIF) 600 mg PO daily × 4 months; **or** Rifabutin (RFB) (dose adjusted based on concomitant ART) × 4 months
Disseminated *Mycobacterium avium* complex (MAC) disease	CD4+ count < 50 cells/μL—after ruling out active MAC infection	Azithromycin 1,200 mg PO once weekly; **or** Clarithromycin 500 mg PO bid; **or** Azithromycin 600 mg PO twice weekly	RFB (dosage adjustment based on concomitant ART); rule out active TB before starting RFB

Table 5.2 Prophylaxis to Prevent First Episode of Opportunistic Disease (cont'd)

Pathogen	Indication	First choice	Alternative
Streptococcus pneumoniae infection	For individuals who have not received any pneumococcal vaccine, regardless of CD4 count, followed by: • if CD4 count ≥200 cells/µL	PCV13 0.5 mL IM × 1 PPV23 0.5 mL IM at least 8 weeks after the PCV13 vaccine	PPV23 0.5 mL IM × 1
	• if CD4 count <200 cells/µL	PPV23 can be offered at least 8 weeks after receiving PCV13 or can wait until CD4 count increased to >200 cells/µL	
	In patients who received polysaccharide pneumococcal vaccination (PPV)	One dose of PCV13 should be given at least 1 year after the last receipt of PPV23	
	Revaccination • If age 19–64 years and ≥5 years since the first PPV23 dose • If age ≥65 years, and if ≥5 years since the previous PPV23 dose	• PPV23 0.5 mL IM × 1 • PPV23 0.5 mL IM × 1	
Influenza A and B virus infection	All HIV-infected patients	Inactivated influenza vaccine 0.5 mL IM annually Live-attenuated influenza vaccine is **contraindicated** in HIV-infected patients	

Table 5.2 Prophylaxis to Prevent First Episode of Opportunistic Disease (cont'd)

Pathogen	Indication	First choice	Alternative
Syphilis	• For individuals exposed to a sex partner with a diagnosis of primary, secondary, or early latent syphilis within past 90 days **or** • For individuals exposed to a sex partner >90 days before syphilis diagnosis in the partner, if serologic test results are not available immediately and the opportunity for follow-up is uncertain	Benzathine penicillin G 2.4 million units IM for 1 dose	For penicillin-allergic patients: • Doxycycline 100 mg PO bid × 14 days **or** • Ceftriaxone 1 g IM or IV daily for 8–10 days **or** • Azithromycin 2 g PO for 1 dose—**not recommended** for MSM or pregnant women
Histoplasma capsulatum infection	CD4+ count ≤ 150 cells/μL and at high risk because of occupational exposure or live in a community with a hyperendemic rate of histoplasmosis (> 10 cases/100 patient-years)	Itraconazole 200 mg PO daily	
Coccidioidomycosis	Positive IgM or IgG serologic test in a patient from a disease-endemic area; and CD4+ count < 250 cells/μL	Fluconazole 400 mg PO daily	

Table 5.2 Prophylaxis to Prevent First Episode of Opportunistic Disease (cont'd)

Pathogen	Indication	First choice	Alternative
Varicella-zoster virus (VZV) infection	Pre-exposure prevention: Patients with CD4+ count ≥ 200 cells/μL who have not been vaccinated, have no history of varicella or herpes zoster, or who are seronegative for VZV Note: routine VZV serologic testing in HIV-infected adults is not recommended Post-exposure prevention: Close contact with a person with chickenpox or herpes zoster; and is susceptible (i.e., no history of vaccination or of either condition, or known to be VZV seronegative)	Pre-exposure prevention: Primary varicella vaccination (Varivax™), 2 doses (0.5 mL SQ each) administered 3 months apart If vaccination results in disease because of vaccine virus, treatment with acyclovir is recommended Post-exposure therapy: Varicella-zoster immune globulin (VariZIG™) 125 IU per 10 kg (maximum of 625 IU) IM, administered as soon as possible and within 10 days after exposure	VZV-susceptible household contacts of susceptible HIV-infected persons should be vaccinated to prevent potential transmission of VZV to their HIV-infected contacts Alternative post-exposure therapy: • Acyclovir 800 mg PO 5×/day for 5–7 days **or** • Valacyclovir 1 g PO tid for 5–7 days These alternatives have not been studied in the HIV population. If antiviral therapy is used, varicella vaccines should not be given until at least 72 hours after the last dose of the antiviral drug.

Table 5.2 Prophylaxis to Prevent First Episode of Opportunistic Disease (cont'd)

Pathogen	Indication	First choice	Alternative
		Note: VariZIG can be obtained only under a treatment IND (800-843-7477, FFF Enterprises). Individuals receiving monthly high-dose IVIG (>400 mg/kg) are likely to be protected if the last dose of IVIG was administered <3 weeks before exposure.	
Human Papillomavirus (HPV) infection	Females aged 13–26 yrs	HPV quadravalent vaccine 0.5 mL IM months 0, 1–2, and 6 **or** HPV bivalent vaccine 0.5 mL IM at months 0, 1–2, and 6	
	Males aged 13–26 years	HPV quadravalent vaccine 0.5 mL IM at months 0, 1–2, and 6	
Hepatitis A virus (HAV) infection	HAV-susceptible patients with chronic liver disease, or who are injection-drug users, or men who have sex with men. Certain specialists might delay vaccination until CD4+ count > 200 cells/μL	Hepatitis A vaccine 1 mL IM × 2 doses at 0 & 6–12 months IgG antibody response should be assessed 1 month after vaccination; non-responders should be revaccinated when CD4+ count >200 cells/μL	For patients susceptible to both HAV and hepatitis B virus (HBV) infection (see below): Combined HAV and HBV vaccine (Twinrix®), 1 mL IM as a 3-dose (0, 1, and 6 months) or 4-dose series (days 0, 7, 21 to 30, and 12 months
Hepatitis B virus (HBV) infection	Patients without chronic HBV or without immunity to HBV (i.e., anti-HBs <10 international units/mL)	Hepatitis B vaccine IM (Engerix-B® 20 μg/mL or Recombivax HB® 10 μg/mL) at 0, 1, and 6 months	

Table 5.2 Prophylaxis to Prevent First Episode of Opportunistic Disease (cont'd)

Pathogen	Indication	First choice	Alternative
	Patients with isolated anti-HBc and negative HBV DNA Early vaccination is recommended before CD4 count falls below 350 cells/μL. However, in patients with low CD4 cell counts, vaccination should not be deferred until CD4 count reaches >350 cells/μL, because some patients with CD4 counts <200 cells/μL do respond to vaccination. In general, patients should be vaccinated, regardless of CD4 cell counts	**or** Combined HAV and HBV vaccine (Twinrix®), 1 mL IM as a 3-dose (0, 1, and 6 months) or 4-dose series (days 0, 7, 21 to 30, and 12 months) Anti-HBs should be obtained one month after completion of the vaccine series	Some experts recommend vaccinating with 40 μg doses of either HBV vaccine
	Vaccine non-responders: Defined as anti-HBs < 10 IU/mL 1 month after a vaccination series For patients with low CD4+ count at the time of first vaccination series, certain specialists might delay revaccination until after a sustained increase in CD4+ count with ART.	Revaccinate with a second vaccine series	Some experts recommend revaccinating with 40 μg doses of either HBV vaccine

Table 5.2 Prophylaxis to Prevent First Episode of Opportunistic Disease (cont'd)

Pathogen	Indication	First choice	Alternative
Malaria	Travel to disease-endemic area	Recommendations are the same for HIV-infected and -uninfected patients. Recommendations are based on region of travel, malaria risks, and drug susceptibility in the region. Refer to the following website for the most recent recommendations based on region and drug susceptibility. http://www.cdc.gov/malaria/.	
Penicilliosis	Patients with CD4 cell counts <100 cells/μL who live or stay for a long period in rural areas in northern Thailand, Vietnam, or Southern China	Itraconazole 200 mg once daily	Fluconazole 400 mg PO once weekly

Definitions of abbreviations: anti-HBc = hepatitis B core antibody; anti-HBs = hepatitis B surface antibody; ART = antiretroviral therapy; bid = twice daily; biw = twice a week; CD4 = CD4 T lymphocyte cell; DOT = directly observed therapy; DS = double strength; HAV = hepatitis A virus; HBV = hepatitis B virus; HPV = human papillomavirus; IgG = immunoglobulin G; IgM = immunoglobulin M; IM = intramuscular; INH = isoniazid; IV= intravenously; IVIG = intravenous immunoglobulin; LTBI = latent tuberculosis infection; MAC = Mycobacterium avium complex; PCP = Pneumocystis pneumonia; PCV13 = 13-valent pneumococcal conjugate vaccine; PO = orally; PPV23 = 23-valent pneumococcal polysaccharides vaccine; SQ = subcutaneous; SS = single strength; TB = tuberculosis; TIW = thrice weekly; TMP-SMX = Trimethoprim-sulfamethoxazole; VZV = varicella zoster virus

Modified from: Guidelines for Prevention and Treatment of Opportunistic Infections in HIV-Infected Adults and Adolescents. Aidsinfo.nih.gov.

P. jirovecii (carinii) pneumonia (PCP)

Without prophylaxis, 80% of AIDS patients develop PCP, and 60–70% relapse within 1 year after the first episode. Prophylaxis with TMP-SMX also reduces the risk for toxoplasmosis and possibly bacterial infections. Among patients with prior non-life-threatening reactions to TMP-SMX, 55% can be successfully rechallenged with 1 SS tablet daily, and 80% can be rechallenged with gradual dose escalation using TMP-SMX elixir (8 mg TMP + 40 mg SMX/mL) given as 1 mL × 3 days, then 2 mL × 3 days, then 5 mL × 3 days, then 1 SS tablet (PO) QD. Primary and secondary prophylaxis may be discontinued if CD4 cell counts increase to > 200/mm³ for 3 months or longer in response to antiretroviral therapy. Prophylaxis should be resumed if the CD4 cell count decreases to < 200/mm³.

Toxoplasmosis
Incidence of toxoplasmosis in seronegative patients is too low to warrant chemoprophylaxis. Primary prophylaxis can be discontinued if CD4 cell counts increase to > 200/mm³ for at least 3 months in response to antiretroviral therapy. Secondary prophylaxis (chronic maintenance therapy) may be discontinued in patients who responded to initial therapy, remain asymptomatic, and whose CD4 counts increase to > 200/mm³ for 6 months or longer in response to antiretroviral therapy. Prophylaxis should be restarted if the CD4 count decreases to < 200/mm³. Some experts would obtain an MRI of the brain as part of the evaluation prior to stopping secondary prophylaxis.

Tuberculosis *(M. tuberculosis)*
Indicated for skin-test or interferon gamma release assay (IGRA)-positive patients, whether current or historical. Also indicated for close (e.g. household) contacts of active cases. Consider prophylaxis for skin-test-negative patients when the probability of prior TB exposure is > 10% (e.g., patients from developing countries, IV drug abusers in some cities, prisoners). However, a trial testing this strategy in the United States did not find a benefit for empiric prophylaxis. Rifamycins interact with PIs, NNRTIs, raltegravir, and maraviroc—use with caution.

M. avium complex (MAC)
Macrolide options (azithromycin, clarithromycin) preferable to rifabutin given greater efficacy, better tolerability, protection against other respiratory tract disease. Among macolide options, azithromycin is generally preferred over clarithromycin (fewer pills, fewer drug-drug interactions, better tolerated). Primary prophylaxis may be discontinued if CD4 cell counts increase to > 100/mm³ and HIV RNA suppresses for 3 months or longer in response to antiretroviral therapy. Resume MAC prophylaxis for CD4 < 100/mm³.

Pneumococcus *(S. pneumoniae)*
Incidence of invasive pneumococcal disease is > 100-fold higher in HIV patients. Efficacy of vaccine seen in multiple observational studies, though not all prospective randomized studies show protection. Vaccine may be offered to HIV pts with CD4 > 200/mm³. Both the 23-valent pneumococcal polysaccharide vaccine and the 13 valent pneumococcal conjugate vaccine are now recommended.

Influenza
Give annually (optimally between October and January). Intranasal live attenuated virus vaccine is contraindicated in immunosuppressed patients.

Hepatitis B
Check antibody response 1–3 months after completion of series. Response rate is lower than in HIV-negative controls. Repeat series if no response, especially if CD4 was low during initial series and has increased due to ART.

Vaccine non-responders: Defined as Anti-HBs < 10 IU/mL 1 month after a vaccination series. For patients with low CD4+ count at the time of first vaccination series, some experts might delay revaccination until after a sustained increase in CD4+ count with ART.

Management of patients with isolated antibody to hepatitis B core (i.e., "core alone") is not well defined—consider screen for HBV DNA to rule out occult chronic HBV prior to vaccination.

Hepatitis A
Response rate is lower than in HIV-negative controls; assess antibody response 1–3 months after vaccination. Some clinicians delay vaccination until CD4 is > 200 cells/mm³.

Measles, mumps, rubella
Single case of vaccine-strain measles pneumonia in severely immuno-compromised adult who received MMR; vaccine is therefore contraindicated in patients with severe immunodeficiency (CD4 < 200/mm³).

H. influenzae
Incidence of H. influenzae disease is increased in HIV patients, but 65% are caused by non-type B strains. Unclear whether vaccine offers protection; not generally recommended.

Travel vaccines*
All considered safe except oral polio, yellow fever, and live oral typhoid–each a live vaccine. Most could probably be given safely to patients with high CD4 cell counts (> 350/mm³), but data are limited.

Varicella zoster virus (VZV)
If vaccination results in disease due to vaccine virus, treatment with acyclovir is recommended.

If exposure occurs and patient is non-immune, consider administration of varicella vaccine and pre-emptive acyclovir, 800 mg 5×/day for 5 days, or valacyclovir 1 g TID × 5d or famciclovir 500 g TID × 5d.

TREATMENT OF OPPORTUNISTIC INFECTIONS

Antiretroviral therapy (ART) and specific antimicrobial prophylaxis regimens have led to a dramatic decline in HIV-related opportunistic infections. Today, opportunistic infections occur predominantly in patients not receiving ART (due to undiagnosed HIV infection or nonacceptance of therapy), or in the period soon after starting ART (due to eliciting a previously absent inflammatory host response, called immune reconstitution inflammatory syndrome (IRIS)). Even when virologic failure occurs in clinical practice, the rate of opportunistic infections in patients compliant with ART remains low, presumably due to continued immunologic response despite virologic failure, a phenomenon that may be linked to impaired "fitness" (virulence) of resistant HIV strains. For patients on or off ART, the absolute CD4 cell count provides the best marker of risk for opportunistic infections.

The precise timing of ART in patients with acute HIV-related OIs has been debated, and hence studied in several clinical trials. Favoring early starting of ART is the critical need to improve immune status, especially in conditions with either no highly effective direct therapy (e.g., PML or cryptosporidiosis) or resulting from HIV itself (e.g., dementia or wasting). Concerns about about drug-drug interactions, pill burden, and the immune reconstitution inflammatory syndrome (IRIS) tip the balance towards deferring treatment until the OI is stabilized. In a randomized clinical trial of patients with opportunistic infections other than TB, the strategy of starting antiretroviral therapy within 2 weeks of the OI diagnosis was compared with deferring therapy until 6–8 weeks later. The results of the study demonstrated a significant reduction in the risk of further AIDS complications or death for the early therapy arm (PLoS One. 2009;4:e5575). In addition, 3 additional studies in HIV-related TB demonstrated clinical benefit for early ART, especially when the CD4 cell count was < 50 cells/mm^3. Early ART may not be beneficial with certain central nervous system infection such as cryptococcal meningitis or tuberculosis meningitis (Clin Infect Dis. 2010;50:1532–1538); one possible explanation is that IRIS in the CNS has more ominous consequences.

Based on the above clinical trials, it is recommended that treatment in patients with acute HIV-related opportunistic infections typically start within 2 weeks of the OI diagnosis. For patients with central nervous system infections, such as cryptococcal or tuberculous meningitis, deferring treatment until 4–6 weeks of anti-infective therapy has been received is recommended. Deferring ART until clinical improvement is also justified for patients with relatively preserved CD4 cell counts who have pulmonary TB or bacterial pneumonia.

Guidelines for treatment of OIs were last updated June 17, 2013 (see aidsinfo.NIH.gov). Specific OI's are listed below in alphabetical order.

Aspergillosis, Invasive

Preferred Therapy, Duration of Therapy, Chronic Maintenance	Alternate Therapy	Other Options/Issues
Preferred therapy Voriconazole 6 mg/kg q12h IV × 1 day, then 4 mg/kg q12h IV, followed by voriconazole PO 200 mg PO q12h after clinical improvement Duration of therapy: until CD4+ count > 200 cells/ μL and with evidence of clinical response	Alternative therapy Amphotericin B deoxycholate 1 mg/kg IV daily **or** Lipid formulation of amphotericin B 5 mg/kg IV daily Caspofungin 70 mg IV × 1, then 50 mg IV daily **or** Anidulafungin 200 mg IV × 1, then 100 mg IV daily **or** Posaconazole 200 mg PO qid, then, after condition improved, 400 mg bid PO	Potential for significant pharmacokinetic interactions between certain ARV agents and voriconazole; they should be used cautiously in these situations. Consider therapeutic drug monitoring and dosage adjustment if necessary.

Clinical Presentation: Pleuritic chest pain, hemoptysis, cough in a patient with advanced HIV disease. Additional risk factors include neutropenia and use of corticosteroids.

Diagnostic Considerations: Diagnosis by bronchoscopy with biopsy/culture. Open lung biopsy (usually video-assisted thorascopic surgery) is sometimes required. Radiographic appearance includes cavitation (sometimes with a characteristic "halo" around a nodule, called the air crescent sign), nodules, sometimes focal consolidation. Dissemination to CNS may occur and manifests as focal neurological deficits. As with HIV-negative patients, elevation in serum galactomannan generally occurs with invasive disease.

Pitfalls: Positive sputum culture for Aspergillus in advanced HIV disease should heighten awareness of possible infection. Watch for drug-drug interactions between voriconazole and antiretrovirals metabolized via the cytochrome p450 system (PIs, NNRTIs).

Therapeutic Considerations: Decrease/discontinue corticosteroids, if possible. If present, treat neutropenia with granulocyte-colony stimulating factor (G-CSF) to achieve absolute neutrophil count > 1000/mm^3. There are insufficient data to recommend chronic suppressive or maintenance therapy.

Prognosis: Poor unless immune deficits can be corrected.

Bacterial Respiratory Diseases

Preferred Therapy, Duration of Therapy, Chronic Maintenance	Alternate Therapy	Other Options/Issues
Preferred empiric outpatient therapy (oral) A beta-lactam plus a macrolide (azithromycin or clarithromycin) *Preferred beta-lactams*: high-dose amoxicillin or amoxicillin/clavulanate *Alternative beta-lactams*: cefpodoxime or cefuroxime, or *for penicillin-allergic patients:* levofloxacin 750 mg PO once daily or moxifloxacin 400 mg PO once daily Duration: 7–10 days (minimum 5 days). Patients should be afebrile for 48–72 h and clinically stable before stopping antibiotics.	Alternative empiric outpatient therapy (oral) A beta-lactam plus doxycycline *Preferred beta-lactams:* high-dose amoxicillin or amoxicillin/clavulanate *Alternative beta-lactams:* cefpodoxime or cefuroxime Alternative empiric therapy for non-ICU inpatient A beta-lactam (IV) plus doxycycline	Fluoroquinolones should be used with caution in patients where TB is suspected but is not being treated Empiric therapy with a macrolide alone is not routinely recommended, because of increasing pneumococcal resistance Patients receiving macrolide for MAC prophylaxis should not receive macrolide monotherapy for empiric treatment of bacterial pneumonia

Bacterial Respiratory Diseases (cont'd)

Preferred Therapy, Duration of Therapy, Chronic Maintenance	Alternate Therapy	Other Options/Issues
Preferred empiric therapy for non-ICU inpatient A beta-lactam (IV) plus a macrolide (azithromycin or clarithromycin) *Preferred beta-lactams*: cefotaxime, ceftriaxone, or ampicillin-sulbactam *for penicillin-allergic patients:* levofloxacin 750 mg PO once daily or moxifloxacin 400 mg PO once daily Preferred empiric ICU inpatient therapy A beta-lactam (IV) plus azithromycin IV or an IV respiratory fluoroquinolone (levofloxacin 750 mg once daily or moxifloxacin 400 mg, once daily) *Preferred beta-lactams*: cefotaxime, ceftriaxone, or ampicillin-sulbactam Preferred empiric *Pseudomonas* therapy (if risks present) An IV antipneumococcal, antipseudomonal beta-lactam plus either ciprofloxacin 400 mg IV q8–12h or levofloxacin 750 mg/day IV once daily *Preferred beta-lactams*: piperacillin-tazobactam, cefepime, imipenem, or meropenem Preferred empiric methicillin-resistant *Staphylococcus aureus* (if risks present) Add vancomycin IV (possibly plus clindamycin) or linezolid alone to above	Alternative empiric ICU therapy *For penicillin-allergic patients:* Aztreonam IV + (levofloxacin 750 mg IV once daily or moxifloxacin 400 mg IV once daily) Alternative empiric Pseudomonas therapy An IV antipneumococcal, antipseudomonal beta-lactam plus an aminoglyscoside plus azithromycin **or** Above beta-lactam plus an aminoglycoside plus (levofloxacin 750 mg IV once daily or moxifloxacin 400 mg IV once daily) *For penicillin-allergic patients:* Replace the beta-lactam with aztreonam	Chemoprophylaxis may be considered for patients with frequent recurrences of serious bacterial respiratory infections Clinicians should be cautious of using antibiotics to prevent recurrences, because of the potential for developing drug resistance and drug toxicities

Clinical Presentation: HIV-infected patients with bacterial pneumonia present similar to those without HIV, with a relatively acute illness (over days) that is often associated with chills, rigors, pleuritic chest pain, and purulent sputum. Patients who have been ill over weeks to months are more likely have PCP, tuberculosis, or a fungal infection. Since bacterial pneumonia can occur at any CD4 cell count, this infection is frequently the presenting symptom of HIV disease, prompting initial HIV testing and diagnosis.

Diagnostic Considerations: The most common pathogens are *Streptococcus pneumoniae*, followed by *Haemophilus influenzae*, *Pseudomonas aeruginosa*, and *Staphylococcus aureus*. The pathogens of atypical pneumonia (*Legionella pneumophila*, *Mycoplasma pneumoniae*, and *Chlamydia pneumoniae*) are rarely encountered, even with extensive laboratory investigation; nonetheless, as with HIV-negative patients, these pathogens should be covered empirically unless a specific alternative diagnosis is made. A lobar infiltrate on chest radiography is a further predictor of bacterial pneumonia. Blood cultures should be obtained preferably before starting antibiotics, as HIV patients have an increased rate of bacteremia compared to those without HIV.

Pitfalls: Sputum gram stain and culture are generally only helpful if collected prior to starting antibiotics, and only if a single organism predominates. HIV patients with bacterial pneumonia may rarely have a more subacute opportunistic infection concurrently, such as PCP or TB. Fluoroquinolones should be used with caution for treatment of suspected bacterial pneumonia if TB is a diagnostic consideration, as they may inadvertently select for quinolone-resistant TB.

Bartonella Infections

Preferred Therapy, Duration of Therapy, Chronic Maintenance	Alternate Therapy	Other Options/Issues
Preferred therapy for bacillary angiomatosis, peliosis hepatis, bacteremia, and osteomyelitis Erythromycin 500 mg PO or IV q6h; **or** Doxycycline 100 mg PO or IV q12h Duration of therapy: at least 3 months CNS infections and severe infections Doxycycline 100 mg PO or IV q12h +/- rifampin 300 mg PO or IV q12h **or** Erythromycin 500 mg PO or IV q6h) +/- RIF 300 mg PO or IV q12h Duration of therapy: at least 3 months	Alternative therapy for bacillary angiomatosis infections, peliosis hepatis, bacteremia, and osteomyelitis Azithromycin 500 mg PO daily Clarithromycin 500 mg PO bid	Severe Jarisch-Herxheimer-like reaction can occur in the first 48 hours of treatment

Bartonella Infections (cont'd)

Preferred Therapy, Duration of Therapy, Chronic Maintenance	Alternate Therapy	Other Options/Issues
Confirmed *Bartonella* Endocarditis: (Doxycycline 100 mg IV q12h + gentamicin 1 mg/kg IV q8h) for 2 weeks, then continue with doxycycline 100 mg IV or PO q12h Duration of therapy: at least 3 months		

Campylobacteriosis

Preferred Therapy, Duration of Therapy, Chronic Maintenance	Alternate Therapy	Other Options/Issues
For mild disease Might withhold therapy unless symptoms persist for several days For mild-to-moderate disease Ciprofloxacin 500–750 mg PO (or 400 mg IV) q12h **or** Azithromycin 500 mg PO daily (Note: Not for patients with bacteremia) For *Campylobacter* bacteremia: Ciprofloxacin 500–750 mg PO (or 400 mg IV) q12h + an aminoglycoside Duration of therapy: Gastroenteritis: 7–10 days (5 days with azithromycin) Bacteremia: ≥14 days Recurrent bacteremia: 2–6 weeks	For mild-to-moderate disease (if susceptible): Levofloxacin 750 mg (PO or IV) q24h **or** Moxifloxacin 400 mg (PO or IV) q24h Add an aminoglycoside to fluoroquinolone in bacteremic patients	Oral or IV rehydration if indicated Antimotility agents should be avoided If no clinical response after 5–7 days, consider follow-up stool culture, alternative diagnosis, or antibiotic resistance There is an increasing rate of fluoroquinolone resistance in the United States (22% resistance in 2009) Antimicrobial therapy should be modified based on susceptibility reports Effective ART may reduce the frequency, severity, and recurrence of campylobacter infections

Therapeutic Considerations: Once improvement has occurred, a switch to oral therapy is generally safe. Patients with advanced HIV disease are at greater risk of bacteremic pneumonia due to gram-negative bacilli, and should be covered empirically for this condition. Preventive therapy (for example daily trimethoprim-sulfa) may be considered for patients with frequent recurrent bacterial respiratory infections.

Prognosis: Response to therapy is generally prompt and overall prognosis is good.

Clinical Presentation: Skin lesions resemble Kaposi's sarcoma. CT of liver shows hepatomegaly and hypodense lesions. Bartonella can rarely present as a CNS mass lesion, similar to toxoplasmosis.

Diagnostic Considerations: Diagnosis by demonstrating organism by stain/culture of skin lesions or by blood culture after lysis-centrifugation.

Pitfalls: Requires lifelong suppressive therapy unless CD4 > 200 with ART. Does not grow in routine cultures.

Therapeutic Considerations: Fluoroquinolones have variable activity in case reports and in vitro; may be considered as alternative therapy. Azithromycin likely to be better tolerated than erythromycin with fewer drug-drug interactions. Long-term suppressive therapy should be given for patients with relapse or reinfection, especially if CD4 cell count remains < 200 cells/mm^3.

Prognosis: Related to extent of infection/degree of immunosuppression.

Clinical Presentation: Acute onset of diarrhea, sometimes bloody; constitutional symptoms may be prominent.

Diagnostic Considerations: Diagnosis by stool culture; bacteremia may rarely occur, so blood cultures also indicated. Suspect campylobacter in AIDS patient with diarrhea and curved gram-negative rods in blood culture. Non-jejuni species may be more strongly correlated with bacteremia.

Therapeutic Considerations: Optimal therapy not well defined. Treat with quinolone or azithromycin; modify therapy based on susceptibility testing. Quinolone resistance can occur and correlates with treatment failure. Imipenem is sometimes used for bacteremia.

Prognosis: Depends on underlying immune status; prognosis is generally good.

Candidiasis (Mucosal)

Preferred Therapy, Duration of Therapy, Chronic Maintenance	Alternate Therapy	Other Options/Issues
Preferred therapy oropharyngeal candidiasis: initial episodes (7–14 day treatment) Fluconazole 100 mg PO daily; **or** Clotrimazole troches 10 mg PO 5 times daily; **or** Miconazole mucoadhesive buccal 50-mg tablet—apply to mucosal surface over the canine fossa once daily (do not swallow, chew, or crush)	Alternative therapy oropharyngeal candidiasis: initial episodes (7–14 day treatment) Itraconazole oral solution 200 mg PO daily; **or** Posaconazole oral solution 400 mg PO bid × 1, then 400 mg daily **or** Nystatin suspension 4–6 mL qid or 1–2 flavored pastilles 4–5 times daily	Chronic or prolonged use of azoles might promote development of resistance Higher relapse rate of esophageal candidiasis seen with echinocandins than with fluconazole use

Candidiasis (Mucosal) (cont'd)

Preferred Therapy, Duration of Therapy, Chronic Maintenance	Alternate Therapy	Other Options/Issues
Preferred therapy esophageal candidiasis (14–21 days) Fluconazole 100 mg (up to 400 mg) PO or IV daily **or** Itraconazole oral solution 200 mg PO daily	Alternative therapy esophageal candidiasis (14–21 days) Voriconazole 200 mg PO or IV bid Posaconazole 400 mg PO bid Caspofungin 50 mg IV daily Micafungin 150 mg IV daily Anidulafungin 100 mg IV × 1, then 50 mg IV daily **or** Micafungin 150 mg IV daily **or** Amphotericin B deoxycholate 0.6 mg/kg IV daily **or** Lipid formulation of amphotericin B 3–4 mg/kg IV daily	Suppressive therapy is usually not recommended unless patients have frequent or severe recurrences. If decision is to use suppressive therapy:
Preferred therapy uncomplicated vulvovaginal candidiasis Oral fluconazole 150 mg for 1 dose **or** Topical azoles (clotrimazole, butoconazole, miconazole, tioconazole, or terconazole) for 3–7 days	Alternative therapy uncomplicated vulvovaginal candidiasis Itraconazole oral solution 200 mg PO daily for 3–7 days	Oropharyngeal candidiasis Fluconazole 100 mg PO daily or tiw Itraconazole oral solution 200 mg PO daily Fluconazole 100–200 mg PO daily Esophageal candidiasis Fluconazole 100–200 mg PO daily Posaconazole 400 mg PO bid
Preferred therapy severe or recurrant vulvovaginal candidiasis Fluconazole 100–200 mg PO daily for ≥7 days **or** Topical antifungal ≥7 days	Alternative therapy fluconazole-refractory oropharyngeal candidiasis or esophageal candidiasis Amphotericin B deoxycholate 0.3 mg/kg IV daily	

Candidiasis (Mucosal) (cont'd)

Preferred Therapy, Duration of Therapy, Chronic Maintenance	Alternate Therapy	Other Options/Issues
	Lipid formulation of amphotericin B 3–5 mg/kg IV daily Anidulafungin 100 mg IV × 1, then 50 mg IV daily Caspofungin 50 mg IV daily Micafungin 150 mg IV daily Voriconazole 200 mg PO or IV BID *Fluconazole-refractory oropharyngeal candidiasis (not esophageal)* Amphotericin B oral suspension 100 mg/mL (not available in U.S.) 1 mL PO QID	<u>Vulvovaginal candidiasis</u> Fluconazole 150 mg PO once weekly
<u>Preferred therapy complicated (severe or recurrent) vulvovaginal candidiasis</u> Fluconazole 150 mg q72h × 2–3 doses Topical antifungal ≥ 7 days		

Oral Thrush *(Candida)*
Clinical Presentation: Dysphagia/odynophagia. More common/severe in advanced HIV disease.
Diagnostic Considerations: Pseudomembranous (most common), erythematous, and hyperplastic (leukoplakia) forms. Pseudomembranes (white plaques on inflamed base) on buccal muscosa/tongue/gingiva/palate scrape off easily, hyperplastic lesions do not. Diagnosis of oral thrush most commonly by clinical appearance. KOH/gram stain of scraping showing yeast/pseudomycelia. Other oral lesions in AIDS patients include herpes simplex, aphthous ulcers, Kaposi's sarcoma, oral hairy leukoplakia.
Pitfalls: Patients may be asymptomatic.
Therapeutic Considerations: Fluconazole is superior to topical therapy in preventing relapses of thrush and treating *Candida* esophagitis. Continuous treatment with fluconazole may lead to fluconazole-resistance, which is best treated initially with itraconazole suspension and, if no response, with IV caspofungin (or other echinocandin) or amphotericin. Chronic suppressive therapy is usually only considered for severely immunosuppressed patients.
Prognosis: Improvement in symptoms are usually seen within 24–48 hours.

Candida Esophagitis
Clinical Presentation: Dysphagia/odynophagia, almost always in the setting of oropharyngeal thrush. Fever is uncommon.
Diagnostic Considerations: Most common cause of esophagitis in HIV disease. For persistent symptoms despite therapy, endoscopy with biopsy/culture is recommended to confirm diagnosis and assess azole-resistance.

Pitfalls: May extend into stomach. Other common causes of esophagitis include CMV, herpes simplex, and aphthous ulcers. Rarely, Kaposi's sarcoma, non-Hodgkin's lymphoma, zidovudine, dideoxycytidine, and other infections may cause esophageal symptoms.

Therapeutic Considerations: Systemic therapy is preferred over topical therapy. Failure to improve rapidly (24–48 hours) on empiric therapy mandates endoscopy to look for other causes, especially herpes viruses/aphthous ulcers. Consider maintenance therapy with fluconazole for frequent relapses, although the risk of fluconazole resistance is increased. Fluconazole resistance is best treated initially with itraconazole suspension and, if no response, with IV echinocandin (caspofungin, micafungin, anidulafungin) or amphotericin. Patients with fluconazole refractory oropharyngeal or esophageal candidiasis who responded to echinocandin should be started on voriconazole or posaconazole for secondary prophylaxis until ART produces immune reconstitution.

Prognosis: Relapse rate is related to degree of immunosuppression.

Chagas Disease (American Trypanosomiasis)

Preferred Therapy, Duration of Therapy, Chronic Maintenance	Alternate Therapy	Other Options/Issues
Preferred therapy for acute, early chronic, and reactivated disease Benznidazole 5–8 mg/kg/day PO in 2 divided doses for 30–60 days (not commercially available in the US, contact the CDC Drug Service at drugservice@cdc.gov or (404) 639–3670, or the CDC emergency operations center at (770) 488–7100)	Alternative therapy Nifurtimox 8–10 mg/kg/day PO for 90–120 days (Contact the CDC Drug Service at drugservice@cdc.gov or (404) 639–3670, or the CDC emergency operations center at (770) 488–7100)	Treatment is effective in reducing parasitemia and preventing clinical symptoms or slowing disease progression. It is ineffective in achieving parasitological cure. Duration of therapy has not been studied in HIV-infected patients Initiation or optimization of ART in patients undergoing treatment for Chagas disease, once the patient is clinically stable

Clostridium difficile Diarrhea/Colitis

Preferred Therapy	Alternate Therapy	Other Options/Issues
Preferred therapy for mild disease Metronidazole 500 mg (PO) q8h°—10–14 days. Avoid use of other antibactericals if possible Preferred therapy for moderate-severe disease (fever, WBC, colitis) Vancomycin 125 mg (PO) q6h°—10–14 days. Avoid use of other antibacterials if possible	Nitazoxanide 500 mg BID × 7–10 days	Severe disease with illeus/toxic mega-colon IV metronidazole Vancomycin per rectum Surgical consultation for possible colectomy

Clinical Presentation: Diarrhea and abdominal pain following antibiotic therapy. Diarrhea may be watery or bloody. Proton pump inhibitors increase the risk. Among antibiotics, clindamycin, quinolones, and beta-lactams are most frequent. Rarely occurs after aminoglycosides, linezolid, doxycycline, TMP-SMX, daptomycin, vancomycin.

Diagnostic Considerations: Most common cause of bacterial diarrhea in United States among HIV patients (Clin Infect Dis 2005;41:1620–7), and increased in those with low CD4 cell counts (AIDS 2013 July 19). Diagnosed with positive *C. difficile* toxin in stool specimen. *C. difficile* stool toxin test is sufficiently sensitive/specific; cultures not useful. After therapy completed, no indication for retesting if the patient is doing well clinically. *C. difficile* virulent epidemic strain is type B1 (toxinotype III), which produces 20-times the amount of toxin A/B compared to less virulent strains.

Pitfalls: *C. difficile* toxin may remain positive in stools for weeks following treatment; do not treat positive stool toxin test unless patient has symptoms.

Therapeutic Considerations: Initiate therapy for mild disease with metronidazole; symptoms usually begin to improve within 2–3 days. For moderate or severe disease, or with evidence of colitis clinically (leukocytosis, fever, colonic thickening on CT scan), vancomycin has become the preferred agent due to concern for the more virulent strain, and based on the results of some studies suggesting vancomycin is more effective. In severe disease, surgical consultation should be obtained; if ileus and/or systemic toxicity occur, then colectomy may be indicated. The duration of therapy should be extended beyond 14 days if other systemic antibiotics must be continued. Relapse occurs in 10–25% of patients, and rates may be higher in patients with HIV due to the frequent need for other antimicrobial therapy. First relapses can be treated with a repeat of the initial regimen of metronidazole or vancomycin. For multiple relapses, a long-term taper of vancomycin is appropriate: week 1, give 125 mg 4x/day; week 2, give 125 mg 2x/day; week 3 , give 125 mg once daily; week 4, give 125 mg every other day; weeks 5 and 6 give 125 mg every 3 days. Fidaxomicin, a non-absorbed macrocyclic antibiotic, was as effective as vancomycin for C diff and associated with fewer relapses; experience in HIV-infected patients is limited. Every effort should be made to resume a normal diet and to avoid other antibacterial therapies. Probiotic treatments (such as lactobacillus or *Saccharomyces boulardii*) have not yet been shown to reduce the risk of relapse in controlled clinical trials. Fecal microbiota therapy (stool transplant) can be considered for multiple relapses (Annals Int Med 2013;158:779–80).

Prognosis: Prognosis with *C. difficile* colitis is related to severity of the colitis.

Coccidioidomycosis

Preferred Therapy, Duration of Therapy, Chronic Maintenance	Alternate Therapy	Other Options/Issues
Preferred therapy for mild infections (focal pneumonia or positive coccidiodal serologic test alone) Fluconazole 400 mg PO daily; **or** Itraconazole 200 mg PO bid	Mild infections (focal pneumonia) for patients who failed to respond to fluconazole or itraconazole: Posaconazole 200 mg PO bid **or** Voriconazole 200 mg PO bid	Certain patients with meningitis may develop hydrocephalus and require CSF shunting

Coccidioidomycosis (cont'd)

Preferred Therapy, Duration of Therapy, Chronic Maintenance	Alternate Therapy	Other Options/Issues
Preferred therapy for severe, nonmeningeal infection (diffuse pulmonary or severely ill patients with extrathoracic disseminated disease): Amphotericin B deoxycholate 0.7–1.0 mg/kg IV daily Lipid formulation amphotericin B 4–6 mg/kg IV daily Duration of therapy: until clinical improvement, then switch to azole Preferred therapy for meningeal infections Fluconazole 400–800 mg PO or IV daily	Alternative therapy for severe nonmeningeal infection (diffuse pulmonary or disseminated disease): acute phase Certain specialists add triazole to amphotericin B therapy and continue triazole once amphotericin B is stopped Alternative therapy for meningeal infections Itraconazole 200 mg PO tid for 3 days, then 200 mg PO bid **or** Posaconazole 200 mg PO bid **or** Voriconazole 200–400 mg PO bid **or** Intrathecal amphotericin B deoxycholate, when triazole antifungals are ineffective	Therapy should be continued indefinitely for patients with diffuse pulmonary or disseminated diseases as relapse can occur in 25%–33% in HIV-negative patients. It can also occur in HIV-infected patients with CD4 counts >250 cells/μL Therapy should be lifelong in patients with meningeal infections as relapse occurred in 80% of HIV-infected patients after discontinuation of triazole therapy Itraconazole, posaconazole, and voriconazole may have significant interactions with certain ARV agents. These interactions are complex and can be bidirectional. Refer to Table 5, http://aidsinfo.nih.gov/contentfiles/lvguidelines/AdultOITablesOnly.pdf, for dosage recommendations. Therapeutic drug monitoring and dosage adjustment may be necessary to ensure triazole antifungal and antiretroviral efficacy and reduce concentration-related toxicities Intrathecal amphotericin B should only be given in consultation with a specialist and administered by an individual with experience with the technique

Coccidioidomycosis (cont'd)

Preferred Therapy, Duration of Therapy, Chronic Maintenance	Alternate Therapy	Other Options/Issues
<u>Maintenance therapy (for all cases)</u> Fluconazole 400 mg PO daily; **or** Itraconazole 200 mg PO bid	Posaconazole 200 mg PO bid **or** Voriconazole 200 mg PO bid	

Clinical Presentation: Typically a complication of advanced HIV infection (CD4 cell count < 200/mm³). Most patients present with disseminated disease, which can manifest as fever, diffuse pulmonary infiltrates, adenopathy, skin lesions (multiple forms—verrucous, cold abscesses, ulcers, nodules), and/or bone lesions. Approximately 10% will have spread to the CNS in the form of meningitis (fever, headache, altered mental status).

Diagnostic Considerations: Consider the diagnosis in any patient with advanced HIV-related immunosuppression who has been in a *C. immitis* endemic area (Southwestern United States, Northern Mexico) and presents with a systemic febrile syndrome. Diagnosis can be made by culture of the organism, visualization of characteristic spherules on histopathology, or a positive complement-fixation antibody (≥ 1:16). In meningeal cases, CSF profile shows low glucose, high protein, and lymphocytic pleocytosis. A coccidiodes urinary antigen test is available (MiraVista Diagnostics) and may provide a more rapid diagnostic strategy.

Pitfalls: Antibody titers are often negative on presentation. CSF profile of meningitis can be similar to TB. CSF fungal cultures may be negative.

Prognosis: Related to extent of infection and degree of immunosuppression. Clinical response tends to be slow, especially with a high disease burden and advanced HIV disease. Meningeal disease is treated with lifelong fluconazole regardless of CD4 recovery.

Clinical Presentation: Often indolent onset of fever, headache, subtle cognitive deficits. Occasional meningeal signs and focal neurologic findings, though non-specific presentation is most common.

Diagnostic Considerations: Diagnosis usually by cryptococcal antigen of serum and/or CSF; India ink stain of CSF is less sensitive. Diagnosis is essentially excluded with a negative serum cryptococcal antigen (sensitivity of test in AIDS patients approaches 100%). If serum cryptococcal antigen is positive, CSF antigen may be negative in disseminated disease without spread to CNS/meninges. Brain imaging is often normal, but CSF analysis is usually abnormal with elevated opening pressure.

Pitfalls: Be sure to obtain a CSF opening pressure, since reduction of increased intracranial pressure is critical for successful treatment. Remove sufficient CSF during the initial lumbar puncture (LP) to reduce closing pressure to < 200 mm H_2O or 50% of opening pressure. Increased intracranial pressure requires repeat daily lumbar punctures until CSF pressure stabilizes; persistently elevated pressure should prompt placement of a lumbar drain or ventriculo-peritoneal shunting. Adjunctive corticosteroids and acetazolamide are not recommended except for the management of severe IRIS.

Therapeutic Considerations: Optimal total dose/duration of amphotericin B prior to fluconazole switch depends on clinical response and rapidity of CSF sterilization (2–3 weeks is reasonable if patient is doing well). Addition of flucytosine to amphotericin B associated with more rapid sterilization of CSF and decreased risk for subsequent relapse. If available, flucytosine levels should be monitored–peak level

Cryptococcal Meningitis

Preferred Therapy, Duration of Therapy, Chronic Maintenance	Alternate Therapy	Other Options/Issues
Preferred induction therapy Liposomal amphotericin B 3–4 mg/kg IV daily + flucytosine 25 mg/kg PO qid. (Note: Flucytosine dose should be adjusted in patients with renal dysfunction.)	Alternative induction therapy Amphotericin B deoxycholate 0.7 mg/kg IV daily + flucytosine 25 mg/kg PO qid **or** Amphotericin B lipid complex 5 mg/kg IV daily + flucytosine 25 mg/kg PO qid	Addition of flucytosine to amphotericin B has been associated with more rapid sterilization of CSF and decreased risk for subsequent relapse
	or Liposomal amphotericin B 3–4 mg/kg IV daily + fluconazole 800 mg PO or IV daily	Patients receiving flucytosine should have either blood levels
Preferred consolidation therapy (after at least 2 weeks of successful induction—defined as significant clinical improvement & negative CSF culture) Fluconazole 400 mg PO daily for 8 weeks	**or** Amphotericin B deoxycholate 0.7 mg/kg IV daily + fluconazole 800 mg PO or IV daily **or** Fluconazole 400–800 mg PO or IV daily + flucytosine 25 mg/kg PO qid	monitored; (peak level 2 hours after dose should not exceed 30–80 μg/mL) or close monitoring of blood counts for development of cytopenia. Dosage should be adjusted in patients with renal insufficiency
Preferred maintenance therapy (after at least 8 weeks of consolidation therapy) Fluconazole 200 mg PO daily for at least 12 months	**or** Fluconazole 1200 mg PO or IV daily	Opening pressure should always be measured when a lumbar puncture (LP) is performed. Repeated LPs or CSF shunting are essential to effectively manage increased intracranial pressure
	Alternative consolidation therapy (after 2 weeks of successful induction therapy) Itraconazole 200 mg PO bid for 8 weeks—less effective than fluconazole	Corticosteroids and mannitol are ineffective in reducing ICP and are NOT recommended
	Alternative maintenance therapy No alternative therapy recommendation	Some specialists recommend a brief course of corticosteroid for management of severe IRIS symptoms

2 hours after dose should not exceed 75 mcg/mL. Flucytosine dose must be reduced in renal insufficiency. Fluconazole is preferred over itraconazole for lifelong maintenance therapy. Consider discontinuation of chronic maintenance therapy in patients who remain asymptomatic with CD4 > 100–200/mm³ for > 6 months due to ART. Two studies have found that early antiretroviral therapy worsened prognosis, possibly due to IRIS (Clin Infect Dis. 2010;50:1532–1538; http://www.niaid.nih.gov/news/newsreleases/2012/Pages/COAT.aspx), one study did not (PLoS One. 2009;4:e5575); our practice is generally to start ART at approximately week two of treatment after the induction phase of amphotericin and flucytosine and some clinical improvement.

Prognosis: Variable. Mortality up to 40%. Adverse prognostic factors include increased intracranial pressure, abnormal mental status.

Cryptosporidiosis

Preferred Therapy, Duration of Therapy, Chronic Maintenance	Alternate Therapy	Other Options/ Issues
Preferred therapy Initiate or optimize ART for immune restoration to CD4+ count >100 cells/µL Symptomatic treatment of diarrhea with anti-motility agents Aggressive oral or IV rehydration & replacement of electrolyte loss	Alternative therapy for cryptosporidiosis No therapy has been shown to be effective without ART. Trial of these agents may be used in conjunction with, but not instead of, ART: Nitazoxanide 500–1000 mg PO bid for 14 days **or** Paromomycin 500 mg PO qid for 14–21 days **or** With optimized ART, symptomatic treatment and rehydration and electrolyte replacement	Tincture of opium may be more effective than loperamide in management of diarrhea

Clinical Presentation: High-volume watery diarrhea with weight loss and electrolyte disturbances, especially in advanced HIV disease.

Diagnostic Considerations: Spore-forming protozoa. Diagnosis by AFB smear of stool demonstrating characteristic oocyte. Malabsorption may occur.

Pitfalls: No fecal leukocytes; organisms are not visualized on standard ova and parasite exams (need to request special stains).

Therapeutic Considerations: Anecdotal reports of antimicrobial success. Nitazoxanide may be effective in some settings, but no increase in cure rate for nitazoxanide if CD4 < 50/mm³. Immune reconstitution in response to antiretroviral therapy is the most effective therapy, and may induce prolonged remissions and cure. Anti-diarrheal agents (Lomotil, Pepto-Bismol) are useful to control symptoms. Hyperalimentation may be required for severe cases.

Prognosis: Related to degree of immunosuppression/response to antiretroviral therapy.

Cytomegalovirus (CMV) Disease

Preferred Therapy, Duration of Therapy, Chronic Maintenance	Alternate Therapy	Other Options/Issues
Preferred therapy for CMV retinitis *For immediate sight-threatening lesions adjacent to the optic nerve or fovea* Intravitreal injections of ganciclovir (2 mg) or foscarnet (2.4 mg) for 1–4 doses over a period of 7–10 days to achieve high intraocular concentration faster Plus one of the listed preferred or alternative systemic therapies Preferred systemic induction therapy • Valganciclovir 900 mg PO bid for 14–21 days *For small peripheral lesions* Administer one of the preferred or alternative systemic therapy	Alternative therapy for CMV retinitis Ganciclovir 5 mg/kg IV q12h for 14–21 days, then 5 mg/kg IV daily; **or** Foscarnet 60 mg/kg IV q8h or 90 mg/kg IV q12h for 14–21 days; **or** Cidofovir 5 mg/kg/week IV for 2 weeks; saline hydration before and after therapy and probenecid 2 g PO 3 hours before the dose followed by 1 g PO 2 hours and 8 hours after the dose (total of 4 g) **Note:** This regimen should be avoided in patients with sulfa allergy because of cross hypersensitivity with probenecid	The choice of initial therapy for CMV retinitis should be individualized, based on location and severity of the lesion(s), level of immunosuppression, and other factors such as concomitant medications and ability to adhere to treatment The ganciclovir ocular implant, which is effective for treatment of CMV retinitis is no longer available. For sight-threatening retinitis, intravitreal injections of ganciclovir or foscarnet can be given to achieve higher ocular concentration faster. The choice of chronic maintenance therapy (route of administration and drug choices) should be made in consultation with an ophthalmologist. Considerations should include the anatomic location of the retinal lesion, vision in the contralateral eye, the patient's immunologic and virologic status and response to ART.
Preferred chronic maintenance therapy (secondary prophylaxis) for CMV retinitis Valganciclovir 900 mg PO daily; **or** Ganciclovir implant (may be replaced every 6–8 months if CD4+ count remains < 100 cells/μL) + valganciclovir 900 mg PO daily until immune recovery	Alternative chronic maintenance (secondary prophylaxis) Ganciclovir 5 mg/kg IV 5–7 times weekly; **or** Foscarnet 90–120 mg/kg IV once daily; **or**	Patients with CMV retinitis who discontinue maintenance therapy should undergo regular eye examinations—optimally every 3 months—for early

Cytomegalovirus (CMV) Disease (cont'd)

Preferred Therapy, Duration of Therapy, Chronic Maintenance	Alternate Therapy	Other Options/Issues
<u>Preferred therapy for CMV esophagitis or colitis</u> Ganciclovir 5 mg/kg IV q12h; may switch to valganciclovir 900 mg PO q12h once the patient can tolerate oral therapy Duration: 21–42 days or until symptoms have resolved Maintenance therapy is usually not necessary, but should be considered after relapses <u>Preferred therapy for documented, histologically confirmed CMV pneumonitis</u> Experience for treating CMV pneumonitis in HIV patients is limited. Use of IV ganciclovir or IV foscarnet is reasonable (doses same as for CMV retinitis) The optimal duration of therapy and the role of oral valganciclovir have not been established. <u>Preferred therapy CMV neurological disease</u> *Treatment should be initiated promptly* Ganciclovir 5 mg/kg IV q12h + foscarnet (90 mg/kg IV q12h or 60 mg/kg IV q8h) to stabilize disease and maximize response, continue until symptomatic improvement The optimal duration of therapy and the role of oral valganciclovir have not been established	Cidofovir 5 mg/kg IV every other week with saline hydration and probenecid as above <u>CMV esophagitis or colitis</u> Foscarnet 90 mg/kg IV q12h or 60 mg/kg q8h for patients with treatment-limiting toxicities to ganciclovir or with ganciclovir resistance **or** Valganciclovir 900 mg PO q12h in milder disease and if able to tolerate PO therapy **or** For mild cases, if ART can be initiated without delay, consider withholding CMV therapy Duration: 21–42 days or until symptoms have resolved	detection of relapse IRU, and then annually after immune reconstitution IRU may develop in the setting of immune reconstitution. <u>Treatment of IRU</u> Periocular corticosteroid or short courses of systemic steroid Initial therapy in patients with CMV retinitis, esophagitis, colitis, and pneumonitis should include initiation or optimization of ART

<u>CMV Retinitis</u>
Clinical Presentation: Blurred vision, scotomata, field cuts common. Often bilateral, even when initial symptoms are unilateral.
Diagnostic Considerations: Diagnosis by characteristic hemorrhagic ("tomato soup and milk") retinitis on funduscopic exam. Consult ophthalmology in suspected cases.
Pitfalls: May develop immune reconstitution vitreitis after starting antiretroviral therapy.

Therapeutic Considerations: Oral valganciclovir is the preferred option for initial and maintenance therapy. Lifelong maintenance therapy for CMV retinitis is required for CD4 counts < 100/mm^3, but may be discontinued if CD4 counts increase to > 100–150/mm^3 for 6 or more months in response to antiretroviral therapy (in consultation with ophthalmologist). Patients with CMV retinitis who discontinue therapy should undergo regular eye exams to monitor for relapse. Ganciclovir intraocular implants might need to be replaced every 6–8 months for patients who remain immunosuppressed with CD4 < 100–150/mm^3. Immune recovery uveitis (IRU) may develop in the setting of immune reconstitution due to ART and be treated by ophthalmologist with periocular corticosteroid, sometimes systemic corticosteroid.

Prognosis: Good initial response to therapy. High relapse rate unless CD4 improves with antiretroviral therapy.

CMV Encephalitis/Polyradiculitis

Clinical Presentation: Encephalitis presents as fever, mental status changes, and headache evolving over 1–2 weeks. True meningismus is rare. CMV encephalitis occurs in advanced HIV disease (CD4 < 50/mm^3), often in patients with prior CMV retinitis. Polyradiculitis presents as rapidly evolving weakness/sensory disturbances in the lower extremities, often with bladder/bowel incontinence. Anesthesia in "saddle distribution" with ↓ sphincter tone possible.

Diagnostic Considerations: CSF may show lymphocytic or neutrophilic pleocytosis; glucose is often decreased. For CMV encephalitis, characteristic findings on brain MRI include confluent periventricular abnormalities with variable degrees of enhancement. Diagnosis is confirmed by CSF CMV PCR (preferred), CMV culture, or brain biopsy.

Pitfalls: For CMV encephalitis, a wide spectrum of radiographic findings are possible, including mass lesions (rare). Obtain ophthalmologic evaluation to exclude active retinitis. For polyradiculitis, obtain sagittal MRI of the spinal cord to exclude mass lesions, and CSF cytology to exclude lymphomatous involvement (can cause similar symptoms).

Therapeutic Considerations: For any established CMV disease, optimization of antiretroviral therapy is important along with initiating anti CMV therapy. Ganciclovir plus foscarnet may be beneficial as initial therapy for severe cases. Consider discontinuation of valganciclovir maintenance therapy if CD4 increases to > 100–150/mm^3 × 6 months or longer in response to antiretroviral therapy.

Prognosis: Unless CD4 cell count increases in response to antiretroviral therapy, response to anti-CMV treatment is usually transient, followed by progression of symptoms.

CMV Esophagitis/Colitis

Clinical Presentation: Localizing symptoms, including odynophagia, abdominal pain, diarrhea, sometimes bloody stools.

Diagnostic Considerations: Diagnosis by finding CMV inclusions on biopsy. CMV can affect the entire GI tract, resulting in oral/esophageal ulcers, gastritis, and colitis (most common). CMV colitis varies greatly in severity, but typically causes fever, abdominal cramping, and sometimes bloody stools.

Pitfalls: CMV colitis may cause colonic perforation and should be considered in any AIDS patient presenting with an acute abdomen, especially if radiography demonstrates free intraperitoneal air.

Therapeutic Considerations: Initial therapy for any CMV disease should include optimization of antiretroviral therapy. Duration of therapy is dependent on clinical response, typically 3–4 weeks. Consider chronic suppressive therapy for recurrent disease. Screen for CMV retinitis.

Prognosis: Relapse rate is greatly reduced with immune reconstitution due to antiretroviral therapy.

Hepatitis B Virus (HBV)

Preferred Therapy, Duration of Therapy, Chronic Maintenance	Alternate Therapy	Other Options/Issues
ART is recommended for all HIV/HBV-co-infected patients regardless of CD4 cell count ART regimen should include 2 drugs that are active against both HBV and HIV, such as [tenofovir 300 mg + emtricitabine 200 mg (or lamivudine 300 mg)] PO once daily (+ additional drug(s) for HIV) Duration: Continue treatment indefinitely	<u>Treatment for patients who refuse or are unable to take ART</u> Assess HBV disease stage and whether HBV treatment should be undertaken. If no indication for treatment of HBV infection, continue to monitor and reassess at a later time. [HBV treatment is indicated for patients with active liver disease, elevated ALT and HBV DNA >2,000 international units/mL or significant liver fibrosis.] **or** Peginterferon alfa-2a 180 µg SQ weekly for 48 weeks **or** Peginterferon alfa-2b 1.5 µg/kg SQ once weekly for 48 weeks If tenofovir cannot be used as part of HIV/HBV therapy (because of existing or high risk of renal dysfunction) Use a fully suppressive ART regimen with entecavir (dose adjustment according to renal function)	Adefovir, emtricitabine, entecavir, lamivudine, or tenofovir should not be used for the treatment of HBV infection in patients who are not receiving combination ART Cross-resistance to emtricitabine or telbivudine should be assumed in patients with suspected or proven lamivudine resistance When changing ART regimens, continue agents with anti-HBV activity because of the risk of IRIS If anti-HBV therapy is discontinued and a flare occurs, therapy should be reinstituted, as it can be potentially life saving

Epidemiology: Hepatitis B virus (HBV) infection is relatively common in patients with HIV, with approximately 60% showing some evidence of prior exposure. Chronic hepatitis B infection interacts with HIV infection in several important ways:

- HBV increases the risk of liver-related death and hepatotoxicity from antiretroviral therapy (Lancet 2002;360:1921–6; Hepatology 2002;35:182–9).
- 3TC, FTC, and tenofovir each have anti-HBV activity. Thus selection of antiretroviral therapy for patients with HBV can have clinical and resistance implications for HBV as well as HIV. This is most notable with 3TC and FTC, as a high proportion of coinfected patients will develop HBV-associated resistance to these drugs after several years of therapy. This resistance reduces response to subsequent non-3TC or FTC anti-HBV therapy.
- Cessation of anti-HBV therapy may lead to exacerbations of underlying liver disease; in some cases, these flares have been fatal (Clin Infect Dis 1999;28:1032–5; Scand J Infectious Diseases 2004;36:533–5).
- Immune reconstitution may lead to worsening of liver status, presumably because HBV disease is immune mediated. This is sometimes associated with loss of HBEAg.
- Entecavir can no longer be recommended for HIV/HBV coinfected patients, as it has anti-HIV activity and may select for HIV resistance mutation M184V (N Engl J Med 2007;356: 2614–21). If needed, it should be used only with a fully suppressive HIV regimen.

Diagnostic Consideration: Obtain HBSAb, HBSAg, and HBCAb at baseline in all patients. If negative, hepatitis B vaccination is indicated. If chronic HBV infection (positive HBSAg) is identified, obtain HBEAg, HBEAb, and HBV DNA levels. As with HCV infection, vaccination with hepatitis A vaccine and counseling to avoid alcohol are important components of preventive care. Isolated Hepatitis B Core Antibody: Some patients with HIV have antibody to hepatitis B core (anti-HBc) but are negative for both HBSAg and HBSAb. This phenomenon appears to be more common in those with HCV coinfection (Clin Infec Dis 2003 36:1602–6). In this scenario, diagnostic considerations include: (1) recently acquired HBV, before development of HBSAb; (2) chronic HBV, with HBSAg below the levels of detection; (3) immunity to HBV, with HBSAb below the levels of detection; (4) false-positive anti-HBV core. As the incidence of HBV is relatively low in most populations and anti-HBc alone is usually a stable phenomenon over years, recent acquisition of HBV is rarely the explanation. We recommend checking HBV DNA in this situation: If positive, this indicates chronic HBV; if negative, then low-level immunity or false-positive anti-HBV core remain as possible explanations; since distinguishing between these possibilities cannot be done, we recommend immunization with the hepatitis B vaccine series. It is useful to measure HBV serologic markers periodically in this population, as improvement in immune status due to ART may lead to increasing titers of HBSAb and subsequently confirm immunity (Clin Infect Dis 2007;45:1221–9).

Therapeutic Considerations: HIV treatment guidelines generally recommend starting antiretroviral therapy in all HBV infected patients, regardless of CD4 cell count. In practice, this means using TDF/FTC (or 3TC) as part of all antiretroviral regimens, as this provides two active drugs against hepatitis B and reduces the risk of inducing FTC or 3TC resistance. Patients being treated with regimens for HBV should be monitored for ALT every 3–4 months. HBV DNA levels provide a good marker for efficacy of therapy and should be added to regular laboratory monitoring. The goal of therapy is to reduce HBV DNA to as low a level as possible, preferably below the limits of detection. The vast majority of patients with HIV/HBV coinfection should be treated with a regimen active against both viruses, with avoidance of single drug treatment of HBV, in particular just 3TC or FTC.

Hepatitis C Virus

Note: Prior to treatment, all patients should have a clinical and laboratory assessment of the degree of liver fibrosis present due to hepatitis C. Given the rapidly changing nature of HCV treatment, in patients with mild-moderate liver disease (e.g., Stage 2 fibrosis or less), current and future treatment options should be carefully considered prior to initiating HCV therapy. The recommendations below should be considered in the context of newly approved treatments in December 2013, and represent the opinions of the authors and not the Opportunistic Infection Guidelines, which did not include these newer drugs.

Preferred Therapy	Alternative Therapy	Comments
<u>Acute HCV infection</u> Treatment should be offered. Because of the high rate of spontaneous clearance, some experts recommend observation for 3–6 months before initiation of therapy, especially for patients with IL28B C/C genotype. Sofosbuvir (SOF) 400 mg PO QD with weight-based ribavirin (RBV) as follows: RBV PO (wt-based dosing): < 75 kg: 600 mg qAM and 400 mg qPM; ≤ 75 kg: 600 mg qAM and 600 mg qPM Duration: 12 weeks	Pegylated interferon (IF) 180 µg or Pegylated IF alfa-2b 1.5 µg/kg) SQ weekly + ribavirin (RBV) PO RBV PO (wt-adjusted dosing): < 75 kg: 600 mg qAM and 400 mg qPM; ≤ 75 kg: 600 mg qAM and 600 mg qPM Duration of therapy: 24–48 weeks	No published experience with SOF in acute HCV; this strategy is under investigation.
<u>Chronic (established) HCV infection</u> **Genotype 1 or 4:** SOF 400 mg QD plus Pegylated interferon (IF) 180 µg or Pegylated IF alfa-2b 1.5 µg/kg) SQ weekly + weight-based ribavirin (RBV) PO Duration: 12 weeks *or*	Sofosbuvir (SOF) 400 mg PO QD with weight-based ribavirin (RBV) PO Duration: 24 weeks	As of December 2013, only sofosbuvir + peg IF/RBV regimens are listed in package insert; SOF + SMP regimen offers interferon-free option with a shorter treatment course. Note that SMP cannot be given with antiretrovirals from the PI or NNRTI class, or with cobicistat, due to drug-drug interactions.

Hepatitis C Virus (cont'd)

Preferred Therapy	Alternative Therapy	Comments
Sofosbuvir 400 mg QD + simeprevir (SMP) 150 mg QD Duration: 12 weeks		
Genotype 2: Sofosbuvir (SOF) 400 mg PO QD with weight-based ribavirin (RBV) PO Duration: 12 weeks		
Genotype 3: Sofosbuvir (SOF) 400 mg PO QD with weight-based ribavirin (RBV) PO Duration: 24 weeks		

Adverse Effects Associated with Interferon and Ribavirin

Agent	Side Effect	Proposed Management
Interferon	Fatigue and flu-like symptoms (fever, chills, muscle aches, headache)	Dose at night so that some initial symptoms can be slept through. Symptoms may not peak until 48–78 hours after weekly dose and can be managed with acetaminophen (maximum 1300 mg/day) or ibuprofen plus good hydration. Fatigue is sometimes a manifestation of thyroid dysregulation or anemia; monitor thyroid function tests and CBC.
	Depression	Interferon can aggravate life-threatening psychiatric conditions. Low threshold for initiating anti-depressant therapy. Patients with a pre-existing history of depression or other psychiatric disease should be followed closely by mental health professionals during HCV treatment.

Adverse Effects Associated with Interferon and Ribavirin (cont'd)

Agent	Side Effect	Proposed Management
	Leukopenia, thrombocytopenia, anemia	Cytopenias are more common in HIV/HCV co-infection. Can treat with G-CSF 300 mcg 3x/week if absolute neutrophil count is < 500/mm^3. If neutropenia persists, decrease dose of interferon. If platelet count falls to < 80,000/mm^3, also consider decreasing interferon dose (some clinicians tolerate counts down to 50,000/mm^3). Low threshold for use of erythropoietin (EPO) 40,000 U/week for anemia or dose reduction of ribavirin.
	Mouth ulcers	Topical viscous lidocaine or sucralfate is helpful in some.
	Gastrointestinal symptoms	Nausea and anorexia are the most common, which may lead to weight loss. Advise patients to eat several small meals daily rather than a few large meals.
	Hair loss	Avoid washing hair too frequently; short layered cuts make the hair look fuller. Reversible after completion of therapy.
Ribavirin	Hemolytic anemia	Manage symptomatic anemia with EPO 40,000 IU SC weekly. Dose reduction recommended for severe anemia—if hemoglobin < 10 g/dl (or Hct < 30%) decrease Ribavirin dose by 200 mg each time and if hemoglobin < 8.5 g/dl (or Hct < 26%) stop ribavirin treatment. Hemolysis may precipitate gout.
	Dyspepsia	Antacids, proton-pump inhibitor.
	Cough	
	Teratogenicity	Pregnancy category X. Women of child-bearing potential must agree to use effective method of birth control.

Epidemiology: Hepatitis C virus (HCV) infection is transmitted primarily through blood exposure; sexual and perinatal transmission are also possible but less efficient. A notable exception is sexually transmitted HCV among HIV-infected gay men. Since modes of transmission of HIV and HCV overlap to some extent, there are high rates of HCV coinfection in HIV—an estimated 16% of HIV patients overall, including 80% or more of IDUs and 5–10% of gay men (Clin Infect Dis 2002;34:831–7). Genotype 1 accounts for 75% of HCV in the United States. HIV accelerates the progression of chronic HCV infection to cirrhosis, liver failure, and hepatocellular carcinoma (J Infect Dis 2001;183:1112–5; Clin Infect Dis 2001;33:562–569). Data are conflicting regarding the independent effect of HCV on HIV disease progression, but several studies have shown a higher rate of antiretroviral therapy-induced hepatotoxicity in those with chronic HCV. In some series, liver failure from HCV is one of the leading causes of death in HIV/HCV coinfected individuals (Clin Infect Dis 2001;32:492–7).

Clinical Presentation: Persistently elevated liver transaminases; usually asymptomatic.

Diagnostic Considerations: All HIV-positive patients should be tested for HCV antibody. If the antibody test is negative but the likelihood of HCV infection is high (IDU, unexplained increase in LFTs), obtain an HCV RNA since false-negative antibody tests may occur, especially in advanced HIV disease (J Clin Microbiol 2000;38:575–7) and since patients with recently-acquired HCV may have a negative HCV antibody due to the window period. Since LFT elevation does not correlate well with underlying HCV activity, other diagnostic strategies are necessary to assess degree of HCV-related liver damage. While liver biopsy is considered the gold standard, many clinicians elect less invasive indirect methods such as fibroelastography (a form of ultrasound that assesses liver stiffness) or algorithms applied to various blood tests (e.g., FibroSure, or AST-to-platelet ratio index). Sexually active men who have sex with men (MSM) are at risk for acquiring HCV; we recommend periodic screening with HCV antibody for those at risk.

Therapeutic Considerations:

HCV therapy is currently in a period of rapid evolution. At the time of this writing, many investigational agents are in the late stages of drug development, with sofosbuvir and simeprevir approved in late 2013, and other treatments expected in 2014–15. As such, treatment recommendations will undergo substantial changes in the near future. Specifically, clinical studies of novel agents in combination have clearly demonstrated that interferon-free regimens can achieve cure rates that are substantially better than existing therapy, with lower toxicity and with shorter courses. One such regimen—sofosbuvir with ribavirin for genotypes 2 and 3—is already FDA approved.

Once Diagnosis is Established. Advise patients to abstain from alcohol and administer vaccinations for hepatitis A and B (if non-immune). Also obtain HCV RNA levels with genotype assessment. HCV RNA levels do not have prognostic significance for underlying degree of liver disease, but higher levels make treatment for cure less likely. Genotype results also correlate with cure rates and for some regimens guide duration of therapy.

Optimal Patient Characteristics for HCV Treatment in HIV include no unstable psychiatric disease or substance abuse; stable HIV disease with undetectable HIV RNA and higher CD4 cell count; receiving an antiretroviral regimen that does not contain drugs that interact with HCV therapies; and adherent to medications, follow-up visits, and blood test monitoring.

For patients beginning interferon-based therapies, they should be fully educated regarding the goals and risks of treatment, with provision of written information about side effects, local support groups, and whom to contact with questions. It is useful to administer the first dose of treatment in the office in order to provide instructions on injection techniques.

Choice of Drug Therapy. The following section discusses individual components that may be part of HCV therapy. Note that the first HCV protease inhibitors, telaprevir and boceprevir, will largely be replaced by sofosbuvir and simeprevir, and are unlikely to be used going forward.

- <u>Pegylated Interferon</u>. Two different formulations of pegylated interferon are available for treatment of HCV infection: (1) peginterferon alfa-2a (Pegasys), supplied as a pre-mixed solution and administered subcutaneously as a fixed dose of 180 mcg once a week; and (2) peginterferon alfa-2b (Peg-Intron), supplied as a powder that is reconstituted in saline and administered subcutaneously as a weight-based dose once a week. Interferon has numerous side effects, the most important of which are listed in Table 5.3.

- <u>Ribavirin</u>. Ribavirin is available in 200-mg capsules. Standard dosing is 400 mg qAM and 600 mg qPM for weight < 75 kg, and 600 mg qAM and 600 mg qPM for weight > 75 kg. Ribavirin causes hemolytic anemia that predictably leads to a measurable decline in hemoglobin; this stabilizes by week 4–8 of treatment. Hemolytic anemia may be exacerbated in patients receiving ZDV; avoid this agent, with preference for tenofovir or abacavir. For symptomatic anemia or patients with coexisting conditions exacerbated by anemia, erythropoietin is used to maintain hemoglobin levels > 10 gm/dL or higher as needed. The typical starting dose of erythropoietin is 40,000 units SQ once a week. ddI is contraindicated during ribavirin administration due to an increased risk of mitochondrial toxicity and hepatic decompensation (Clin Infect Dis 2004;38:e79–e80). d4T should also be avoided because of its potential for inducing mitochondrial toxicity itself. Another common side effect of ribavirin is GI distress, which can overlap with a similar effect of interferon. Ribavirin is pregnancy category × (potent teratogen), and can only be used in sexually active women of childbearing potential if they are using 2 forms of birth control. Pregnancy should be avoided until at least 6 months after stopping ribavirin.

- The anti-HCV protease inhibitors boceprevir and telaprevir were approved in 2011 by the US Food and Drug Administration for the treatment of hepatitis C monoinfection. Small studies in HIV/HCV coinfected patients supported the use in HIV/HCV coinfected patients as well. Common side effects of telaprevir include rash, anemia, GI upset, taste disturbance, and anorectal discomfort; boceprevir has many of the same side effects, with a lower rate of rash but a higher rate of anemia. Given the significant side effects, high pill burden, and potential drug-drug interactions between boceprevir and telaprevir, most clinicians believe these agents should no longer be used in HIV/HCV coinfected patients unless there are no other options.

- <u>Simeprevir</u> is the newest HCV protease inhibitor with several advantages over telaprevir and boceprevir, including once-daily dosing and fewer side effects. It is approved for genotype 1 HCV in combination with peg-IF and ribavirin. Simeprevir is only to be given during the first 12 weeks of treatment; total treatment duration is 24 weeks for treatment-naïve or prior relapsers, and 48 weeks for those who were null responders. Response rates are diminished in those who have a baseline Q80K polymorphism in the protease enzyme. The most common side effects are rash, pruritus, and photosensitivity. Simeprevir interacts with many antiretroviral agents, including all protease inhibitors, NNRTIs, and the PK booster cobicistat; it should not be used with these drugs.

- <u>Sofosbuvir</u> is a nucleotide HCV polymerase inhibitor with activity against all HCV genotypes. Administered as one 400 mg tablet daily, sofosbuvir has few significant side effects and no notable significant drug-drug interactions with HIV therapies. As such, until there are further options, it should be a component of all HCV treatment in HIV/HCV coinfected patients. It has been FDA approved for treatment of genotype 1 or 4 in combination with peg IF/RBV for 12 weeks; for genotype 2 with RBV alone for 12 weeks; or for genotype 3 with RBV for 24 weeks. (For those who cannot take interferon, the FDA has also approved treatment for genotype 1 with sofosbuvir and ribavirin for 24 weeks, though response rates are somewhat lower than the interferon-based option.) Notably, one small study found that cure rates with sofosbuvir and simeprevir were 90% or higher with a variety of strategies, including just these two drugs for 12 weeks. This is not an FDA-approved regimen, but might be an off-label option for some patients provided there are no significant drug-drug interactions with the HIV regimen.

<u>Monitoring</u>. The monitoring plan for HIV/HCV coinfected patients consists of both safety and efficacy evaluations (Table 5.3).

Table 5.3. Monitoring Plan During. Treatment for HCV Infection with Interferon and Ribavirin based treatment duration varies depending on patient characteristics and choice of additional active drug **(see Table at start of Hepatitis C section and text for details).**

	Weeks of Treatment								
	Baseline	2	4	8	12	16	20	24	24–48
CBC	X	X	X	X	X	X	X	X	q4 weeks
LFTs + metabolic panel	X		X	X	X	X	X	X	q4 weeks
HCV RNA	X		X[¶]		X			X	q12 weeks
HIV RNA + CD4 profile	X				X[†]			X	q12 weeks
TSH	X				X			X	q12 weeks
Depression	X	X	X	X	X	X	X	X	ongoing
Ophthalmologic exam	X[‡]				X			X	q12 weeks
PT	X					X			q12 weeks
Pregnancy test	Perform at regular intervals if appropriate								

† Anticipate decrease in absolute cell count but stable CD4%.
‡ Necessary for patients with a history of retinopathy; IFN package insert recommends screening for all patients prior to treatment. Many clinicians choose to defer the initial exam and monitor for disturbances in vision and loss of color perception.

Adapted from: Brown, et al. Clinician's Guide to HIV/HCV Coinfection, 2004.

If HCV RNA is undetectable at the end of therapy, this is considered an "end of treatment" response. Additional measurements should be obtained at weeks 4, 12, and 24 after stopping treatment. An undetectable HCV RNA at week 24 posttreatment is the current standard for assessing a "sustained virologic response" (SVR), which can be equated with cure; most studies suggest that a negative HCV RNA at week 12 is also suggestive of cure. Importantly, patients cured of HCV are susceptible to reacquisition and should be cautioned about resuming high-risk behavior.

Herpes Simplex Virus (HSV) Disease

Preferred Therapy, Duration of Therapy, Chronic Maintenance	Alternate Therapy	Other Options/Issues
Preferred therapy for orolabial lesions and initial or recurrent genital HSV Valacyclovir 1 g PO bid, famciclovir 500 mg PO bid, or acyclovir 400 mg PO tid Duration of therapy: Orolabial HSV: 5–10 days Genital HSV: 5–14 days Preferred therapy for severe mucocutaneous HSV infections Initial therapy acyclovir 5 mg/kg IV q8h After lesions began to regress, change to PO therapy as above. Continue therapy until lesions have completely healed		
Preferred therapy for acyclovir-resistant mucocutaneous HSV infections Foscarnet 80–120 mg/kg/day IV in 2–3 divided doses until clinical response	Alternative therapy for acyclovir-resistant mucocutaneous HSV infections IV cidofovir (dosage as in CMV retinitis) **or** Topical trifluridine **or** Topical cidofovir **or** Topical imiquimod	Patients with HSV infections can be treated with episodic therapy when symptomatic lesions occur, or with daily suppressive therapy to prevent recurrences Topical formulations of neither trifluridine nor cidofovir are commercially available in the US

Herpes Simplex Virus (HSV) Disease (cont'd)

Preferred Therapy, Duration of Therapy, Chronic Maintenance	Alternate Therapy	Other Options/Issues
Suppressive therapy (For patients with frequent or severe recurrences of genital herpes) Valacyclovir 500 mg PO bid Famciclovir 500 mg PO bid Acyclovir 400 mg PO bid Continue indefinitely regardless of CD4+ cell count.	Duration of therapy: 21–28 days or longer	Extemporaneous compounding of topical products can be prepared using trifluridine ophthalmic solution and the intravenous formulation of cidofovir

Herpes Simplex (genital/oral)

Clinical Presentation: Painful, grouped vesicles on an erythematous base that rupture, crust, and heal within 2 weeks. Lesions may be chronic, severe, ulcerative with advanced immunosuppression.

Diagnostic Considerations: Diagnosis by viral culture of swab from lesion base/roof of blister; alternative diagnostic techniques include Tzanck prep or immunofluorescence staining.

Pitfalls: Acyclovir prophylaxis is not required in patients receiving ganciclovir or foscarnet.

Therapeutic Considerations: In refractory cases, consider acyclovir resistance and treat with foscarnet. Topical trifluridine ophthalmic solution (Viroptic 1%) may be considered for direct application to small, localized areas of refractory disease; clean with hydrogen peroxide, then debride lightly with gauze, apply trifluridine, and cover with bacitracin/polymyxin ointment and non-adsorbent gauze; topical cidofovir (requires compounding) also may be tried. Chronic suppressive therapy with oral acyclovir, famciclovir, or valacyclovir may be indicated for patients with frequent recurrences, dosing similar to HIV-negative patients.

Prognosis: Responds well to treatment except in severely immunocompromised patients, in whom acyclovir resistance may develop.

Herpes Encephalitis (HSV-1)

Clinical Presentation: Acute onset of fever and change in mental status.

Diagnostic Considerations: EEG is abnormal early (< 72 hours), showing unilateral temporal lobe abnormalities. Brain MRI is abnormal before CT scan, which may require several days before a temporal lobe focus is seen. Definitive diagnosis is by CSF PCR for HSV-1 DNA. Profound decrease in sensorium is characteristic of HSV meningoencephalitis. CSF may have PMN predominance and low glucose levels, unlike other viral causes of meningitis. A different clinical entity is HSV meningitis, which is usually associated with HSV-2 and can recur with lymphocytic meningitis. HSV encephalitis is surprisingly rare in HIV patients, but when it occurs, residual neurologic deficits are common; by contrast, HSV meningitis (usually in association with genital HSV outbreaks) has an excellent prognosis.

Pitfalls: Rule out non-infectious causes of encephalopathy. Surprisingly, HSV encephalitis is a relatively rare cause of encephalitis in patients with HIV.

Therapeutic Considerations: Treat as soon as possible since neurological deficits may be mild and reversible early on, but severe and irreversible later.

Prognosis: Related to extent of brain injury and early antiviral therapy.

HHV-8 Infection*

Preferred Therapy, Duration of Therapy, Chronic Maintenance	Alternate Therapy	Other Options/Issues
Initiation or optimization of ART should be done for all patients with KS, PEL, or MCD Preferred therapy for visceral KS, disseminated cutaneous KS, and PEL Chemotherapy + ART Oral valganciclovir or IV ganciclovir might be useful as adjunctive therapy in PEL		Patients who receive rituximab for MCD may experience subsequent exacerbation or emergence of KS
Preferred therapy for MCD Valganciclovir 900 mg PO bid for 3 weeks; **or** Ganciclovir 5 mg/kg IV q12h for 3 weeks **or** Valganciclovir 900 mg PO bid + zidovudine 600 mg PO q6h for 7–21 days	Alternative therapy for MCD Rituximab, 375 mg/m^2 given weekly × 4–8 weeks, may be an alternative to or used adjunctively with antiviral therapy	

* (Kaposi's Sarcoma [KS], primary effusion lymphoma [PEL], multicentric Castleman's disease [MCD])

Histoplasma capsulatum

Preferred Therapy, Duration of Therapy, Chronic Maintenance	Alternate Therapy	Other Options/Issues
Preferred therapy for moderately severe to severe disseminated disease *Induction therapy* (for 2 weeks or until clinically improved) Liposomal amphotericin B at 3 mg/kg IV daily Maintenance therapy Itraconazole 200 mg PO TID for 3 days, then BID Preferred therapy for less severe disseminated disease *Induction and maintenance therapy* Itraconazole 200 mg PO tid for 3 days, then 200 mg PO bid Duration of therapy: at least 12 months	Alternative therapy moderately severe to severe disseminated disease *Induction therapy* (for 2 weeks or until clinically improved) Amphotericin B lipid complex 3 mg/kg IV daily **or** Amphotericin B cholesteryl sulfate complete 3 mg/kg IV daily Alternatives to itraconazole for maintenance therapy or treatment of less severe disease Voriconazole 400 mg PO bid for 1 day, then 200 mg bid **or**	Itraconazole, posaconazole, and voriconazole may have significant interactions with certain ARV agents. These interactions are complex and can be bi-directional. Refer to Table 5, http://aidsinfo.nih.gov/contentfiles/lvguidelines/AdultOITablesOnly.pdf for dosing recommendations. Therapeutic drug monitoring and dosage adjustment may be necessary to ensure triazole antifungal and ARV efficacy and reduce concentration-related toxicities.

Histoplasma capsulatum (cont'd)

Preferred Therapy, Duration of Therapy, Chronic Maintenance	Alternate Therapy	Other Options/Issues
Preferred therapy for meningitis *Induction therapy* (4–6 weeks) Liposomal amphotericin B 5 mg/kg/day *Maintenance therapy* Itraconazole 200 mg PO bid to tid for ≥ 1 year and until resolution of abnormal CSF findings Preferred therapy for long-term suppression therapy In patients with severe disseminated or CNS infection and in patients who relapse despite appropriate therapy Itraconazole 200 mg PO daily	Posaconazole 400 mg PO bid Fluconazole 800 mg PO daily Meningitis No alternative therapy recommendation Long-term suppression therapy Fluconazole 400 mg PO daily	Random serum concentrations of itraconazole + hydroxyitraconazole should be > 1 μg/mL Clinical experience with voriconazole or posaconazole in is limited. Acute pulmonary histoplasmosis in HIV-infected patients with CD4+ count > 300 cells/μL should be managed as non-immunocompromised host

Clinical Presentation: Two general forms: Mild disease with fever/lymph node enlargement (e.g., cervical adenitis), or severe disease with fever, wasting—also may have diarrhea/meningitis/GI ulcerations.

Diagnostic Considerations: Diagnosis by urine/serum histoplasmosis antigen, sometimes by culture of bone marrow/liver or isolator blood cultures. May occur in patients months to years after having lived/moved from an endemic area.

Pitfalls: Relapse is common after discontinuation of therapy in patients with advanced immunosuppression. Cultures may take 7–21 days to turn positive. Itraconazole has many drug-drug interactions with antiretrovirals, especially PIs.

Therapeutic Considerations: Initial therapy depends on severity of illness on presentation. Extremely sick patients should be started on amphotericin B deoxycholate, with duration of IV therapy dependent on response to treatment. Mildly ill patients can be started on itraconazole. Regardless of disease severity, itraconazole levels should be obtained to ensure adequate absorption. Serum concentrations of itraconazole + hydroxyitraconazole should be > 1 μg/mL. All patients require chronic suppressive therapy, with possible discontinuation for immune reconstitution with CD4 counts > 100/mm³ for at least 6 months. HIV patients with CD4 > 500/mm³ and acute pulmonary histoplasmosis might not require therapy, but a short course of itraconazole (4–8 weeks) is reasonable to prevent systemic spread.

Prognosis: Usually responds to treatment, except in fulminant cases.

Human Papillomavirus (HPV) Disease

Preferred Therapy, Duration of Therapy, Chronic Maintenance	Alternate Therapy	Other Options/Issues
Treatment of condyloma acuminata (genital warts)		
Patient-applied therapy Podofilox 0.5% solution or 0.5% gel—apply to all lesions bid × 3 consecutive days, followed by 4 days of no therapy, repeat weekly for up to 4 cycles; **or** Imiquimod 5% cream—apply to lesion at bedtime and remove in the morning on 3 nonconsecutive nights weekly for up to 16 weeks. Each treatment should be washed with soap and water 6–10 hours after application **or** Sinecatechins 15% ointment—apply to affected areas tid for up to 16 weeks, until warts are completely cleared and not visible	Provider-applied therapy Cryotherapy (liquid nitrogen or cryoprobe)—apply until each lesion is thoroughly frozen; repeat every 1–2 weeks. Some providers allow the lesion to thaw, then freeze a second time in each session. **or** Trichloroacetic acid or bicloroacetic acid cauterization—80%–90% aqueous solution, apply to each lesion, repeat weekly for up to 6 weeks until lesions are no longer visible **or** Surgical excision or laser surgery to external or anal warts **or** Podophyllin resin 10%–25% suspension in tincture of benzoin—apply to all lesions (up to 10 cm²), then wash off a few hours later, repeat weekly for up to 6 weeks until lesions are no longer visible	HIV-infected patients may have larger or more numerous warts and may not respond as well to therapy for genital warts when compared to HIV-uninfected individuals. Topical cidofovir has activity against genital warts, but the product is not commercially available Intralesional interferon-alpha is usually not recommended because of high cost, difficult administration, and potential for systemic side effects The rate of recurrence of genital warts is high, despite treatment There is no consensus on the treatment of oral warts. Many treatments for anogenital warts cannot be used in the oral mucosa. Surgery is the most common treatment for oral warts that interfere with function or for aesthetic reasons

Isospora belli Infection

Preferred Therapy, Duration of Therapy, Chronic Maintenance	Alternate Therapy	Other Options/Issues
Preferred therapy for acute infection: TMP-SMX (160 mg/800 mg) PO (or IV) qid for 10 days; **or** TMP-SMX (160 mg/800 mg) PO (or IV) bid for 7–10 days Can start with bid dosing first and increase daily dose and/or duration (up to 3–4 weeks) if symptoms worsen or persist IV therapy may be used for patients with potential or documented malabsorption Preferred chronic maintenance therapy (secondary prophylaxis) In patients with CD4+ count < 200/μL, TMP-SMX (160 mg/800 mg) PO tiw	Alternative therapy for acute infection Pyrimethamine 50–75 mg PO daily plus leucovorin 10–25 mg PO daily; **or** Ciprofloxacin 500 mg PO bid × 7 days as a second line alternative Alternative chronic maintenance therapy (secondary prophylaxis) TMP-SMX (160 mg/800 mg) PO daily or (320 mg/1600 mg) tiw **or** Pyrimethamine 25 mg PO daily + leucovorin 5–10 mg PO daily **or** Ciprofloxacin 500 mg tiw as a second line alternative	Fluid and electrolyte management in patients with dehydration Nutritional supplementation for malnourished patients Immune reconstitution with ART may result in fewer relapses

Genital/Perianal Warts (Condyloma Acuminata)

Clinical Presentation: Single/multiple verrucous genital lesions ± pigmentation usually without inguinal adenopathy.

Diagnostic Considerations: Diagnosis by clinical appearance. Genital warts are usually caused by HPV types 11, 16. Anogenital warts caused by HPV types 16, 18, 31, 33, 35 are associated with cervical neoplasia.

Pitfalls: Most HPV infections are asymptomatic.

Therapeutic Considerations: First-line therapy is ablative (cryotherapy or cauterization); if no response to standard treatment, attempt to treat with surgery or cidofovir. Intralesional interferon-alfa generally is not recommended.

Prognosis: The rate of recurrence of anogenital warts is high despite treatment.

Clinical Presentation: Severe chronic diarrhea without fever/fecal leukocytes.

Diagnostic Considerations: Spore-forming protozoa *(Isospora belli)*. Oocyst on AFB smear of stool larger that cryptosporidium (20–30 microns vs. 4–6 microns). More common in HIV patients from tropical areas. Less common than cryptosporidium or microsporidia. Malabsorption may occur with severe cases. Can be associated with eosinophilia.

Pitfalls: Multiple relapses are possible.

Therapeutic Considerations: Chronic suppressive therapy may be required if CD4 cell count does not increase.

Prognosis: Related to degree of immunosuppression/response to antiretroviral therapy.

Comments: Immune reconstitution with ART results in fewer relapses.

Leishmaniasis, Cutaneous

Preferred Therapy, Duration of Therapy, Chronic Maintenance	Alternate Therapy	Other Options/Issues
Preferred therapy for acute infection Liposomal amphotericin B 2–4 mg/kg IV daily for 10 days or interrupted schedule (e.g., 4 mg/kg on days 1–5, 10, 17, 24, 31, 38) to achieve total dose of 20–60 mg/kg; **or** Sodium stibogluconate 20 mg/kg IV or IM daily for 3–4 weeks Chronic maintenance therapy May be indicated in immunocompromised patients with multiple relapses	Alternative therapy for acute infection Oral miltefosine (can be obtained via a treatment IND) **or** Topical paromomycin **or** Intralesional sodium stibogluconate **or** Local heat therapy No data exist for any of these agents in HIV-infected patients; choice and efficacy dependent on species of *Leishmania*	

Leishmaniasis, Visceral

Preferred Therapy, Duration of Therapy, Chronic Maintenance	Alternate Therapy	Other Options/Issues
Preferred therapy for initial infection Liposomal amphotericin B 2–4 mg/kg IV daily × 10 days; or interrupted schedule (e.g., 4 mg/kg on days 1–5, 10, 17, 24, 31, 38) to achieve total dose of 20–60 mg/kg	Alternative therapy for initial infection Other lipid formulation of amphotericin B, dose and schedule as in preferred therapy **or**	ART should be initiated or optimized For sodium stibogluconate, contact the CDC Drug Service at (404) 639-3670 or drugservice@cdc.gov

Leishmaniasis, Visceral (cont'd)

Preferred Therapy, Duration of Therapy, Chronic Maintenance	Alternate Therapy	Other Options/Issues
Preferred chronic maintenance therapy (secondary prophylaxis)— especially in patients with CD4+ count < 200 cells/μL Liposomal amphotericin B 4 mg/kg every 2–4 weeks **or** Amphotericin B lipid complex 3 mg/kg every 21 days	Amphotericin B deoxycholate 0.5–1.0 mg/kg IV daily for total dose of 1.5–2.0 grams; **or** Sodium stibogluconate (pentavalent antimony) 20 mg/kg body weight IV or IM daily for 28 days **or** Miltefosine 100 mg PO daily for 4 weeks (available in the United States under a treatment IND) Alternative chronic maintenance therapy (secondary prophylaxis) Sodium stibogluconate 20 mg/kg IV or IM every 4 weeks	

Malaria

Preferred Therapy, Duration of Therapy, Chronic Maintenance	Alternate Therapy	Other Options/Issues
Because *Plasmodium falciparum* malaria can progress within hours from mild symptoms or low-grade fever to severe disease or death, all HIV-infected patients with confirmed or suspected *P. falciparum* infection should be hospitalized for evaluation, initiation of treatment, and observation. Treatment recommendations for HIV-infected patients are the same as HIV-uninfected patients. Choice of therapy is guided by the degree of parasitemia, the species of *Plasmodium*, the patient's clinical status, region of infection, and the likely drug susceptibility of the infected species, and can be found at http://www.cdc.gov/malaria.	When suspicion for malaria is low, antimalarial treatment should not be initiated until the diagnosis is confirmed.	For treatment recommendations for specific regions, clinicians should refer to the following web link: http://www.cdc.gov/malaria/ or call the CDC Malaria Hotline: (770) 488-7788: M–F 8 AM–4:30 PM ET, or (770) 488-7100 after hours

Microsporidiosis

Preferred Therapy, Duration of Therapy, Chronic Maintenance	Alternate Therapy	Other Options/Issues
Initiate or optimize ART; immune restoration to CD4+ count > 100 cells/μL is associated with resolution of symptoms of enteric microsporidiosis		Severe dehydration, malnutrition, and wasting should be managed by fluid support and nutritional supplement
Preferred therapy for gastrointestinal infections caused by *Enterocytozoon bienuesi* Initiate or optimize ART; immune restoration to CD4+ count >100 cells/μL is associated with resolution of symptoms of enteric microsporidiosis. Manage severe dehydration, malnutrition, and wasting by fluid support and nutritional supplement.	Alternative therapy for gastrointestinal infections caused by *E. bienuesi* Fumagillin 60 mg/day and TNP-470 (a synthetic analog of fumagillin) may be effective, but neither is available in the United States. Nitazoxanide 1,000 mg bid with food for 60 days—effects might be minimal for patients with low CD4+ count	Antimotility agents can be used for diarrhea control if required
Preferred therapy for disseminated (not ocular) and intestinal infection attributed to microsporidia other than *E. bienuesi* and *Vittaforma corneae* Albendazole 400 mg PO bid, continue until CD4+ count > 200 cells/μL for > 6 months after initiation of ART	Alternative therapy for disseminated disease Itraconazole 400 mg PO daily plus albendazole 400 mg PO bid for disseminated disease attributed to *Trachipleistophora* or *Anncaliia*	
For ocular infection Topical fumagillin bicylohexylammonium (Fumidil B) 3 mg/mL in saline (fumagillin 70 μg/mL) eye drops—2 drops q2h for 4 days, then 2 drops qid (investigational use only in US) plus albendazole 400 mg PO bid for management of systemic infection Therapy should be continued until resolution of ocular symptoms and CD4 count increase to >200 cells/μL for >6 months in response to ART		

Clinical Presentation: Most commonly, intermittent chronic diarrhea without fever/fecal leukocytes; also can disseminate and cause disease in other organs (eyes, lungs).

Diagnostic Considerations: Spore-forming protozoa (S. intestinalis, E. bieneusi). Diagnosis by modified trichrome or fluorescent antibody stain of stool. Microsporidia can rarely disseminate to sinuses/cornea. Severe malabsorption may occur.

Pitfalls: Microsporidia cannot be detected by routine microscopic examination of stool due to small size.

Therapeutic Considerations: Key to successful resolution is optimizing ART to improve immune function. Albendazole is less effective for E. bieneusi than S. intestinalis, but speciation is usually not possible. Consider treatment discontinuation for CD4 > 200/mm³ if patient remains asymptomatic (no signs or symptoms of microsporidiosis). If ocular infection is present, continue treatment indefinitely.

Prognosis: Related to degree of immunosuppression/response to antiretroviral therapy.

Mycobacterium avium Complex (MAC) Disease

Preferred Therapy, Duration of Therapy, Chronic Maintenance	Alternate Therapy	Other Options/Issues
Preferred therapy for disseminated MAC At least 2 drugs as initial therapy with Clarithromycin 500 mg PO bid + ethambutol 15 mg/kg PO daily (Azithromycin 500–600 mg + ethambutol 15 mg/kg) PO daily if drug interaction or intolerance precludes the use of clarithromycin **or** Duration: at least 12 months of therapy, can discontinue if no signs and symptoms of MAC disease and sustained (>6 months) CD4+ count >100 cells/µL in response to ART	Alternative therapy for disseminated MAC (e.g., when drug interactions or intolerance precludes the use of clarithromycin) Addition of a third or fourth drug should be considered for patients with advanced immunosuppression (CD4+ count < 50 cells/µL), high mycobacterial loads (> 2 log CFU/mL of blood), or in the absence of effective ART Options include: Amikacin 10–15 mg/kg IV daily; **or** Streptomycin 1 gm IV or IM daily; **or** RFB 300 mg PO daily (dosage adjustment may be necessary based on drug interactions) **or**	Testing of susceptibility to clarithromycin and azithromycin is recommended NSAIDs may be used for patients who experience moderate to severe symptoms attributed to ART-associated immune reconstitution inflammatory syndrome (IRIS) If IRIS symptoms persist, short term (4–8 weeks) of systemic corticosteroid (equivalent to 20–40 mg of prednisone) can be used

Mycobacterium avium Complex (MAC) Disease (cont'd)

Preferred Therapy, Duration of Therapy, Chronic Maintenance	Alternate Therapy	Other Options/Issues
Chronic maintenance therapy (secondary prophylaxis) Same as treatment drugs and regimens Duration: Lifelong therapy, unless in patients with sustained immune recovery on ART	Levofloxacin 500 mg PO daily; **or** Moxifloxacin 400 mg PO daily	

Clinical Presentation: Typically presents as a febrile wasting illness in advanced HIV disease (CD4 < 50/mm³). Focal invasive disease is possible, especially in patients with advanced immunosuppression after starting antiretroviral therapy. Focal disease likely reflects restoration of pathogen-specific immune response to subclinical infection ("immune reconstitution inflammatory syndrome" [IRIS]), and typically manifests as fever with lymphadenitis (mesenteric, cervical, thoracic) or rarely disease in the spine mimicking Pott's disease. Immune reconstitution syndrome usually occurs within weeks to months after starting antiretroviral therapy for the first time, but may occur a year or more later.

Diagnostic Considerations: Diagnosis by isolation of organism from a normally sterile body site (blood, lymph node, bone marrow, liver biopsy). Lysis centrifugation (DuPont isolator) is the preferred blood culture method. Anemia/↑ alkaline phosphatase are occasionally seen.

Pitfalls: Isolator blood cultures may be negative, especially in immune reconstitution inflammatory syndrome initially.

Therapeutic Considerations: Some studies suggest benefit for addition of rifabutin 300 mg (PO) QD, others do not. Rifabutin may require dosage adjustment with NNRTIs and PIs (see p. 119). Monitor carefully for rifabutin drug toxicity (arthralgias, uveitis, leukopenia). Treat IRIS initially with NSAIDs; if symptoms persist, systemic corticosteroids (prednisone 20–40 mg daily) for 4–8 weeks can be used. Some patients will require a more prolonged course of corticosteroids with a slow taper over months. Azithromycin is often better tolerated than clarithromycin and has fewer drug-drug interactions. Optimal long-term management is unknown, though most studies suggest that treatment can be discontinued in asymptomatic patients with > 12 months of therapy and CD4 > 100/mm³ for > 6 months.

Prognosis: Depends on immune reconstitution in response to antiretroviral therapy. Adverse prognostic factors include high-grade bacteremia or severe wasting.

Mycobacterium tuberculosis

Preferred Therapy, Duration of Therapy, Chronic Maintenance	Alternate Therapy	Other Options/Issues
After collecting specimen for culture and molecular diagnostic tests, empiric treatment should be initiated and continued in HIV-infected individuals with clinical and radiographic presentation suggestive of TB		Adjunctive corticosteroid improves survival for TB meningitis and pericarditis
Treatment of drug-susceptible active TB disease	**Treatment for drug-resistant active TB**	See text for drug, dose, and duration recommendations. RIF is not recommended for patients receiving HIV PI because of its induction of PI metabolism
Initial phase (2 months) Isoniazid (INH)† + [rifampin (RIF) or rifabutin (RFB)] + pyrazinamide (PZA) + ethambutol EMB)	Resistant to INH RIF or RFB) + EMB + PZA + (moxifloxacin or levofloxacin) for 2 months; followed by (RIF or RFB) + EMB + (moxifloxacin or levofloxacin) for 7 months	RFB is a less potent CYP3A4 inducer than RIF and is preferred in patients receiving PIs.
Continuation Phase INH + (RIF or RFB) daily (5–7 times/week) or tiw		Once weekly rifapentine can result in development of rifamycin resistance in HIV-infected patients and is not recommended
Total duration of therapy (for drug-susceptible TB) Pulmonary TB: 6 months Pulmonary TB and culture-positive after 2 months of TB treatment: 9 months	Resistant to rifamycins +/- other drugs Regimen and duration of treatment should be individualized based on resistance pattern, clinical and microbiological responses, and in close consultation with experienced specialists	Therapeutic drug monitoring should be considered in patients receiving rifamycin and interacting ART. Paradoxical IRIS that is not severe can be treated with NSAIDs without a change in TB or HIV therapy
Extra-pulmonary TB w/CNS infection: 9–12 months		
Extra-pulmonary TB w/bone or joint involvement: 6 to 9 months Extra-pulmonary TB in other sites: 6 months		For severe IRIS reaction, consider prednisone and taper over 4 weeks based on clinical symptoms
Total duration of therapy should be based on number of doses received, not on calendar time		For example: If receiving RIF: prednisone 1.5 mg/kg/day for 2 weeks, then 0.75 mg/kg/day for 2 weeks. If receiving RFB: prednisone 1.0 mg/kg/day for 2 weeks, then 0.5 mg/kg/day for 2 weeks

Mycobacterium tuberculosis (cont'd)

Preferred Therapy, Duration of Therapy, Chronic Maintenance	Alternate Therapy	Other Options/Issues
		A more gradual tapering schedule over a few months may be necessary for some patients

† All patients receiving INH should receive pyridoxine 25–50 mg PO daily

Clinical Presentation: May present atypically. HIV patients with high (> 500/mm³) CD4 cell counts are more likely to have a typical pulmonary presentation, but patients with advanced HIV disease may have a diffuse interstitial pattern, hilar adenopathy, or a normal chest x-ray. Tuberculin skin testing (TST) and interferon gamma release assays (IGRAs) are helpful if positive, but unreliable if negative due to impaired immune response.

Diagnostic Considerations: In many areas, TB is one of the most common HIV-related respiratory illnesses. In other areas, HIV-related TB occurs infrequently except in immigrants or patients arriving from highly TB endemic areas. Maintain a high Index of suspicion for TB in HIV patients with unexplained fevers/pulmonary infiltrates.

Pitfalls: Extrapulmonary and pulmonary TB often coexist, especially in advanced HIV disease.

Therapeutic Considerations: Treatment by directly observed therapy (DOT) is strongly recommended for all HIV patients. If patients have cavitary disease or either positive sputum cultures or lack of clinical response at 2 months, total duration of therapy should be increased up to 9 months or longer depending on clinical response. For CNS disease (meningitis or mass lesions), corticosteroid should be initiated as early as possible (along with TB treatment) and continued for 6–8 weeks. If hepatic transaminases are elevated (AST ≥ 3 times normal) before treatment initiation, treatment options include: (1) standard therapy with frequent monitoring; (2) rifamycin (rifampin or rifabutin) + EMB + PZA for 6 months; or (3) INH + rifamycin + EMB for 2 months, then INH + rifamycin for 7 months. Once-weekly rifapentine is not recommended for HIV patients. Non-severe immune reconstitution inflammatory syndrome (IRIS) may be treated with nonsteroidal anti-inflammatory drugs (NSAIDs); severe cases should be treated with corticosteroids. In all cases of IRIS, antiretroviral therapy should be continued if possible. Monitor carefully for signs of rifabutin drug toxicity (arthralgias, uveitis, leukopenia). In general, ART regimens should avoid protease inhibitors due to interactions with rifamycins; raltegravir, dolutegravir, or efavirenz (in combination with 2 NRTIs) would be safer options. The optimal timing of ART in the setting of HIV-related TB has recently been clarified by several pivotal studies. ART should be started within 2 weeks of TB treatment when the CD4 cell count is below 50/µL and by 8 to 12 weeks for those with higher CD4 cell counts. The optimal timing for patients with TB meningitis, regardless of CD4 cell count, is less certain, but ART should be started within the first 2 to 8 weeks of diagnosis.

Prognosis: Usually responds to treatment. Relapse rates are related to the degree of immunosuppression and local risk of re-exposure to TB.

Penicilliosis

Preferred Therapy, Duration of Therapy, Chronic Maintenance	Alternate Therapy	Other Options/Issues
Acute infection in severely ill patients Liposomal amphotericin B 3–5 mg/kg/day IV for 2 weeks; followed by itraconazole 200 mg PO bid for 10 weeks, followed by chronic maintenance therapy (as below)	Acute infection in severely ill patients Voriconazole 6 mg/kg IV q12h for 1 day, then 4 mg/kg IV q12h for at least 3 days, followed by 200 mg PO bid for a maximum of 12 weeks, followed by maintenance therapy For mild disease Voriconazole 400 mg PO bid for 1 day, then 200 mg bid for a maximum of 12 weeks, followed by chronic maintenance therapy	ART should be initiated simultaneously with treatment for penicilliosis to improve treatment outcome. Itraconazole and voriconazole may have significant interactions with certain ARV agents. These interactions are complex and can be bidirectional. Refer to Table 5 in http://aidsinfo.nih.gov/contentfiles/lvguidelines/AdultOITablesOnly.pdf for dosage recommendations
Mild disease Itraconazole 200 mg PO bid for 8 weeks followed by chronic maintenance therapy (as below) Chronic maintenance therapy (secondary prophylaxis) Itraconazole 200 mg PO daily		Therapeutic drug monitoring and dosage adjustment may be necessary to ensure triazole antifungal and ARV efficacy and reduce concentration-related toxicities.

Penicilliosis (*Penicillium marneffei*)

Clinical Presentation: Papules, pustules, nodules, ulcers, or abscesses. Mostly seen in advanced HIV/AIDS in residents/visitors of Southeast Asia or Southern China.

Diagnostic Considerations: Diagnosis by demonstrating organism by stain/culture in tissue. specimen. An early presumptive diagnosis can be made several days before the results of fungal cultures are available by microscopic examination of the Wright-stained samples of skin scrapings, bone marrow aspirate, or lymph-node biopsy specimens. Many intracellular and extracellular basophilic, spherical, oval, and elliptical yeast-like organisms can be seen, some with clear central septation, which is a characteristic feature of *P. marneffei*.

Pitfalls: Lesions commonly become umbilicated and resemble molluscum contagiosum.

Therapeutic Considerations: ART should be administered according to standard of care in the community. Requires lifelong suppressive therapy with itraconazole unless CD4 increases to > 100 for ≥ 6 months in response to ART.

Prognosis: Dependent on degree of immune recovery secondary to ART. Without HIV treatment, prognosis is poor, as most affected patients have advanced immunosuppression.

Pneumocystis Pneumonia (PCP)

Preferred Therapy, Duration of Therapy, Chronic Maintenance	Alternate Therapy	Other Options/Issues
Preferred treatment for moderate to severe PCP Trimethoprim-sulfamethoxazole (TMP-SMX): [15–20 mg TMP and 75–100 mg SMX]/kg/day IV administered q6h or q8h, may switch to PO after clinical improvement Duration of therapy: 21 days	Alternative therapy for moderate to severe PCP Pentamidine 4 mg/kg IV daily infused over ≥ 60 minutes, certain specialists reduce dose to 3 mg/kg IV daily because of toxicities; **or** Primaquine 30 mg (base) PO daily plus (clindamycin 600 mg q6h IV or 900 mg IV q8h) or (clindamycin 300 mg PO q6h or 450 mg PO q8h)	Indications for corticosteroids PaO_2 < 70 mmHg at room air or alveolar-arterial O_2 gradient > 35 mmHg Prednisone doses (beginning as early as possible and within 72 hours of PCP therapy):
Preferred treatment for mild to moderate PCP Same daily dose of TMP-SMX as above, administered PO in 3 divided doses; **or** TMP-SMX (160 mg/800 mg or DS) 2 tablets PO tid Duration of therapy: 21 days	Alternative therapy for mild-to-moderate PCP Dapsone 100 mg PO daily and TMP 5 mg/kg/day PO tid **or** Primaquine 30 mg (base) PO daily plus (clindamycin 300 mg PO q6h or 450 mg PO q8h) **or** Atovaquone 750 mg PO bid with food	Days 1–5: 40 mg PO bid Days 6–10: 40 mg PO daily Days 11–21: 20 mg PO daily IV methylprednisolone can be administered as 75% of prednisone dose
Preferred secondary prophylaxis TMP-SMX (160 mg/800 mg or DS) 1 tablet PO daily; **or** TMP-SMX (80 mg/400 mg or SS) 1 tablet PO daily	Secondary prophylaxis, after completion of PCP treatment TMP-SMX (160 mg/800 mg or DS) 1 tablet PO tiw **or** Dapsone 100 mg PO daily; **or** Dapsone 50 mg PO daily + pyrimethamine 50 mg PO weekly + leucovorin 25 mg PO weekly; **or** Dapsone 200 mg PO + pyrimethamine 75 mg PO + leucovorin 25 mg PO weekly; **or**	Benefits of corticosteroid if started after 72 hours of treatment is unknown, but a majority of clinicians will use it in patients with moderate to severe PCP Whenever possible, patients should be tested for G6PD deficiency before use of dapsone or primaquine. Alternative therapy should be used in patients found to have G6PD deficiency.

Pneumocystis Pneumonia (PCP) (cont'd)

Preferred Therapy, Duration of Therapy, Chronic Maintenance	Alternate Therapy	Other Options/Issues
	Aerosolized pentamidine 300 mg every month via Respirgard II™ nebulizer; **or** Atovaquone 1,500 mg PO daily; **or** Atovaquone 1,500 mg + pyrimethamine 25 mg + leucovorin 10 mg, each PO daily	Patients who are receiving pyrimethamine/sulfadiazine for treatment or suppression of toxoplasmosis do not require additional PCP prophylaxis. If TMP-SMX is discontinued because of a mild adverse reaction, reinstitution should be considered after the reaction resolves. The dose can be increased gradually (desensitization), reduced, or the frequency modified. TMP-SMX should be permanently discontinued in patients with possible or definite Stevens-Johnson Syndrome or toxic epidermal necrosis.

Clinical Presentation: Fever, cough, dyspnea; often indolent presentation. Physical exam is usually normal. Chest x-ray is variable, but commonly shows a diffuse interstitial pattern. Elevated LDH and exercise desaturation are highly suggestive of PCP.

Diagnostic Considerations: Definitive diagnosis is made by observing the organism on stained specimens of respiratory secretions, obtained by induced sputum or bronchoscopy. Check ABG if O_2 saturation is abnormal or respiratory rate is increased. Serum 1, 3 beta-glucan is usually elevated and may provide additional supportive evidence for the diagnosis of PCP (Clin Infect Dis. 2011 Jul 15;53(2):197–202).

Pitfalls: Slight worsening of symptoms is common after starting therapy, especially if not treated with steroids. Benefits of corticosteroid if started after 72 hours of treatment is unknown, but majority of clinicians will still use it if clinically warranted even after 72 hours. Do not overlook superimposed bacterial pneumonia or other secondary infections, especially while on pentamidine.

Patients receiving second-line agents for PCP prophylaxis—in particular aerosolized pentamidine—may present with atypical radiographic findings, including apical infiltrates, multiple small-walled cysts, pleural effusions, pneumothorax, or single/multiple nodules.

Therapeutic Considerations: Outpatient therapy is possible for mild-moderate disease, but only when close follow-up is assured. Adverse reactions to TMP-SMX (rash, fever, GI symptoms, hepatitis, hyperkalemia, leukopenia, hemolytic anemia) occur in 25–50% of patients, many of whom will need a second-line regimen to complete therapy (e.g., trimethoprim-dapsone or atovaquone). Unless an adverse reaction to TMP-SMX is particularly severe (e.g., Stevens-Johnson syndrome or other life-threatening problem), TMP-SMX may later be considered for PCP prophylaxis, since prophylaxis requires a much lower dose (only 10–15% of treatment dose). Patients being treated for severe PCP with TMP-SMX who do not improve after one week may be switched to pentamidine or clindamycin plus primaquine, although there are no prospective data to confirm this approach. In general, patients receiving antiretroviral therapy when PCP develops should have their treatment continued, since intermittent antiretroviral therapy can lead to drug resistance. For newly diagnosed or antiretroviral-naïve HIV patients, antiretroviral therapy should be started as soon as feasible, preferably within 2 weeks. Steroids should be tapered, not discontinued abruptly. Adjunctive steroids increase the risk of thrush/herpes simplex infection, but probably not CMV, TB, or disseminated fungal infection. Patients should be tested for G6PD deficiency prior to use of primaquine and dapsone.

Prognosis: Usually responds to treatment. Adverse prognostic factors include ↑ A-a gradient, hypoxemia, ↑ LDH.

Progressive Multifocal Leukoencephalopathy (PML)

Preferred Therapy, Duration of Therapy, Chronic Maintenance	Alternate Therapy	Other Options/Issues
There is no specific antiviral therapy for JC virus infection. The main treatment approach is to reverse the immunosuppression caused by HIV.		Corticosteroids may be used for PML-IRIS characterized by contrast enhancement, edema or mass effect, and with clinical deterioration
Initiate antiretroviral therapy in ART-naïve patients		
Optimize ART in patients who develop PML in phase of HIV viremia on antiretroviral therapy		

Clinical Presentation: Hemiparesis, ataxia, aphasia, other focal neurologic defects, which may progress over weeks to months. Usually alert without headache or seizures on presentation.

Diagnostic Considerations: Demyelinating disease caused by reactivation of the latent papovavirus JC virus. Diagnosis by clinical presentation and MRI showing patchy demyelination of white matter, usually without enhancement. Any region of the CNS may be involved, most commonly the occipital lobes (with hemianopia), frontal and parietal lobes (hemiparesis and hemisensory deficits), and cerebellar peduncles and deep white matter (dysmetria and ataxia). JC virus PCR of CSF is useful for non-invasive diagnosis. In confusing or atypical presentation, biopsy may be needed to distinguish PML from other opportunistic infections, CNS lymphoma, or HIV encephalitis/encephalopathy.

Pitfalls: Primary HIV-related encephalopathy may have a similar appearance on MRI.

Therapeutic Considerations: The only effective therapy is antiretroviral therapy with immune reconstitution. Treatment should be started promptly if the patient is not on therapy. Some patients experience worsening neurologic symptoms once ART is initiated due to immune reconstitution induced inflammation. ART should be continued, with consideration of adjunctive steroids especially if neuroimaging shows evidence of inflammation (enhancement or edema). Randomized controlled trials have evaluated cidofovir and vidarabine—neither is effective nor recommended.

Prognosis: Rapid progression of neurologic deficits over weeks to months is common. Best chance for survival is immune reconstitution in response to antiretroviral therapy, although some patients will have progressive disease despite immune recovery. (J Infect Dis 2009;199:77)

Salmonellosis

Preferred Therapy, Duration of Therapy, Chronic Maintenance	Alternate Therapy	Other Options/Issues
All HIV-infected patients with salmonellosis should be treated due to the high risk of bacteremia in these patients		Oral or IV rehydration if indicated.
Preferred therapy for *Salmonella* gastroenteritis with or without symptomatic bacteremia Ciprofloxacin 500–750 mg PO bid (or 400 mg IV q12h, if susceptible)	Alternative therapy for *Salmonella* gastroenteritis with or without symptomatic bacteremia Levofloxacin 750 mg (PO or IV) q24h **or** Moxifloxacin 400 mg (PO or IV) q24h **or** TMP, 160 mg-SMX 800 mg (PO or IV) q12h **or** Ceftriaxone 1 g IV q24h **or** Cefotaxime 1 g IV q8h	Antimotility agents should be avoided The role of long-term secondary prophylaxis for patients with recurrent *Salmonella* bacteremia is not well established. Must weigh the benefit against the risks of long-term antibiotic exposure.
Duration of therapy: *For gastroenteritis without bacteremia:* • If CD4 count <200 cells/μL: 7–14 days • If CD4 count <200 cells/μL: 2–6 weeks		Effective ART may reduce the frequency, severity, and recurrence of *Salmonella* infections.
For gastroenteritis with bacteremia: • If CD4 count <200/μL: 14 days; longer duration if bacteremia persists or if the infection is complicated (e.g., if metastatic foci of infection are present) • If CD4 count <200 cells/μL: 2–6 weeks		

Salmonellosis (cont'd)

Preferred Therapy, Duration of Therapy, Chronic Maintenance	Alternate Therapy	Other Options/Issues
Secondary prophylaxis should be considered for: Patients with recurrent Salmonella gastroenteritis +/- bacteremia **or** Patients with CD4 <200 cells/µL with severe diarrhea		

Clinical Presentation: Patients with HIV are at markedly increased risk of developing salmonellosis. Three different presentations may be seen: (1) self-limited gastroenteritis, as typically seen in immunocompetent hosts; (2) a more severe and prolonged diarrheal disease, associated with fever, bloody diarrhea, and weight loss; or (3) *Salmonella* septicemia, which may present with or without gastrointestinal symptoms.

Diagnostic Considerations: The diagnosis is established through cultures of stool and blood. Given the high rate of bacteremia associated with *Salmonella* gastroenteritis—especially in advanced HIV disease—blood cultures should be obtained in any HIV patient presenting with diarrhea and fever.

Pitfalls: A distinctive feature of *Salmonella* bacteremia in patients with AIDS is its propensity for relapse (rate > 20%).

Therapeutic Considerations: The mainstay of treatment is a fluoroquinolone; greatest experience is with ciprofloxacin, but newer quinolones (moxifloxacin, levofloxacin) may also be effective. For uncomplicated salmonellosis in an HIV patient with CD4 > 200/mm^3, 1–2 weeks of treatment is reasonable to reduce the risk of extraintestinal spread. For patients with advanced HIV disease (CD4 < 200/mm^3) or who have *Salmonella* bacteremia, at least 2–6 weeks of treatment is required. Chronic suppressive therapy, given for several months or until antiretroviral therapy-induced immune reconstitution ensues, is indicated for patients who relapse after cessation of therapy. Consider using ZDV as part of the antiretroviral regimen (ZDV is active against salmonella).

Prognosis: Usually responds well to treatment. Relapse rate in AIDS patients in the pre-antiretroviral therapy era with bacteremia was > 20%.

Shigellosis

Preferred Therapy, Duration of Therapy, Chronic Maintenance	Alternate Therapy	Other Options/Issues
Preferred therapy for Shigella infection Ciprofloxacin 500–750 mg PO (or 400 mg IV) q12h	Levofloxacin 750 mg (PO or IV) q24h **or** Moxifloxacin 400 mg (PO or IV) q24h **or**	Therapy is indicated both to shorten the duration of illness and to prevent spread of infection. Oral or IV rehydration if indicated.

Shigellosis (cont'd)

Preferred Therapy, Duration of Therapy, Chronic Maintenance	Alternate Therapy	Other Options/Issues
Duration of therapy: 　Gastroenteritis: 7–10 days 　Bacteremia: ≥14 days 　Recurrent infections: 　up to 6 weeks	TMP 160 mg-SMX 800 mg (PO or IV) q12h (Note: *Shigella* infections acquired outside of the United States have high rates of TMP-SMX resistance) **or** Azithromycin 500 mg PO daily for 5 days (Note: not recommended for patients with bacteremia)	Antimotility agents should be avoided. If no clinical response after 5–7 days, consider follow-up stool culture, alternative diagnosis, or antibiotic resistance. Effective ART may reduce the frequency, severity, and recurrence of *Shigella* infections.

Clinical Presentation: Acute onset of bloody diarrhea/mucus.

Diagnostic Considerations: Diagnosis by demonstrating organism in stool specimens. Shigella ulcers in colon are linear, serpiginous, and rarely lead to perforation. More common in gay men.

Therapeutic Considerations: Shigella dysentery is more acute/fulminating than amebic dysentery. Shigella has no carrier state, unlike entamoeba. Shigella infections acquired outside of United States have high rates of TMP-SMX resistance. Therapy is indicated to shorten the duration of illness and to prevent spread of infection.

Prognosis: Good if treated early. Severity of illness related to shigella species: *S. dysenteriae* (most severe) > *S. flexneri* > *S. boydii/S. sonnei* (mildest).

Toxoplasma gondii Encephalitis

Preferred Therapy, Duration of Therapy, Chronic Maintenance	Alternate Therapy	Other Options/Issues
Acute infection Pyrimethamine 200 mg PO × 1, followed by weight-based therapy: If weight <60 kg, pyrimethamine 50 mg PO once daily + sulfadiazine 1000 mg PO q6h + leucovorin 10–25 mg PO once daily If weight ≥60 kg, pyrimethamine 75 mg PO once daily + sulfadiazine 1,500 mg PO q6h + leucovorin 10–25 mg PO once daily Leucovorin dose can be increased to 50 mg daily or bid)	Acute infection Pyrimethamine (leucovorin)* + clindamycin 600 mg IV or PO q6h; **or** TMP-SMX (5 mg/kg TMP and 25 mg/kg SMX) IV or PO bid; **or** Atovaquone 1,500 mg PO bid with food (or nutritional supplement) + sulfadiazine 1,000–1,500 mg PO q6h; (weight-based dosing, as in preferred therapy) **or**	Adjunctive corticosteroids (e.g., dexamethasone) should be administered when clinically indicated only for treatment of mass effect attributed to focal lesions or associated edema; discontinue as soon as clinically feasible

Toxoplasma gondii Encephalitis (cont'd)

Preferred Therapy, Duration of Therapy, Chronic Maintenance	Alternate Therapy	Other Options/ Issues
Duration for acute therapy At least 6 weeks; longer duration if clinical or radiologic disease is extensive or response is incomplete at 6 weeks Chronic maintenance therapy: Pyrimethamine 25–50 mg PO daily + sulfadiazine 2,000–4,000 mg PO daily (in 2–4 divided doses) + leucovorin 10–25 mg PO daily Preferred chronic maintenance therapy Pyrimethamine 25–50 mg PO daily plus sulfadiazine 2,000–4,000 mg PO daily (in two to four divided doses) plus leucovorin 10–25 mg PO daily	Atovaquone 1,500 mg PO bid with food; **or** Pyrimethamine (leucovorin)* plus azithromycin 900–1200 mg PO daily Alternative chronic maintenance therapy/secondary prophylaxis Clindamycin 600 mg PO q8h + pyrimethamine 25–50 mg PO daily + leucovorin 10–25 PO daily **or** Atovaquone 750–1,500 mg PO bid +/- [(pyrimethamine 25 mg PO daily plus leucovorin 10 mg PO daily) or sulfadiazine 2,000–4,000 mg PO] daily *Pyrimethamine and leucovorin doses are the same as for preferred therapy.	Anticonvulsants should be administered to patients with a history of seizures and continued through the acute treatment; but should not be used prophylactically If clindamycin is used in place of sulfadiazine, additional therapy must be added to prevent PCP

* Pyrimethemine and leucovorin doses—same as in "Preferred therapy" for toxoplasmosis

Clinical Presentation: Wide spectrum of neurologic symptoms, including sensorimotor deficits, seizures, confusion, ataxia. Fever/headache are common.

Diagnostic Considerations: Diagnosis by characteristic radiographic appearance and response to empiric therapy in a for *T. gondii* seropositive patient.

Pitfalls: Use leucovorin (folinic acid) 10 mg (PO) daily with pyrimethamine-containing regimens, not folate/folic acid. Radiographic improvement may lag behind clinical response.

Therapeutic Considerations: Alternate agents include atovaquone, azithromycin, clarithromycin, minocycline (all with pyrimethamine if possible). Decadron 4 mg (PO or IV) q6h is useful for edema/mass effect. Intravenous TMP-SMX useful for critically ill or neurologically compromised patients who cannot take oral therapy. Chronic suppressive therapy can be discontinued if patients are free from signs and symptoms of disease and have a CD4 cell count > 200/mm^3 for > 6 months due to ART. In some centers, TMP-SMX has become the preferred initial therapy given its widespread availability, low cost, and ease of dosing compared with pyrimethamine and sulfadiazine.

Prognosis: Usually responds to treatment if able to tolerate drugs. Clinical response is evident by 1 week in 70%, by 2 weeks in 90%. Radiographic improvement is usually apparent by 2 weeks. Neurologic recovery is variable.

Treponema pallidum (Syphilis)

Preferred Therapy, Duration of Therapy, Chronic Maintenance	Alternate Therapy	Other Options/Issues
Preferred therapy early stage (primary, secondary, and early latent syphilis) Benzathine penicillin G 2.4 million units IM for 1 dose Preferred therapy late-latent disease (> 1 year or of unknown duration, CSF examination ruled out neurosyphilis) Benzathine penicillin G 2.4 million units IM weekly for 3 doses Preferred therapy late-stage (tertiary–cardiovascular or gummatous disease) Benzathine penicillin G 2.4 million units IM weekly for 3 doses (Note: rule out neurosyphilis before initiation of benzathine penicillin, and obtain infectious diseases consultation to guide management) Preferred therapy neurosyphilis (including otic and ocular disease) Aqueous crystalline penicillin G, 18–24 million units per day, administered as 3–4 million units IV q4h or by continuous IV infusion for 10–14 days +/- benzathine penicillin G 2.4 million units IM weekly for 3 doses after completion of IV therapy	Alternative therapy early stage (primary, secondary, and early latent syphilis) *For penicillin-allergic patients:* Doxycycline 100 mg PO bid for 14 days; **or** Ceftriaxone 1 g IM or IV daily for 10–14 days; **or** Azithromycin 2 g PO for 1 dose (Note: azithromycin is not recommended for MSM or pregnant women) Alternative therapy late-latent disease (without CNS involvement) *For penicillin-allergic patients:* Doxycycline 100 mg PO bid for 28 days Alternative therapy neurosyphilis Procaine penicillin 2.4 million units IM daily plus probenecid 500 mg PO qid for 10–14 days +/- benzathine penicillin G 2.4 million units IM weekly for 3 doses after completion of above; **or** *For penicillin-allergic patients:* Desensitization to penicillin is the preferred approach; if not feasible, ceftriaxone 2 g IV daily for 10–14 days	The efficacy of non-penicillin alternatives has not been evaluated in HIV-infected patients and should be undertaken only with close clinical and serologic monitoring Combination of procaine penicillin and probenecid is not recommended for patients with history of sulfa allergy The Jarisch-Herxheimer reaction is an acute febrile reaction accompanied by headache and myalgias that might occur within the first 24 hours after therapy for syphilis. This reaction occurs most frequently in patients with early syphilis, high non-treponemal titers, and prior penicillin treatment.

Epidemiology: Syphilis is highly prevalent among some groups with high rates of HIV, notably gay men. Studies have shown that syphilis facilitates HIV transmission, and case reports/series suggest that syphilis in HIV-infected patients is associated with multiple and slower resolving primary chancres, higher titer RPR, slower decline of RPR titers, higher rate of serologic failure, increased frequency of CSF abnormalities and CSF-VDRL positivity, higher incidence of ocular disease, and higher rates of relapse after treatment (Sex Transm Dis 2001;28:158–65; N Engl J Med 1997 Jul;337:307–14; Ann Intern Med 1990;113:872).

Clinical Presentation: The causative organism of syphilis is *Treponema pallidum*, which cannot be cultured in routine clinical laboratories. As a result, the diagnosis of syphilis depends on recognizing the clinical stages and use of serologic tests:

- Primary syphilis: Following an incubation period of 2–6 weeks, primary syphilis presents as a papule that later ulcerates to form a syphilitic chancre. These are generally painless and may occur on any mucosal surface. Non-tender regional adenopathy may also be present. Serologic tests for syphilis (RPR or VDRL) can be negative early in primary syphilis, so empiric treatment is indicated in suspected cases, with follow-up testing necessary to confirm the disease.

- Secondary syphilis: Approximately 60–90% of patients with untreated primary syphilis will develop secondary syphilis as a manifestation of *T. pallidum* dissemination. The time course is typically within 6 months of infection acquisition, and the clinical manifestations are highly variable. The most common manifestation of secondary syphilis is a non-pruritic macular-papular rash over the entire body, including the palms and soles. Other symptoms and laboratory abnormalities can include condyloma lata (white genital lesions similar in appearance to condyloma acuminata), mucous patches (shallow ulcerations on the oral or genital mucosa), fever, malaise, lymphadenopathy, anorexia, hepatitis, and diminished vision secondary to uveitis.

- Latent syphilis: Defined by a reactive serologic test in the absence of active symptoms, latent syphilis is divided into "early-latent" (< 1 year after exposure) and "late-latent" (> 1 year after exposure). Patients who are unable to give an accurate exposure date are classified as "latent syphilis of unknown duration" and treated as late-latent disease.

- Tertiary (late) syphilis: This develops in 25–40% of patients untreated for earlier disease, usually months to years later. Tertiary syphilis can cause CNS disease, cardiovascular disorders, and gummatous lesions involving the skin and bones. Cardiovascular and gummatous syphilis have become extremely rare, but CNS syphilis still occurs with some frequency and can present in various ways. *Acute syphilitic meningitis* and *meningovascular syphilis* occur relatively early after exposure (typically within the first 1–5 years), sometimes during dissemination of the organism with secondary syphilis. By contrast, *parenchymatous syphilis* usually occurs decades later, and includes general paresis, tabes dorsalis, and focal lesions due to CNS gummas.

Diagnostic Considerations: Diagnostic strategies for syphilis are the same as in HIV-negative patients, and rely mostly on serologic studies since the organism cannot be cultured. Darkfield microscopy on fluid obtained from chancres or condyloma lata may demonstrate the characteristic spiral-shaped organism; however, this technique is of limited utility since it cannot be used in the absence of obvious lesions, and most clinicians do not have access to a darkfield microscope.

As a result, a positive serologic test for syphilis (RPR or VDRL or T pallidum ELISA) followed by a positive confirmatory test (MHA-TP, FTA-ABS, or TP-PA) is the most common way to diagnose syphilis in patients with (or without) HIV. Although case reports have cited unusually high titers, false negative results, and delayed onset of seropositivity in patients with HIV infection, no alternative testing strategy is routinely recommended. <u>Neurosyphilis</u> is diagnosed via clinical presentation and CSF examination. In symptomatic neurosyphilis, presenting complaints may include cognitive dysfunction, motor or sensory deficits, cranial nerve palsies, ophthalmic or auditory symptoms, and symptoms or signs of meningitis. Diagnostic criteria for neurosyphilis by CSF examination vary, but one commonly used definition is a CSF white blood cell count > 20 cells/mcL or a reactive CSF VDRL. (Although considered highly sensitive, the FTA-ABS test of the spinal fluid is not specific and can be used only to rule out disease.) The diagnosis of neurosyphilis is challenging since the CSF VDRL (the most specific test) is positive in only 30–70%, even in HIV-negative-patients. Furthermore, HIV itself may induce cellular responses independent of syphilis, and clinical manifestations are extremely varied. As a result, there is some debate about which patients with HIV and syphilis should undergo lumbar puncture (LP). One study of 326 HIV-infected patients with syphilis who underwent LP found that 65 (20%) met criteria for neurosyphilis by CSF exam; the risk was substantially higher if the CD4 cell count was ≤ 350 or the RPR was ≥ 1:32 (J Infect Dis 2004;189:369–76). Based on this study, the diagnostic approach shown in Table 5.4 is reasonable.

Therapeutic Considerations: The treatment of syphilis is generally the same as for HIV-negative patients, with penicillin as the mainstay of therapy. The criteria for treatment response are the same in HIV-infected and HIV-negative individuals. Specifically, the RPR or VDRL titer should decline ≥ 4-fold by one year after treatment for early syphilis and by 2–3 years after treatment for latent syphilis. (For HIV patients with early syphilis, there is an increased rate of treatment failure when using serologic criteria; therefore, our practice is to include an RPR as part of monitoring labs performed every 3–4 months unless the titer has reverted to negative.) Failure to achieve ≥ 4-fold decline in titer should prompt investigation of reinfection or a CSF examination to exclude neurosyphilis. For patients with neurosyphilis, follow-up CSF examinations are performed every 6 months until CSF pleocytosis has normalized; if still abnormal 2 years after treatment, consider retreatment with intravenous penicillin. In general, non-penicillin therapies for syphilis have had limited evaluation in HIV patients; hence these cases warrant close clinical and laboratory follow-up. Procaine penicillin/ probenecid options may not be used in patients with sulfa allergy.

Table 5.4. Need for Lumbar Puncture (LP) in HIV-Infected Patients with Syphilis

Stage of Syphilis	Recommendation
Primary, secondary, or early latent	No LP; if RPR > 1:32 or CD4 < 350, be especially vigilant for lack of response
Late-latent or syphilis of unknown duration	Perform LP (some clinicians only LP for RPR > 1:32 or CD4 < 350)
Positive RPR and confirmatory test with neurologic, ophthalmic, or auditory symptoms/signs	Perform LP

Varicella-Zoster Virus (VZV) Disease

Preferred Therapy, Duration of Therapy, Chronic Maintenance	Alternate Therapy	Other Options/Issues
Varicella (chickenpox) *Uncomplicated cases* Valacyclovir 1,000 mg PO tid for 5–7 days, or famciclovir 500 mg PO tid × 5–7 days *Severe or complicated cases* Acyclovir 10–15 mg/kg IV q8h × 7–10 days May switch to oral acyclovir, famciclovir, or valacyclovir after defervescence if no evidence of visceral involvement Herpes zoster (shingles) *Acute localized dermatomal* Valacyclovir 1g PO tid for 7–10 days or famciclovir 500 mg PO tid for 7–10 days, longer duration should be considered if lesions are slow to resolve *Extensive cutaneous lesion or visceral involvement* Acyclovir 10–15 mg/kg IV q8h until clinical improvement is evident Switch to oral therapy (valacyclovir 1,000 mg TID or famciclovir 500 mg TID, or acyclovir 800 mg PO 5x daily) after clinical improvement is evident, to complete a 10–14 day course Progressive outer retinal necrosis (PORN) (Ganciclovir 5 mg/kg +/- foscarnet 90 mg/kg) IV q12h + (ganciclovir 2 mg/0.05 mL +/- foscarnet 1.2 mg/0.05 mL) intravitreal injection biw Initiate or optimize ART Acute retinal necrosis (ARN) Acyclovir 10 mg/kg IV q8h + ganciclovir 2 mg/0.05 mL intravitreal injection biw x 1-2 doses × 10–14 days, followed by valacyclovir 1,000 mg PO tid × 6 weeks	Primary Varicella infection (chickenpox) *Uncomplicated cases (for 5-7 days)* Acyclovir 800 mg PO 5 times/day Herpes zoster (shingles) *Acute localized dermatomal* For 7–10 days; consider longer duration if lesions are slow to resolve Acyclovir 800 mg PO 5 times/day	Involvement of an experienced ophthalmologist with management of VZV retinitis is strongly recommended Duration of therapy for VZV retinitis is not well defined, and should be determined based on clinical, virologic, and immunologic responses and ophthalmologic responses. Optimization of ART is recommended for serious and difficult-to-treat VZV infections (e.g., retinitis, encephalitis)

Clinical Presentation: Primary varicella (chickenpox) presents as widely disseminated clear vesicles on an erythematous base that heal with crusting and sometimes scarring. Zoster usually presents as painful tense vesicles on an erythematous base in a dermatomal distribution. In patients with HIV, primary varicella is more severe/prolonged, and zoster is more likely to involve multiple dermatomes/disseminate. VZV can rarely cause acute retinal necrosis, which requires close consultation with ophthalmology.

Diagnostic Considerations: Diagnosis is usually clinical. In atypical cases, immunofluorescence can be used to distinguish herpes zoster from herpes simplex.

Pitfalls: Extend treatment beyond 7–10 days if new vesicles are still forming after initial treatment period. Corticosteroids for dermatomal zoster are not recommended in HIV-positive patients.

Therapeutic Considerations: IV therapy is generally indicated for severe disease/cranial nerve zoster.

Prognosis: Usually responds slowly to treatment.

Chapter 6

Complications of HIV Infection*

* Also see Chapter 5 for Opportunistic Infections and Chapters 3 and 9 for Drug-Induced Adverse Effects

HEMATOLOGIC COMPLICATIONS

A. **Thrombocytopenia.** May be the first and only sign of HIV infection. Treatment is only required for platelet count < 20,000/mm³, active bleeding, or planned procedures. Causes include medications, alcohol, idiopathic thrombocytopenic purpura (ITP), thrombotic thrombocytopenic purpura (TTP), and advanced HIV disease ± marrow infiltration with secondary opportunistic infections (usually accompanied by pancytopenia).

1. **Idiopathic Thrombocytopenic Purpura (ITP).** Can occur at any stage of HIV disease and sometimes emerges as antiretroviral therapy induces an immune response. Consultation with a hematologist is advised for platelet count < 20,000 or if rapid recovery of platelet count is required.

   a. **Preferred therapy.** Combination antiretroviral therapy. Although ZDV is the best studied agent for ITP treatment, alternative combination regimens may be effective as well.

   b. **If rapid control of platelet count is needed.** IVIG 1–2 gm/kg total dose, over 2–5 days. Duration of response is typically 3–4 weeks. <u>Alternative</u>: Anti-RH D globulin (WinRho) 50–75 µg/kg IV (effective only in RH-positive, non-splenectomized patients). Causes mild hemolysis. Duration of response is similar to IVIG, and may work in some patients who do not respond to IVIG.

   c. **Miscellaneous alternative therapies.** Prednisone 1 mg/kg daily, with taper as tolerated; danazol 400–800 mg (PO) QD; dapsone 100 mg (PO) QD (if not G6PD-deficient); alpha-interferon 3 million units 3×/week; splenectomy. Some anecdotal evidence for use of vincristine, splenic irradiation, anti-cd20 antibody (Rituximab).

2. **Thrombotic Thrombocytopenic Purpura (TTP).** Manifests as microangiopathic hemolytic anemia associated with renal insufficiency and neurologic symptoms. TTP is a **medical emergency**—if it is suspected based on clinical grounds and examination of blood smear, consult hematologist immediately. Standard treatment is prednisone 60–100 mg (PO) QD (or IV equivalent) plus plasmapheresis.

B. **Anemia.** Anemia is associated with a lower quality of life; several studies also suggest it is independently associated with reduced survival (Clin Infect Dis 1999;29:44–9).

1. **Etiology**

   a. **Decreased RBC production (low reticulocyte count)**

      • **Direct effect of HIV** (usually CD4 < 100/mm³); responds well to initiation of antiretroviral therapy.

      • **Infiltration of bone marrow:** in particular MAC—suspect in a patient with advanced AIDS who has fever, weight loss, and anemia out of proportion to drop in other cell lines; can also be due to lymphoma.

- **Iron deficiency (women)**
- **B12 or folate deficiency:** a high MCV is usually related to a side effect of NRTIs (especially ZDV), but need to rule out B12 and folate deficiency, which appears to be more common among patients with HIV.
- **Certain infections:** <u>Parvovirus B19</u>: infects and inhibits early RBC precursors, with characteristic bone marrow showing giant pronormoblasts; diagnosed by viral DNA by PCR of blood (not by serology); treated with IVIG. <u>MAC</u>: diagnosed by isolator blood cultures or bone marrow biopsy; treated as described on p. 112.
- **Drugs:** ZDV (most common in advanced HIV disease, but can occur at any stage; other antiretroviral agents rarely cause anemia); ganciclovir and valganciclovir (lower WBC also); TMP-SMX; amphotericin; interferon.

b. **Increased RBC destruction (high reticulocyte count)**
- **Drug-induced:** Dapsone and primaquine if patient is G6PD deficient; ribavirin as part of HCV therapy (causes dose-related hemolytic anemia), which may further compromise fatigue associated with HCV therapy.
- **TTP** (described on p. 128)

2. **Evaluation.** As a minimum work-up, evaluate clinical status, stage of HIV disease, stool for occult blood, CBC/differential, RBC indices, reticulocyte count, iron, TIBC, creatinine, LFTs, B12, folate. Bone marrow aspiration is indicated when above work-up and history fail to identify a cause.

3. **Treatment.** If no reversible cause of anemia is identified, or if the cause cannot be removed (for example, ribavirin-associated anemia during HCV treatment), consider erythropoietin (EPO) for patients with Hgb < 10 gm/dL or HCT < 30. Start with 40,000 units (SQ) once weekly with iron supplementation; if at 4 weeks, Hgb has increased by > 1 gm/dL, continue same dose until Hgb reaches 11–12 gm/dL. Dose can then be reduced to 10,000 units (SQ) once weekly to maintain Hgb at this level. Higher levels have been associated with increased risk of thromboembolic events in non-HIV populations. For non-responders, 60,000 units (SQ) once weekly may be effective. Supplemental iron should also be given.

C. **Neutropenia.** As with anemia, neutropenia is much more common in advanced HIV disease. The risk of infection is increased with lower absolute neutrophil counts (ANC), especially when < 500/mm^3.

1. **Etiology**

   a. **Direct effect of HIV.** Responds well to initiation of antiretroviral therapy.

   b. **Drugs.** ZDV, ganciclovir and valganciclovir (ZDV and ganciclovir given together can cause particularly severe neutropenia), pyrimethamine, TMP-SMX at PCP treatment doses, interferon (pegylated interferon more likely to cause neutropenia than standard interferon), flucytosine. Uncommon causes include other NRTIs, ribavirin, amphotericin, TMP-SMX at dose used for PCP prophylaxis, pentamidine, rifabutin. TMP-SMX given at doses used for PCP prophylaxis rarely is the sole cause of neutropenia; if neutropenia does not improve after a trial of an alternative prophylactic regimen, TMP-SMX can be restarted.

   c. **Infections.** MAC, CMV, disseminated fungal diseases (e.g., histoplasmosis).

2. **Treatment.** Only indicated if ANC is consistently < 750/mm³ (some cite 500/mm³). After underlying causes are corrected, consider G-CSF (Neupogen) 150–300 μg (SQ) every 1–7 days. Start with 3×/week dosing, then titrate dose to maintain ANC > 1000/mm³.

D. **Eosinophilia**
   1. **Etiology**
      a. **Direct effect of HIV.** Sometimes seen with no apparent cause, especially in advanced HIV disease.

      b. **Drug allergy.** Most commonly to TMP-SMX and other sulfonamides.

      c. **Parasitic infection (rare).** Most HIV-related parasitic infections (e.g., toxoplasmosis, cryptosporidiosis) do not cause eosinophilia. Rare exceptions include *Isospora belli* and strongyloidiasis (if patient from endemic area).

   2. **Treatment.** Consider withdrawal of offending agent if associated with other allergic phenomena. Check stool for ova and parasites, strongyloides serology.

ONCOLOGIC COMPLICATIONS

Malignancies definitely associated with HIV infection include Kaposi's sarcoma, non-Hodgkin's lymphoma, Hodgkin's disease, lung cancer, squamous cell carcinomas (cervical, anal, head and neck), and soft tissue sarcoma (in children). Possible associated malignancies include seminoma, lung cancer, and multiple myeloma. Prolonged survival due to ART has led to a greater appreciation of the increased incidence of non-AIDS malignancies in HIV patients (Ann Intern Med 2008 May 20;148:728);risk appears related to CD4 cell count (AIDS 2008 Oct 18;22:2143).

A. **Kaposi's Sarcoma.** Infection with HHV-8 is a critical viral cofactor; interaction between host immunosuppression, genetic factors, and this virus determine a patient's risk. In North America, Australia, and Western Europe, Kaposi's sarcoma occurs most commonly in gay/bisexual men. The incidence has diminished markedly since the introduction of potent antiretroviral therapy. In developing countries (especially in certain parts of Africa), Kaposi's sarcoma is more evenly distributed among men and women.

   1. **Presentation.** Usually presents as violaceous nodules and plaques on the skin; oral cavity and other mucosal surfaces may be involved. With more advanced immunosuppression, visceral involvement (lungs, gastrointestinal tract) can be life-threatening. Invasion of local lymphatics can lead to chronic edema of the limbs, face, and genitals, with increased risk of bacterial superinfection.

2. **Treatment.** Initiation of antiretroviral therapy is often sufficient to cause regression of disease. For disease that progresses despite antivirals, options include local measures (intralesional chemotherapy, radiation therapy) and systemic chemotherapy (liposomal anthracyclines are especially effective). Occasionally clinical disease may temporarily worsen soon after starting ART as a manifestation of the immune reconstitution inflammatory syndrome (IRIS); in these cases, ART should be continued and systemic chemotherapy considered or intensified.

B. **Non-Hodgkin's Lymphoma (NHL).** In patients with HIV infection, NHL is most commonly a manifestation of advanced immunosuppression (CD4 < 100/mm³) though a minority of cases occur with relatively preserved immune function. Some data suggest that duration of uncontrolled viremia also is a risk factor for NHL.

1. **Presentation.** Clinical presentation reflects extranodal involvement of the disease: typically, gastrointestinal tract (45%), bone marrow (20%), and CNS (20–30%). Often multiple sites are involved simultaneously. Of note, the patient with AIDS who has diffuse adenopathy and fever will more likely have a systemic infection (most commonly *M. avium* complex, histoplasmosis, cryptococcus) rather than lymphoma. Although the incidence of NHL has declined since the introduction of potent antiretroviral therapy, it has done so to a lesser degree than other opportunistic infections. As a result, NHL in some centers is responsible for a higher proportion of AIDS-related complications compared with the pre-antiretroviral era.

2. **Treatment.** Generally involves full-dose chemotherapy (e.g., CHOP), with use of recombinant growth factors (G-CSF, erythropoietin) as needed to support cell lines. Initiation of antiretroviral therapy concurrently with chemotherapy may improve outcome by reducing infectious complications and improving recovery time of bone marrow function. It is important to avoid the use of antiviral agents that may have overlapping toxicities with the prescribed chemotherapy (e.g., avoid d4T or ddI when patients are receiving systemic vincristine therapy, as this increases the risk of peripheral neuropathy; avoid ZDV since this may further suppress the bone marrow).

C. **Primary CNS Lymphoma.** Usually a manifestation of advanced HIV disease, with the vast majority of patients having a CD4 cell count < 50/mm³.

1. **Presentation.** The typical presentation is one of focal neurologic deficits or seizures, reflecting focal lesion(s) in the brain. MRI findings typically show lesions with irregular enhancement, sometimes involving the corpus callosum and crossing the midline; mass effect is generally evident. Appearance of primary CNS lymphoma is similar to that of CNS toxoplasmosis; in the latter, lesions are often greater in number, but radiographic abnormalities overlap significantly.

2. **Diagnosis.** If a patient with advanced AIDS presents with focal enhancing lesion(s) on MRI or CT scan and is either toxoplasmosis seronegative or taking TMP-SMX for toxoplasmosis prophylaxis, then primary CNS lymphoma is the most likely diagnosis. While noninvasive testing such as thallium SPECT scan, PET scan, and CSF studies for

cytology and Epstein-Barr virus DNA (by PCR) can sometimes be helpful, the definitive diagnosis is generally made through stereotactic brain biopsy. Of note, Epstein-Barr virus PCR of the CSF in HIV patients without characteristic CNS mass lesions has a very low specificity for CNS lymphoma; the test should not be routinely ordered (Clin Infect Dis 2004 Jun 1;38[11]:1629–32).

3. **Treatment.** The prognosis of primary CNS lymphoma remains quite poor, especially for patients who fail antiretroviral therapy. Treatment with steroids and radiation therapy is palliative. Rare patients have experienced sustained remissions after initiating antiretroviral therapy and achieving a significant improvement in immune function.

D. **Cervical Cancer.** Compared to HIV-negative women, the incidence of cervical cancer in HIV-infected women is higher and the disease may be more aggressive. Cervical cancer is strongly associated with HPV infection and progressive immunosuppression. A diagnosis of cervical cancer along with a positive HIV serology is considered AIDS defining. Recommendations for screening include a Pap smear twice the first year after HIV diagnosis, and yearly thereafter if normal. This strategy is associated with a low risk of invasive cervical cancer, comparable to HIV-negative women.

E. **Anal Cancer.** The incidence of anal cancer in HIV-infected MSM is approximately 80 times that of the general population. As with cervical cancer, anal cancer is strongly associated with HPV infection. Although screening for anal cancer using anal Pap smears could identify precancerous lesions much as with cervical cancer, it has not yet been proven that this screening strategy will reduce the incidence of anal cancer. As such, routine screening is not formally recommended in the OI prevention guidelines, but is recommended in the Primary Care Guidelines, with the caveat that the evidence supporting the screening is weak. Pending results of ongoing studies, a reasonable strategy is as follows:

1. At a minimum, perform annual periodic visual inspection and a digital rectal exam.

2. Perform anal Pap smear for any anorectal complaints; some recommend annual testing on all HIV-positive gay men.

3. For atypical cells of uncertain significance, repeat anal Pap smear in 6–12 months.

4. For squamous intraepithelial lesion (SIL), refer to a colorectal surgeon or other specialist for anoscopy and/or anal colposcopy with biopsy.

ENDOCRINE COMPLICATIONS

A. **Disorders of Adrenal Function.** Although adrenal gland involvement has been documented in up to two-thirds of patients with AIDS on postmortem examination, clinically relevant adrenal insufficiency is rare (~ 3% of patients with AIDS) and is generally a manifestation of late-stage AIDS. Currently the most common cause of adrenal function pathology is iatrogenic, when corticosteroids given by any route (including injected, inhaled, topical) interact with ritonavir or cobicistat.

1. **Etiology.** Potential causes of primary adrenal dysfunction include destruction of the adrenal gland from opportunistic infections (especially CMV), neoplasms (Kaposi's sarcoma, lymphoma), hemorrhage, and infarction. More commonly, adrenal insufficiency results from the adverse effect of medications, including ketoconazole (decreased steroidogenesis), rifampin/rifabutin (enhanced cortisol metabolism), and corticosteroids/megestrol acetate (suppressed pituitary secretion of corticotropin due to intrinsic glucocorticoid activity; latter may actually induce Cushing's syndrome with prolonged use). A relatively common cause of cortisol excess is the use of inhaled (especially fluticasone) or intra-articular steroids with ritonavir. Ritonavir blocks the metabolism of many corticosteroids, leading to increased exposure and iatrogenic Cushing's syndrome. Conversely, stopping the inhaled steroid can cause adrenal insufficiency (J Clin Endocrinol Metab 2005;90:4394–8). If possible, inhaled or injectable steroids should be avoided in patients receiving boosted PIs or cobicistat. Among inhaled steroids, beclomethasone appears to be the safest (J AIDS 2013; 63:355–61).

2. **Diagnosis.** Hypercortisolism should be considered in any patient if they have received corticosteroids by any route and are receiving a boosted PI or cobisistat. Typical symptoms may include fatigue, irritability, sleep disturbance, muscle weakness, facial fullness, erectile dysfunction, with new-onset hypertension and labs demonstrating hyperglycemia. The diagnosis is confirmed with a low AM cortisol and ACTH. Adrenal insufficiency should be suspected in a patient with advanced HIV disease or recent therapy with steroid-interfering medications who presents with hypotension, profound weakness, or electrolyte abnormalities (hyponatremia, hyperkalemia). Evaluation consists of measurement of a.m. cortisol; if normal and the diagnosis is still suspected, perform a corticotropin stimulation test. If the diagnosis is still suspected despite a normal corticotropin stimulation test, referral to an endocrinologist is warranted since some patients with AIDS have peripheral resistance to glucocorticoid action.

3. **Treatment.** Patients with basal low cortisol levels, even if asymptomatic, require replacement therapy (prednisone 5 mg [PO] at bedtime). For corticotropin hyporesponsiveness, steroid supplementation for stressing conditions (e.g., surgery, intercurrent illness) is indicated. For life-threatening situations, immediate treatment with dexamethasone 4 mg (IV) is indicated; this will not impair the diagnostic utility of the corticotropin stimulation test. Patients with cortisol excess syndromes should have the exogenous steroid discontinued, and be closely monitored for adrenal insufficiency.

B. **Hypogonadism.** Men with HIV infection are more likely to be hypogonadal than HIV-negative controls. The frequency of this abnormality increases with progressive immunodeficiency and may reach 50% in patients with AIDS. In general, there is no detectable underlying etiology. HIV-related hypogonadism is associated with weakness, weight loss, decreased libido, and impaired quality of life. Replacement therapy can improve many of these symptoms, especially when combined with a resistance exercise program. While low testosterone levels have also been observed in HIV-infected women, replacement therapy is experimental. Treatment for men consists of testosterone gel 5 mg QD, testosterone transdermal patch, or injectable testosterone cypionate/enanthate 200 mg every other week. Potential side effects include acne, gynecomastia, and testicular atrophy. Monitor prostate specific antigen annually for patients on replacement therapy.

C. Thyroid Disease. The thyroid gland is rarely involved in disseminated opportunistic infections (e.g., extrapulmonary pneumocystis). Chronically ill patients with HIV may have low T3, but TSH is generally normal. Immune response to antiretroviral therapy may unmask subclinical Grave's disease, leading to clinical hyperthyroidism. Treatment of Grave's disease consists of radioactive thyroid ablation or an anti-thyroid medication (e.g., methimazole) as directed by an endocrinologist. Beta-blockers can be used to ameliorate the symptoms of hyperthyroidism. On rare occasions, autoimmune thyroiditis may emerge as a manifestation of the immune reconstitution inflammatory syndrome.

D. Pancreatitis. Clinical presentation is similar to HIV-negative patients, with nausea, vomiting, abdominal pain.

    1. Etiology

        a. Medications: The HIV-related medications that commonly were implicated as causes of pancreatitis (didanosine stavudine, and pentamidine), are rarely used today. Less common causes include other NRTIs, TMP-SMX, and protease inhibitors when accompanied by very high triglyceride levels.

        b. Opportunistic infections. Most commonly identified opportunistic infection to cause pancreatitis is CMV. Can rarely be caused by TB, MAC, intestinal protozoa (cryptosporidia, microsporidia), widely disseminated toxoplasmosis.

        c. Non-HIV–related. Alcohol, obesity, gallstones.

    2. Treatment. Discontinue potentially offending drug; treat identified cause.

E. Hyperglycemia. Patients with HIV appear to be at higher risk of developing insulin resistance and diabetes mellitus than HIV-negative controls. Potential contributing factors include lipodystrophy syndrome (especially subcutaneous fat loss) and medications (most notably indinavir and the NRTI stavudine).

    1. Diagnosis. For patients on antiretroviral therapy, monitor serum glucose every 3–6 months as part of safety labs. If elevated or abnormal, consider a fasting glucose, insulin level, and hemoglobin A1C. A fasting blood glucose > 126 mg/dL or a glucose level > 200 mg/dL two hours after administration of 75 gm of glucose is diagnostic of diabetes mellitus.

    2. Treatment. If the patient is on a protease inhibitor and has an undetectable HIV RNA and no history of NRTI resistance, consider substituting an NNRTI (e.g., efavirenz, rilpivirine, nevirapine) or raltegravir for the protease inhibitor. Alternatively, there is evidence that atazanavir may be least likely to lead to insulin resistance, and hence can be substituted for other protease inhibitors. If the patient is not on a protease inhibitor and fasting hyperglycemia persists, follow established guidelines for treatment of diabetes mellitus in the general population, including weight loss, dietary modification, and exercise. When medical therapy is required, consider the use of insulin-sensitizing agents such as metformin 500 mg (PO) q12h or pioglitazone

15–30 mg (PO) QD. In small studies, metformin therapy in patients with HIV has led to improvements in insulin sensitivity, reduction in waist circumference, and decreased blood pressure; potential adverse effects include diarrhea, progression of lipoatrophy, and (rarely) lactic acidosis. Pioglitazone in one study improved insulin sensitivity and subcutaneous fat stores, and appears to be safer in HIV patients than rosiglitazone, which has been associated with hyperlipidemia.

F. Hypoglycemia. Pentamidine induces hypoglycemia by lysing pancreatic islet cells. Monitor fingerstick glucose levels daily while patients receive this therapy. Prolonged, repeated use of pentamidine may result in diabetes mellitus from irreversible damage to islet cells, leading to insulin deficiency.

G. Ovarian Complications. Amenorrhea is common in women with advanced AIDS who have significant weight loss. Menses may resume with weight gain and improvement in clinical status accompanying antiretroviral therapy.

H. Bone Disease

   1. Osteonecrosis. This complication has been reported in association with HIV infection since the late 1980s, but it appears to be more common since the introduction of effective antiretroviral therapy (J AIDS 2006;42:286–92). It is not clear if the increased incidence is due simply to prolonged survival, or to a direct toxic effect of antiretroviral medications. The most commonly involved sites are the femoral heads, followed by the humeral heads, femoral condyles, proximal tibia, and small bones of the hands and wrists. Most patients will have traditional underlying risk factors, such as a history of corticosteroid use, hyperlipidemia, alcohol abuse, or a hypercoagulable state. The relationship to any specific form of antiretroviral therapy has not been conclusively demonstrated (HIV Med 2004 Nov;5[6]:421–6).

   a. Diagnosis. Consider osteonecrosis in a patient with refractory hip pain, especially if there are underlying risk factors (see above). If plain film imaging is negative, proceed to MRI, which is more sensitive. Bilateral imaging is indicated since the disease is often bilateral.

   b. Treatment. Conservative management with physical therapy is recommended initially. If pain persists, refer to an orthopedic surgeon for consideration of hip stabilization/hip replacement.

   2. Osteoporosis. Osteopenia and osteoporosis have been reported in 22–50% and 3–21% of patients receiving chronic antiretroviral therapy, respectively. Low bone mineral density appears to be substantially more common in patients with HIV than those who are HIV negative (AIDS 2006 Nov 14;20[17]:2165–74). Spontaneous fractures have also been reported, although the risk is low. Initiation of ART is generally associated with a decline in bone mineral density that then stabilizes; this decrease is greater with tenofovir-containing regimens (J Infect Dis. 2011 Jun;203(12): 1791–801.)

   a. Diagnosis. Some sources recommend screening for all men older than 50, all postmenopausal women, and for patients with a history of fracture (Clin Infect Dis. 2010 Oct 15;51(8):937–46). The appropriate screening test is regional DEXA scanning. Secondary causes of osteopenia and osteoporosis should be evaluated, including thyrotoxicosis, hyperparathyroidism, hypogonadism, weight loss, alcohol intake, and certain medications (especially corticosteroids). Smoking cessation should be strongly encouraged.

b. Treatment. All patients should receive adequate diet, and if needed, supplements of calcium and vitamin D. If osteoporosis is demonstrated on DEXA scan (t-score of −2.5 or lower), consider biphosphonate therapy. Both alendronate and zoledronate have been tested in prospective clinical studies (J Acquir Immune Defic Syndr 2005 Apr 1;38[4]:426–31; J Clin Endocrinol Metab 2007 Apr;92[4]:1283–8).

GASTROINTESTINAL TRACT COMPLICATIONS

A. Anorexia

   1. Etiology. Commonly associated with advanced HIV disease, possibly due to high cytokine (especially TNF) levels that correlate with high titer HIV RNA. Other causes include depression, medications, opportunistic infections (especially MAC), and lactic acidosis (related to mitochondrial toxicity).

   2. Treatment. Megecetrol acetate (Megace) liquid suspension 400–800 mg (PO) QD improves appetite, quality of life (Ann Intern Med 1994 Sep 15;121[6]:400–8). Weight gain that results is generally fat, not lean body mass. Side effects include hypogonadism, DVT, gynecomastia. Megecetrol has corticosteroid properties, and therefore can lead to Cushings-like state (prolonged use) or adrenal insufficiency (when drug is withdrawn). Prolonged use should be avoided; if required, dose should be tapered gradually. Dronabinol (Marinol) 2.5 mg q12h stimulates appetite and reduces nausea. Dronabinol is a synthetic delta-9-tetrahydrocannabinol (THC), the active ingredient in marijuana. The main side effect is oversedation. Patients should start with a dose at bedtime and then increase to q12h as tolerated.

B. Nausea/Vomiting

   1. Etiology

      a. Medications. Direct effect of antiretroviral medications (especially PIs, ZDV, abacavir hypersensitivity), medication-related pancreatitis (see above), or lactic acidosis from NRTIs.

      b. Opportunistic infections. Intestinal protozoa (e.g., cryptosporidiosis, isospora, giardiasis—all usually accompanied by diarrhea), CMV esophagitis/gastritis, GI tract involvement of MAC.

      c. Others. Gastric lymphoma, CNS process producing mass effect (toxoplasmosis or lymphoma) or raised intracerebral pressure (cryptococcal meningitis).

   2. Treatment. Address underlying etiology. If felt to be due to the direct effect of antiretrovirals, choose an alternate regimen if safe from the virologic perspective (e.g., substitute tenofovir for ZDV, efavirenz for PI). If underlying cause cannot be treated or removed, or for temporary relief of symptoms, therapeutic options include: prochlorperazine (Compazine) 10 mg (PO) or 25 mg (PR) q12h prn; metoclopramide (Reglan) 10 mg (PO) q6h prn; trimethobenzamide (Tigan) 250 mg (PO) q6h prn; lorazepam 0.5–1.0 mg (PO or IV) q6h prn; ondansetron (Zofran) 4–8 mg (PO) q8h prn or 32 mg (IV or IM) as a single dose; dronabinol (Marinol) 2.5–5.0 mg (PO) q12h. Patients with HIV are at increased risk for phenothiazine-related dystonia, which may occur with prochlorperazine, metoclopramide, and trimethobenzamide. Treat dystonia with diphenhydramine (Benadryl) 50 mg (PO or IV) × 1 dose.

C. Diarrhea
1. Etiology
a. Infection. <u>Acute diarrhea</u>: salmonella, shigella, campylobacter, *C. difficile*, giardiasis, cyclospora; <u>subacute/chronic diarrhea</u>: giardiasis, cryptosporidia, microsporidia, isospora, CMV.

b. Medication-related. Especially nelfinavir, all ritonavir-boosted PIs, full-dose ritonavir (rarely used), buffered version of ddI; can be part of abacavir hypersensitivity syndrome. Medication-related diarrhea is rarely associated with weight loss or fever (abacavir excluded). Risk of ritonavir-related diarrhea appears to be dose related—several comparative studies have shown lower rates of diarrhea when the total daily dose is 100 mg rather than 200 mg.

2. Treatment.
Treat underlying cause (see Chapter 5). If PI-related, consider changing to an alternative PI that is less likely to cause diarrhea (e.g., atazanavir/ritonavir or darunavir/ritonavir), or to an NNRTI (efavirenz or nevirapine) integrase inhibitor. To avoid resistance, NNRTI replacement should only be considered when the HIV RNA is < 50 copies/mL, and preferably when there is no history of treatment failure that would lead to NRTI resistance. If diarrhea persists or if medication changes are not possible, offer symptomatic therapy with psyllium 1 tsp q12h–24h, loperamide 2 mg q6h prn, calcium 500 mg q12h; pancreatic enzymes 1–2 tabs with each meal, diphenoxylate/atropine (Lomotil) 1–2 tabs q8h prn, or octreotide 100–500 µg (SQ) q12h. Crofelemer 125 mg PO bid may be helpful in certain patients, in particular those with PI-related diarrhea.

D. Oral or Esophageal Ulcers
1. Presentation.
Intensely painful ulcers of various size; esophageal ulcers cause severe dysphagia. May occur at any stage of HIV disease (including primary infection), but more common with progressive immunosuppression (CD4 < 100, associated neutropenia). Most common diagnosis is idiopathic aphthous ulcers; other causes include CMV, HSV, histoplasmosis, lymphoma. For first-time presentation, culture for HSV and refer for biopsy to exclude other causes.

2. Treatment.
For idiopathic aphthous ulcers, start with symptom relief, followed by application of local steroids, followed by either systemic steroids or thalidomide. Lesions sometimes respond to immune reconstitution from antiretroviral therapy

along with resolution of neutropenia (adjunctive therapy with G-CSF may hasten healing). Therapeutic modalities include:

a. Symptom reduction with viscous lidocaine (2%).

b. Topical fluocinonide (Lidex) 0.05% ointment mixed 1:1 with Orobase; apply q6h as needed.

c. Dexamethasone 0.5/5M elixir mouth rinse q8h–12h.

d. Local corticosteroid injections by oral surgeon.

e. Prednisone 40–60 mg/day × 1–2 weeks, tapered as tolerated over 1–2 weeks or longer as needed.

f. Thalidomide 200 mg (PO) at bedtime × 4–6 weeks, followed by 100 mg (PO) at bedtime twice weekly. Side effects include sedation, constipation, peripheral neuropathy. Severe teratogenicity of thalidomide requires that physicians register with company-sponsored monitoring program before prescribing (see http://www.thalomid.com/steps_program.aspx). Women of childbearing age must use at least two forms of contraception and have regular pregnancy tests while receiving thalidomide. Informed consent in package insert must be signed before therapy is initiated.

E. HIV Cholangiopathy

1. Presentation. Presents with right upper quadrant pain, fever, and sometimes jaundice. Laboratory evaluation invariably demonstrates increased alkaline phosphatase. Generally occurs with severe immunosuppression (CD4 < 100/mm^3). Imaging with ultrasound or ERCP shows dilated or prominent intrahepatic and extrahepatic ducts. Papillary stenosis may also be present.

2. Etiology. Differential diagnosis include cholelithiasis, acalculous cholecystitis, infiltrative infectious or neoplastic diseases of the liver. Screen for infectious etiology, including stool for ova/parasites and/or ERCP aspirates for cryptosporidia, microsporidia, cyclospora, CMV.

3. Treatment. Symptomatic improvement is sometimes seen with endoscopic guided sphincterotomy or stenting. Treat underlying infectious process, if identified.

RENAL COMPLICATIONS

A. HIV-Associated Nephropathy. A form of progressive glomerulosclerosis, leading to massive proteinuria and progressive renal dysfunction. Over 80% of cases occur in African-Americans. Renal biopsy shows extensive collapsing glomerulosclerosis, tubular ectasia, and tubulo-interstitial disease. Occurs most commonly with low CD4 cell counts (< 100/mm^3), but may occur at any level of immunosuppression. Very uncommon with undetectable HIV RNA (Clin Infect Dis 2006;43:377–80).

1. **Presentation.** Clinical presentation varies from asymptomatic to symptoms of hypoalbuminemia and renal failure (edema, fatigue, anemia). Hypertension generally is absent. Renal ultrasound demonstrates enlarged or normal-sized kidneys. The cardinal laboratory feature is proteinuria > 1 g/day, usually with rapidly progressive renal failure evolving over weeks to months to end-stage renal disease requiring dialysis.

2. **Diagnostic Considerations.** Biopsy should be considered to rule out other causes of progressive renal disease, such as HCV-associated renal disease, medication-associated toxicity (see below), or a non-HIV-related cause.

3. **Treatment.** Effective options include antiretroviral therapy (case reports suggest PI-based therapy may lead to resolution of disease), ACE inhibitors, and high-dose corticosteroids (60 mg prednisone QD × 1 month followed by gradual taper) (Kidney International 2000;58:1253). Since high-dose steroids are associated with further immune suppression and other complications, a reasonable approach is to begin with antiretroviral therapy plus an ACE inhibitor (e.g., captopril 6.25 mg q8h).

B. **Medication-Related Renal Disease.** HIV-related medications most likely to cause nephrotoxicity are listed below. (See antiretroviral drug summaries in Chapter 9 for dosing in renal insufficiency.)

1. **Tenofovir.** Can rarely cause tubular injury, leading to increased creatinine. Sometimes accompanied by Fanconi's syndrome, with phosphate wasting and acidosis. Renal toxicity is more likely to occur in those with underlying renal disease or advanced HIV infection (Clin Infect Dis 2005;15:1194–8; J Infect Dis 2008;197:102). Risk of TDF-related renal disease higher when given with boosted PIs. (J Infect Dis. 2008 Jan 1;197(1):102–8) and a similar incidence is likely when tenofovir is coadministered with cobicistat. Use calculated creatinine clearance (Cockgroft-Gault equation or MDRD) to assess renal function; in renal impairment, consider alternatives to tenofovir. If tenofovir is required despite decreased GFR, reduce dose as recommended in the package insert.

2. **Atazanavir and indinavir.** Both medications can cause nephrolithiasis, and some studies have linked atazanavir to an increased risk of decreased renal function. As indinavir is no longer widely used, this complication is most likely to occur with atazanavir. For severe nephrolithiasis or other renal complication, strongly consider changing the patient to an alternative PI. As atazanavir may also cause nephrolithiasis, the best alternative option would be darunavir/ritonavir.

3. **Pentamidine.** Can cause renal failure in up to 50% of patients; other adverse effects include electrolyte/mineral wasting and hypoglycemia. Risk is related to cumulative dose; monitor creatinine, electrolytes, glucose, calcium, and phosphate during therapy.

4. **Foscarnet.** Induces dose-related renal failure as well as wasting of potassium, calcium, and phosphate. Dose adjustment is necessary for reduced creatinine clearance. Supplement potassium, calcium, and phosphorus as needed.

5. **Cidofovir.** Associated with dose-related renal toxicity, which can be reduced by concomitant administration of probenecid and hydration. Check serum creatinine and urine for protein prior to each dose; if creatinine is > 2 gm/dL or there is more than 2+ proteinuria, do not administer further cidofovir as renal toxicity may be irreversible.

6. **Amphotericin B.** Dose-dependent renal toxicity is common. Liposomal preparations are less nephrotoxic.

7. **Trimethoprim-sulfamethoxazole (TMP-SMX).** May cause hyperkalemia through amiloride-like effect from trimethoprim, especially when used at high doses for PCP treatment. Sulfonamide component can rarely cause crystal nephropathy (reversible with hydration).

8. **Acyclovir.** High-dose IV administration can crystalize in kidney and cause acute renal failure. Risk can be reduced with adequate hydration, and renal dysfunction usually responds to hydration and cessation of drug.

C. **HCV-Associated Renal Disease.** Often a manifestation of HCV-associated mixed cryoglobulinemia.
   1. **Presentation.** Patients may present with palpable purpura or other dermatologic signs, along with hematuria, proteinuria, and sometimes renal failure. Other related laboratory findings include HCV RNA in plasma, cryoglobulins in blood, and low complement; renal biopsy shows HCV-related immune complexes.
   2. **Treatment.** Therapy directed at hepatitis C (PEG-interferon plus ribavirin) can lead to improvement in renal disease and other manifestations of cryoglobulinemia.

D. **Heroin Nephropathy.** Can coexist with other forms of renal failure listed above. Results from glomerular injury, presumably from toxic effects of heroin or other contaminants. Distinguished from HIV-associated nephropathy by a slower rate of progression, small (as opposed to large) kidneys on ultrasound, and less proteinuria. Treatment consists of cessation of drug use.

E. **Inhibition of Tubular Secretion of Creatinine.** Several HIV-related drugs block tubular secretion of creatinine, leading to a rapid but small increase in serum creatinine. These drugs include cobicistat, dolutegravir, and TMP-SMX in particular; ritonavir and rilpivirine also induce this effect to a lesser extent. The increase is typically small (< 0.2 mg/dL), occurs shortly after starting treatment, and is not progressive or associated with an actual decline in glomerular function.

CARDIAC COMPLICATIONS

A. **HIV-Related Cardiomyopathy** (JAMA 2008;299:324–31). Biventricular reduction in ejection fraction, with pathologic features typical of myocarditis and/or immune-mediated cardiomyopathy. Prevalence varies widely depending on definition; echocardiogram may show reduced ejection fraction in up to 50% of patients with AIDS, but symptomatic cardiomyopathy occurs in only 1–3%. More common with progressive immunodeficiency, especially when CD4 cell count < 100.

1. **Etiology.** Usually idiopathic. Differential diagnosis includes several causes, not mutually exclusive: HIV itself, secondary infection (CMV, toxoplasmosis, coxsackie, adenovirus, Chagas), disordered immune response leading to autoimmune myocarditis, nutritional deficiencies (selenium, carnitine), drug toxicity (NRTI-associated mitochondrial toxicity, alcohol, doxorubicin).

2. **Presentation.** Presents as left ventricular failure, with dyspnea, congestive heart failure, elevated jugular venous pressure, a prominent S_3 on exam. Chest x-ray typically demonstrates an enlarged heart, and echocardiogram shows marked biventricular dysfunction with reduced ejection fraction. Diagnosis is made after exclusion of other common causes of low EF (alcohol, poor nutrition, myocardial ischemia). Cardiac biopsy is rarely useful.

3. **Treatment.** Patients should receive antiretroviral therapy plus usual therapies for heart failure (diuretics, beta-blockers, ACE inhibitors are often quite effective in reducing symptoms). For manifestations of disseminated CMV disease or a positive blood CMV viral load, empiric CMV treatment with valganciclovir 900 mg (PO) q12h × 3 weeks. Although case reports have shown improvement in ejection fraction after cessation of NRTIs, this is a much less common cause of cardiomyopathy than HIV itself.

B. Pericarditis/Pericardial Effusion

1. **Etiology.** Pericardial fluid may be due to HIV itself or a complicating malignancy/opportunistic infection. The most common malignancy is lymphoma, where an effusion may be the first manifestation of an extranodal high-grade B-cell lymphoma; Kaposi's sarcoma causes effusions generally only when the disease is widespread elsewhere. In addition, numerous common and opportunistic infections have been reported to cause pericarditis in HIV patients, including pyogenic bacteria (especially *S. aureus* and *S. pneumoniae*), TB, atypical mycobacteria, cryptococcal disease, disseminated histoplasmosis, and CMV.

2. **Presentation and Diagnosis.** Often diagnosed incidentally through enlarged cardiac silhouette and subsequent echocardiogram. May be asymptomatic or cause chest pain, dyspnea, cardiac tamponade, pericardial friction rub. Pericardiocentesis is indicated for large or symptomatic effusions, with fluid sent for cultures (routine, fungal, mycobacterial) and cytology.

3. **Treatment.** Directed at underlying condition. If idiopathic pericarditis, consider starting antiretroviral therapy, and manage symptoms with NSAIDs and corticosteroids (as in HIV-negative patients).

C. Tricuspid Valve Endocarditis

1. **Etiology.** Injection drug users (IDUs) with HIV, particularly those with lower CD4 cell counts, are at substantially higher risk for endocarditis than HIV-negative IDUs (J Infect Dis 2002;185:1761–6). *Staphylococcus aureus* is the most common pathogen. In one series, rates of infection included *S. aureus* (73%), coagulase-negative *Staphylococcus* species (1%), *Staphylococcus* species not otherwise classified (7%), *Streptococcus*

species (13%), *Pseudomonas* species (2%), *Bacillus* species (2%), and other organisms (2%). Most urban centers are experiencing an increasing rate of MRSA.

2. **Presentation and Diagnosis.** Patients typically present with fever, weight loss, and sometimes pulmonary symptoms (dyspnea, chest pain) reflective of septic emboli arising from an infected tricuspid valve. Physical examination usually reveals a heart murmur ± evidence of peripheral septic emboli. Chest x-ray may show multiple septic emboli, some with cavitation. An echocardiogram should be performed to assess for valvular vegetations. Diagnosis is confirmed when a patient with the above clinical presentation has positive blood cultures for an organism known to be associated with endocarditis.

3. **Treatment.** While a short course (2 weeks) of therapy has been effective in HIV-negative IDUs with tricuspid endocarditis, this regimen cannot be recommended in HIV-positive patients. Recommended regimens include:

   - Methicillin-sensitive *S. aureus*: Nafcillin 2 gm (IV) q4h × 28 days plus gentamicin 1 mg/kg (IV) q8h × 3–5 days or until blood cultures clear.

   - Methicillin-resistant *S. aureus* or beta-lactam allergy: Vancomycin 1 gm (IV) q12h × 28 days plus gentamicin 1 mg/kg (IV) q8h × 3–5 days or until blood cultures clear. Alternative to vancomycin is daptomycin (IV) 6 mg/kg QD × 4 weeks.

   - Unable or unwilling to receive IV therapy: Ciprofloxacin 750 mg (PO) q12h plus rifampin 300 mg (PO) q12h × 4 weeks. This regimen cannot be used with PIs due to rifampin-PI interaction. Linezolid 600 mg (PO) q12h × 4 weeks can be used as an alternative (limited data).

PULMONARY COMPLICATIONS

A. **Pulmonary Hypertension** (JAMA 2008;299:324–31). Idiopathic elevation of pulmonary pressures is sometimes seen in HIV infection. The pathological process is similar to primary pulmonary hypertension (i.e., hypertrophy of vascular endothelium). Pulmonary hypertension is more common in women and can occur at any CD4 cell count.

   1. **Presentation.** Dyspnea on exertion, palpitations, chest pain. Exam may reveal elevated JVP and precordial heave. Diagnosis is supported by echocardiogram and doppler studies showing right ventricular hypertrophy and elevated PA pressures. Most sensitive test is right heart catheterization, where pressures will exceed 30 mmHg. Recurrent pulmonary emboli should be excluded as a possible cause.

   2. **Treatment.** Epoprostenol (FloLan) by continuous infusion. Requires placement of a permanent central venous catheter. Diuretics also help relieve symptoms. Anticoagulation is generally indicated. Sildenafil is also used as an adjunct to therapy. There are mixed reports on whether antiretroviral therapy improves hemodynamics or outcome.

B. **Lymphocytic Interstitial Pneumonitis (LIP).** An idiopathic form of diffuse lung disease that is more common in children. Tends to occur with moderate immunosuppression (CD4 cell count 200–400/mm³) and mimics PCP.

1. **Presentation and Diagnosis.** Cough, dyspnea on exertion, exercise oxygen desaturation. Usually afebrile. Chest x-ray and chest CT show diffuse bilateral reticulonodular infiltrates. Differentiated from PCP by generally higher CD4 cell counts and lower LDH. Diagnosed by bronchioalveolar lavage (BAL) with biopsy, which will exclude PCP and yield the characteristic histopathology of LIP (patchy lymphocytic infiltration and no microorganisms on special stains).

2. **Treatment.** Antiretroviral therapy can either improve LIP or worsen it through enhanced immune activity. Prednisone usually achieves rapid reduction in dyspnea, but tapering dose may be accompanied by a relapse of symptoms.

C. **Emphysema.** Cigarette smoking is associated with a more rapid progression to bullous emphysema in patients with HIV compared to HIV-negative controls. Clinical presentation and treatment are the same as for the general population.

D. **Pulmonary Kaposi's Sarcoma.** Generally occurs only in patients with advanced HIV disease and extensive Kaposi's sarcoma elsewhere.

1. **Presentation and Diagnosis.** Chest x-ray demonstrates nodules, masses, and/or pleural effusions. Diagnosed by visual inspection of the airway during bronchoscopy, where typical violaceous plaques may be observed.

2. **Treatment.** Antiretroviral therapy may lead to dramatic improvement in even severe Kaposi's sarcoma, although temporary flares due to immune reconstitution have been reported. Concomitant systemic chemotherapy is also generally required.

HEENT COMPLICATIONS

A. **Aphthous Ulcers.** See p. 137.

B. **Oral Hairy Leukoplakia**

1. **Presentation.** Presents as ribbed, "corduroy"-like white patches on the side of the tongue. More common with increased immunosuppression (CD4 < 200/mm³). Usually painless. Distinguished from oral thrush in that oral hairy leukoplakia does not rub off with tongue depressor. Caused by Epstein-Barr virus.

2. **Treatment.** No treatment is needed unless the patient is symptomatic. Antiretroviral therapy often leads to resolution. Other treatment options include acyclovir 800 mg (PO) 5×/day or famciclovir 500 mg (PO) q12h or valacyclovir 1,000 mg (PO) q8h until resolution. Topical application of podophyllin is sometimes effective.

C. **Salivary Gland Enlargement**

1. **Presentation.** Can occur at any stage of HIV infection and usually worsens with disease progression. Often accompanied by xerostomia. Biopsy shows lymphoid infiltration, possibly due to HIV itself; may be part of diffuse infiltrative lymphocytosis

syndrome (DILS), which can be accompanied by involvement of the lungs, kidneys, and peripheral nerves. For progressive parotid enlargement, a CT scan is recommended to differentiate solid from cystic enlargement. Differential diagnosis includes infectious parotitis, which presents more acutely with fever and local pain.

2. **Treatment.** Antiretroviral therapy is the preferred approach; will lead to improvement in a majority of cases. Other forms of treatment include repeated aspiration of fluid-filled cysts when symptomatic, local measures for dry mouth (sugarless gum, artificial saliva), and prednisone 40 mg (PO) QD × 1 week followed by gradual taper over 1–2 weeks.

D. Lymphoepithelial Cysts

1. **Presentation.** Presents as enlarged cervical cysts that can mimic lymphadenopathy. Can occur at any CD4 cell count. A biopsy is needed to rule out lymphoma, other malignancies (notably squamous cell carcinoma), opportunistic infections. Cause is unknown.

2. **Treatment.** Antiretroviral therapy often causes dramatic reduction in size of cysts.

E. Gingivitis/Periodontitis

1. **Presentation.** Presents as painful gums with easy bleeding, along with erythematous and receding gingiva. May be the initial manifestation of underlying HIV disease. Severity correlates with stage of immunosuppression. Caused by oral anaerobic bacteria (usually polymicrobial), and exacerbated by poor local oral hygiene, smoking, alcoholism.

2. **Treatment.** Improve local hygiene, (brush, floss, antibacterial mouth rinse). Curettage by dentist/periodontist may be helpful. For severe cases, treat for 7–10 days with metronidazole 500 mg (PO) q8h or clindamycin 300 mg (PO) q6h or amoxicillin-clavulanate 850 mg (PO) q12h.

MUSCULOSKELETAL COMPLICATIONS

A. HIV Arthropathy

1. **Presentation.** Presents as painful arthropathy, often involving multiple joints. Pain out of proportion to physical findings. Cause is unknown.

2. **Treatment.** NSAIDs, other pain relievers.

B. Reiter's Syndrome

1. **Presentation.** Asymmetrical polyarthritis involving the large joints of lower extremities. Arthritis is seen in conjunction with urethritis, skin lesions (circinate balanitis, keratoderma blennorrhagica), ocular disease. May also occur after gastroenteritis. Appears to occur with greater frequency among HIV patients, usually in association with HLA-B27.

2. **Diagnosis.** Differential diagnosis includes septic arthritis; if joint effusions are present, arthrocentesis with cultures/gram stain is indicated. Urethral swab for chlamydia and gonorrhea is also recommended.

3. **Treatment.** Consider treatment of urethritis with empiric chlamydia therapy with azithromycin 1 g (PO) × 1 dose. Other measures include NSAIDs and referral to rheumatology for possible immunosuppressive therapy (prednisone, methotrexate, TNF antagonists).

C. **Pyomyositis.** Focal infection of muscle often occurring at site of injections, trauma.
   1. **Presentation.** Presents as localized pain, swelling, fever. Usually caused by *Staphylococcus aureus* including MRSA less commonly other pyogenic bacteria, e.g., streptococci, gram-negative rods. More common with advanced HIV immunosuppression (CD4 cell count < 100).
   2. **Diagnosis.** Imaging of suspected area with CT followed by diagnostic aspiration for gram stain/culture.
   3. **Treatment.** Antibiotics directed at causative pathogen (usually an anti-staphylococcal penicillin or vancomycin). May also require surgical incision/drainage.

D. **HIV Myopathy and NRTI-Related Myopathy.** These two conditions may present similarly.
   1. **Presentation.** Patients present with myalgias, muscle tenderness, weakness, and elevated CPK levels. Proximal leg muscles are most commonly involved. Condition can occur at any stage of HIV disease.
   2. **Diagnosis.** Some experts recommend a biopsy to distinguish between HIV and NRTI-related myopathy. In the former, there is a more prominent inflammatory infiltrate; the latter usually shows evidence of mitochondrial myopathy. NRTI-related myopathy is most commonly associated with zidovudine.
   3. **Treatment.** For symptomatic HIV-related myopathy, corticosteroids at high doses (prednisone 1 mg/kg/day) are recommended. Once improvement occurs, this should be tapered over several weeks. For NRTI-related myopathy, change to a regimen that either avoids NRTIs entirely or switches to those NRTIs with lower mitochondrial toxicity (abacavir, emtricitabine, lamivudine, tenofovir).

E. **Rhabdomyolysis.** Extensive muscle necrosis with myoglobinuria and acute renal failure. May occur as part of medication toxicity (to older NRTIs such as ZDV, d4T, ddI, or rarely to raltegravir) or to HIV itself. Management is by withdrawal of possibly offending agents and hydration—hemodialysis if necessary.

NEUROLOGIC COMPLICATIONS

A. **Distal Sensory Neuropathy.** Caused by HIV itself and/or neurotoxic effects of medications, in particular the di-deoxy NRTIs (d4T, ddI, ddC).
   1. **Presentation.** Typically presents as pain, aching, burning, or tingling of the distal extremities (toes/feet more commonly than fingers/hands). Pain is often worse at

night. Principal risk factors include the stage of HIV disease and exposure to the above listed drugs, especially when used in combination.

2. **Diagnosis and Evaluation.** Usually clinical, based on patient history. Reduced pin-prick and vibration sense in the involved extremities support the diagnosis, but symptoms often precede objective physical findings. Attempt to identify contributing/other causes, including B_{12} deficiency, syphilis, CMV, multiple myeloma, other neurotoxic agents (dapsone, INH, vincristine; avoid using these drugs if possible with d4T or ddl). If presentation is confusing, refer for EMG and nerve conduction studies, which will show an axonal neuropathy.

3. **Treatment.** Withdraw offending agents, in particular d4T and ddl; symptoms may persist or even worsen for several weeks after cessation of these drugs, and severe neuropathy may be irreversible. Many of the patients currently in care with neuropathy received d4T and/or ddl in the past, and have residual nerve damage. Antiretroviral therapy should be continued and one of several therapies used for neuropathic symptoms can be administered:
   - NSAIDs or acetaminophen for mild pain
   - Avoid tight-fitting shoes, extremes of temperature
   - Gabapentin 300 mg at bedtime; increase up to 1200 mg divided q6–8h as needed
   - Nortriptyline 10 mg at bedtime; increase up to 75 mg at bedtime as tolerated
   - Lamictal 25 mg q12h; increase up to 150 mg q12h as tolerated
   - Topical therapy: capsaicin (may make symptoms worse), lidocaine patches
   - Acupuncture
   - Severe pain may require chronic long-acting narcotic pain relievers (e.g., methadone, MS-Contin, transdermal fentanyl).

B. **Other Forms of Neuropathy**
   1. **Types**
      a. **Acute inflammatory demyelinating neuropathy (AIDP, Guillain-Barré syndrome).** Ascending motor weakness usually without sensory involvement. Reported in early and late stage HIV. May evolve into a chronic form with waxing and waning symptoms. Treatment consists of steroids, plasmapheresis, IVIG. Prognosis is variable for all—tends to be best for mononeuritis especially if due to acute HIV infection.
      b. **Mononeuritis multiplex.** Scattered, asymmetrical, motor and sensory deficits (e.g., facial weakness, foot drop). Reported in acute and chronic HIV. Some cases ascribed to CMV in advanced HIV (CD4 < 50/mm³). Treatment consists of steroids, IVIG. If caused by CMV, treat with valganciclovir at standard doses.
      c. **HIV-associated neuromuscular weakness syndrome.** Rare complication of NRTI-therapy (especially d4T), presenting as progressive ascending paralysis in association with lactic acidosis. When severe, mechanical ventilation may be

required. Treatment consists of withdrawal of NRTIs, especially d4T. Residual neurologic impairment is common after recovery.

   d. Progressive polyradiculopathy. Complication of advanced HIV disease that typically presents with lower extremity weakness, anaesthesia in a "saddle" distribution (perineal area), and/or bowel and bladder dysfunction. Most common causes include CMV polyradiculitis (p. 92) and lymphoma. Diagnostically, obtain an MRI of the lumbosacral spine to exclude a mass lesion, then proceed to CSF exam. If due to CMV, the usual CSF finding is increased WBC (predominantly polys), increased protein, and positive CMV PCR. If due to lymphoma, the CSF shows increased protein and lymphoma cells on cytology. For CMV polyradiculitis, treat × 3–4 weeks or until improvement with either ganciclovir 5 mg/kg (IV) q12h or valganciclovir 900 mg (PO) q12h or foscarnet 90 mg/kg (IV) q12h; for severe cases, some advocate ganciclovir plus foscarnet. For lymphoma, treat with chemotherapy plus radiation.

2. **Prognosis.** Prognosis is variable for all forms of neuropathy but tends to be best for mononeuritis, especially if due to acute HIV infection.

C. **HIV-Associated Dementia (AIDS dementia, HIV encephalitis/encephalopathy).** Typical presentation at onset consists of short-term memory loss, often with apathy or withdrawal from usual activities. As the disease progresses, cognitive impairment worsens, and speech, motor, and gait disturbances develop. Seizures and akinetic mutism are late-stage manifestations. The incidence of this complication has decreased dramatically since the widespread introduction of combination antiretroviral therapy in 1996. Progression of dementia is gradual (usually over months) and can be arrested/ reversed with potent antiretroviral therapy. A more rapidly progressive form has also been reported. HIV dementia almost always occurs in the late stages of HIV disease (CD4 < 100/mm^3, HIV RNA > 100,000 copies/mL), but on rare occasions occurs with relatively preserved immune function and low plasma HIV RNA. In the latter case, relatively high HIV RNA levels are often present in the CSF.

1. **Diagnosis.** Diagnosis is based on a combination of clinical, laboratory, and imaging criteria, as well as exclusion of alternative causes (depression, adverse drug effects, neurosyphilis, CMV encephalitis). HIV-associated dementia should be suspected in a patient with advanced HIV disease and subacute to chronic cognitive impairment, especially short-term memory loss. Administration of the four-step HIV-dementia scale (AIDS Reader 2002;12:29) may help quantify the extent of deficits. MRI shows cerebral atrophy and often non-enhancing white matter abnormalities that can be indistinguishable from progressive multifocal leukoencephalopathy (PML). CSF exam is usually abnormal, with elevated protein and low-level lymphocytic pleocytosis. When HIV RNA in the CSF is measured, it is usually detectable at 1,000 copies/mL or higher; an undetectable CSF HIV RNA is unusual in HIV dementia and suggests an alternative diagnosis.

2. **Treatment.** Potent antiretroviral therapy is the mainstay of therapy and can lead to dramatic improvement, especially in treatment-naïve individuals. Selection of

drugs with higher penetration into the CNS is theoretically preferable (Arch Neurol 2008 Jan;65[1]:65–70), although there are no definitive clinical data to support this approach over choosing alternative agents. As a result, the primary goal should be to choose a regimen with a high likelihood of achieving virologic suppression. In a patient who has failed antiretroviral therapy, treatment is based on blood resistance testing to maximize antiviral potency.

PSYCHIATRIC COMPLICATIONS

Psychiatric illness is more common in patients with HIV than in those with other medical illnesses of comparable severity. Potential explanations include pre-existing psychiatric illness which predisposes to high-risk behavior for HIV acquisition (substance abuse, sexual addiction), extreme grief reactions from having a stigmatized illness, or neurotoxic effects of HIV manifesting as psychiatric illness. For all psychiatric illnesses, consider starting antiretroviral therapy even if there are otherwise no indications, as therapy is associated with improved neuropsychiatric function. Carefully review package inserts and drug interaction tables at www.aidsinfo.nih.gov prior to prescribing any psychotropic agent.

A. Depression

    1. Presentation and Diagnosis. Common symptoms include depressed mood, decreased interest in work/leisure activities, blunted affect, sleep disturbances, alterations in appetite, forgetfulness, and diminished concentration. Key differential is HIV dementia, but depressed mood is usually not a prominent feature of dementia. Among antiretroviral agents, efavirenz is the drug most strongly linked to depression. Consider changing to an different option from the list of Preferred or Recommended initial regimens if a patient develops depression while receiving efavirenz.

    2. Treatment. SSRIs or tricyclic antidepressants are the mainstays of therapy, as for HIV-negative patients. In general, start with low-doses of all agents and titrate up as needed. Always check treatment guidelines for potential drug interactions with antiretroviral agents (aidsinfo.nih.gov). If rapid onset of response is needed, stimulants such as methylphenidate or dextroamphetamine may be tried. MAO inhibitors are contraindicated due to drug interactions.

B. Mania. HIV may produce an unusual form of mania as a manifestation of HIV encephalopathy.

    1. Presentation. These patients usually have CD4 cell counts < 200/mm^3. It is distinguished from non-HIV-related bipolar disease in that there is no family history of bipolar illness and onset may occur at any age. Symptoms include expansive mood, grandiosity, and diminished sleep.

    2. Treatment. Treatment should be undertaken with the assistance of a psychiatrist. Options include lithium 300 mg (PO) q8h or valproic acid 250 mg (PO) q12h or carbamazepine 200 mg (PO) q12h.

C. Insomnia

1. Etiology. Sleep disturbance may be a symptom of an underlying medical condition (hepatic encephalopathy, HIV dementia), a psychiatric illness (depression, mania, substance abuse, anxiety), or a medication side effect (efavirenz, corticosteroids).

2. Treatment. Attempt to identify/treat underlying causes, including "poor sleep hygiene" (excessive caffeine, alcohol, other stimulants). For patients with a history of substance abuse, avoid if possible the chronic use of benzodiazepines, which have addictive potential. As an alternative, trazodone 50–100 mg (PO) at bedtime can be very effective. Short-term insomnia due to anxiety or jet lag can be treated with benzodiazepines such as zolpidem (Ambien) 2.5–5.0 mg (PO) at bedtime or lorazepam 1.0 mg (PO) at bedtime.

DERMATOLOGIC COMPLICATIONS

A. Viral Infections

1. Herpes Simplex Infection. Oral/anogenital diseases occur more frequently and are more severe in patients with HIV. Infection may also occur on non-mucosal surfaces (e.g., skin), especially when the patient is severely immunocompromised.

    a. Diagnosis. Characteristic vesicles on an erythematous base. Ulcerations may occur in primary disease and more advanced HIV-related immunosuppression. A viral culture for HSV is the diagnostic test of choice and is quite sensitive, especially early during the outbreak and prior to starting anti-herpes therapy.

    b. Treatment. See p. 112.

2. Varicella-Zoster Infection. Herpes zoster is much more common (20- to 50-fold increased risk) in HIV patients than in age-matched HIV-negative controls and may be first sign of underlying HIV infection. AIDS patients are at increased risk for chronic non-healing zoster, which can last for several weeks. Appearance may also be atypical, with nodular rather than vesicular lesions.

    a. Diagnosis. Diagnosed by clinical appearance. DFA test of a lesion can help distinguish zoster from HSV if the diagnosis is unclear.

    b. Treatment. See p. 125.

3. Molluscum Contagiosum

    a. Presentation. Manifests as clusters of white, umbilicated papules outside the groin/perineal area. Rarely seen except with severe immunosuppression (CD4 < 100/mm³); the number/size of lesions increase as immunosuppression progresses.

    b. Diagnosis. Diagnosed by clinical appearance. Biopsy is rarely necessary, but when performed shows large inclusions known as "molluscum bodies." Etiologic virus (a pox virus) cannot be cultured in clinical practice.

   c. **Treatment.** Effective antiretroviral therapy can often lead to dramatic, spontaneous improvement. If this is not possible, or for more immediate control, local cryosurgery, or other ablative methods can be effective.

4. **Oral Hairy Leukoplakia (OHL).** See p. 143.

5. **Warts.** Cutaneous and genital warts are extremely common in HIV disease, and in severe cases are disfiguring and difficult to treat. Although usually more severe with progressive HIV disease, in some patients they remain a debilitating problem even with good response to antiretroviral therapy.

   a. **Diagnosis.** Generally a clinical diagnosis. In severe or refractory cases, biopsy is sometimes needed to exclude underlying squamous cell carcinoma.

   b. **Treatment**

     i. **Genital warts.** Imiquimod 5% cream 3×/week at bedtime, wash off in AM. Alternative: podofilox q12h application with cotton swab for 3 days followed by 4 days without treatment, then repeat. Local inflammation is common with both measures. Provider applied therapies include cryotherapy, podophyllin resin (severe or bulky cases).

     ii. **Cutaneous warts.** As in HIV-negative patients, spontaneous resolution may occur, especially in relatively immunocompetent patients. Therapy is otherwise similar as in HIV-negative patients, with multiple ablative therapies available (cryotherapy, liquid nitrogen, salicylic acid, bichloracetic acid, curettage). Refractory cases should be referred to a dermatologist for intralesional therapy or wide excision.

B. **Bacterial Infections**

1. **Staphylococcal Infections.** May cause staphylococcal folliculitis, a pruritic condition associated with small papules. Larger collections of soft tissue staph infection can cause furunculosis or subcutaneous abscesses (more common with advanced HIV-related immunosuppression.) In most parts of the United States, MRSA is the most common cause of purulent soft tissue infection.

   a. **Diagnosis.** Clinical appearance. Culture to exclude MRSA.

   b. **Treatment.** For furunculosis, which is often due to MRSA, treat empirically and modify according to sensitivities; doxycycline or TMP-SMX 1 DS (PO) BID or clindamycin 300 mg PO TID are often effective; vancomycin 1 gm IV q12H or linezolid 600 mg (PO) BID are recommended for severe cases. If organism is MSSA, dicloxacillin 500 mg QID or cephalexin 500 mg QID are options. Large furuncles or soft tissue collections must be surgically drained (Antimicrob Agents Chemother 2007 Nov;51[11]:4044–8). For multiple recurrences, consider decontamination strategies:

     i. **Antibacterials:** Mupirocin nasal ointment anterior nares BID, Bactrim 1 DS BID, ± rifampin 300 mg PO BID—all for 7–10 days (do not use rifampin with protease inhibitors).

  ii. Household contacts (including pets) cultured/treated.

  iii. Local measures
- Keep cuts/abrasions covered.
- Bathe for 10 minutes; 1 tsp bleach/gallon of water.
- Using a bath sponge, lather armpits, groin, anus, and under the breasts with chlorhexidine topical antiseptic (Hibiclens scrub) after draining bath water.
- Shower Hibiclens off.

  iv. Frequent laundering of towels, sheets, clothing.

2. **Bacillary Angiomatosis.** A cutaneous manifestation of *Bartonella quintanna* and *Bartonella henselae* infection (cat scratch bacillus). Presents as a dome-shaped and often pedunculated papule or papules in a patient with severe immunosuppression. Appearance can mimic Kaposi's sarcoma. Organism can also cause hepatic disease (peliosis hepatitis), fever, encephalopathy, endocarditis. Clinical syndromes due to bartonella infection have become extremely rare since the availability of potent antiretroviral therapy.

  a. Diagnosis. Characteristic appearance and biopsy, with pathology showing the characteristic bacillus on Warthin-Starry and Dieterle stains. Organism can be cultured, but laboratory needs to be alerted so special media can be used. Serologies also may be helpful.

  b. Treatment. Azithromycin 250–500 mg (PO) qd or clarithromycin 500 mg (PO) q12h or doxycycline 100 mg (PO) q12h. Treatment duration is determined by recovery of immune system in response to antiretroviral therapy.

3. **Syphilis.** See p. 122.

C. Fungal Infections
1. **Disseminated and Invasive Fungal Infections.** All disseminated fungal infections can cause skin lesions. Most characteristic are molluscum-like lesions with cryptococcal disease, erythema nodosum with coccidioides, and nodular skin lesions with blastomycosis.

2. **Tinea Corporis, Cruris, or Pedis (jock itch, athlete's foot).** Extensive erythematous plaques with severe pruritus.

  a. Diagnosis. Characteristic appearance, with KOH slide preparation showing branched, septated hyphae.

  b. Treatment. Topical therapy with over-the-counter preparations, or by prescription with one of several topical antifungals, including clotrimazole, ciclopirox, or butenafine q12h. For severe disease, use fluconazole 100–200 mg (PO) qd × 7–14 days or terbinafine 250 mg (PO) qd × 14 days.

3. **Candidiasis.** In addition to mucosal infections, *Candida* can cause disease in the skin and nails. In the skin, it is often seen in intertriginous areas (groin, under breasts),

where it causes a pruritic papular eruption that can coalesce to form large plaques. Web spaces of the fingers and toes may also be involved. Heat and moisture in these areas encourage candidal growth.

a. **Diagnosis.** Clinically suspected with papular, sometimes pustular eruption in intertriginous areas. A KOH slide shows yeast and pseudohyphae of *Candida*.

b. **Treatment.** Topical therapy with antifungals, such as clotrimazole q12h × 14 days. More severe cases may require systemic therapy with fluconazole 100–200 mg (PO) qd × 7–14 days. It is also important to maintain good hygiene, attempt to aerate and dry involved areas, and avoid tight clothing.

D. **Miscellaneous Skin Conditions.** All can be the first sign of underlying HIV infection.

1. **Seborrheic Dermatitis.** Presents as waxy erythematous and sometimes flakey plaques with scale, usually on face and scalp. Usually worsens with progressive immunodeficiency. May be caused by the yeast *Pityrosporum ovale*. Antiretroviral therapy usually leads to improvement. Symptomatic treatment consists of ketoconazole cream q12h × 7 14 days or a low-potency topical steroid (e.g., hydrocortisone cream 2.5% q12h × 7–14 days). For refractory cases where higher-potency steroids may be indicated, referral to a dermatologist is recommended.

2. **Psoriasis.** Severity of psoriasis correlates with the degree of immunosuppression. HIV can sometimes unmask a prior history of mild disease. May be accompanied by arthritis. Antiretroviral therapy is often useful. Other treatments as per HIV-negative patients.

3. **Eosinophilic Folliculitis.** An erythematous, papular, severely pruritic eruption, usually on the upper trunk and face. Appearance is similar to bacterial folliculitis, but the rash is unresponsive to antibacterials and biopsy demonstrates an eosinophilic infiltrate. The process becomes more difficult to treat as HIV disease progresses; rubbing/scratching can lead to ulcerations, prurigo nodularis, secondary staph infections. In darker-skinned individuals, this can ultimately lead to disfiguring post-inflammatory hyperpigmentation.

a. **Diagnosis.** Skin biopsy is required.

b. **Treatment.** The disease is characterized by its refractory nature and frequent relapses. Individual treatments may work well in some individuals but not in others. Options include ART, oral/topical corticosteroids, isotretinoin, and phototherapy. Antiretroviral therapy will ultimately lead to improvement in most patients. However, some individuals go through a paradoxical worsening due to a heightened inflammatory response, which can be difficult to distinguish from an adverse drug reaction and can sometimes last for weeks to months. Prednisone 70 mg (PO) qd, tapered by 5–10 mg/d, is also helpful. Intermittent therapy of 60 mg (PO) qd × 2–3 days may be useful to control flares after discontinuation. Potent topical corticosteroids q12h–q8h × 10–14 days can be effective but should not be used on the face. Isotretinoin (Accutane) 1 mg/kg/d or 40 mg (PO) q12h is also of value, with duration determined by response to therapy (associated with skin dryness). Ultraviolet B phototherapy may be used 3×/week until improvement, then maintenance as needed.

4. **Xerosis/Ichthyosis.** Manifests as dry, flaky, and extremely pruritic skin. Worsens as HIV disease progresses, and exacerbated by some antiretrovirals, particularly indinavir. Treatment consists of antiretroviral therapy (avoid indinavir) and emollients (e.g., Aquaphor, Eucerin, Cetaphil). Short-duration (7–14 days) topical steroids may also be considered for dry/inflamed skin.

Chapter 7

HIV Infection and Pregnancy

HIV AND PREGNANCY

Antiretroviral therapy reduces the risk of perinatal transmission by lowering maternal HIV RNA and by providing pre- and post-exposure prophylaxis for the infant. The risk of perinatal infection has dropped from 25–30% without intervention to 2% or lower with combination antiretroviral therapy (MMWR Morb Mortal Wkly Rep 2005;55:592-7), especially when ART reduces HIV RNA to below the levels of detection. Although the risk of vertical transmission correlates with maternal viral load, there is no maternal viral load below which the risk of transmission is zero (J Infect Dis 2001; 183:539-45). As a result, combination therapy is indicated for all pregnant women, regardless of baseline HIV RNA or CD4 cell count.

Treatment recommendations for pregnant women are updated based on clinical studies and data collected by the Antiretroviral Pregnancy Registry (www.apregistry.com/index.htm). The most recent version of the US Public Health Service Task Force treatment guidelines was updated July 31, 2012 and is available at aidsinfo.nih.gov. The National Perinatal HIV Hotline (1-888-448-8765) provides free clinical consultation on all aspects of perinatal HIV care. This service is particularly useful in settings where clinicians may not see a large volume of HIV-infected pregnant women.

In settings where safe, affordable and feasible alternatives are available and culturally acceptable, breastfeeding is not recommended for HIV-infected women. By contrast, in many resource-limited settings, breastfeeding is preferred, with data now strongly supporting the benefits of ongoing ART to the mother in preventing HIV transmission to the newborn during the breastfeeding period (N Engl J Med. 2010 Jun 17;362(24):2282-94).

INITIAL EVALUATION

Initial evaluation of the HIV-infected pregnant woman requires assessment of the considerations shown in Table 7.1.

Table 7.1. Initial Evaluation of HIV-Infected Pregnant Women

- Degree of immunodeficiency (defined by current and past CD4 cell counts)
- Risk for disease progression and perinatal transmission (determined by HIV RNA)
- If HIV RNA is detectable, whether an antiretroviral resistance is present (determined by resistance testing; previous tests should also be reviewed)
- Need for opportunistic infection prophylaxis
- Baseline hematologic, metabolic, renal, and hepatic parameters
- Complete history of past and current antiretroviral therapy regimens
- Presence of co-infections that might require treatment or special care of the newborn (syphilis, gonorrhea, chlamydia, genital herpes simplex, hepatitis B, hepatitis C)
- Assessment of supportive care needs

REPRODUCTIVE OPTIONS FOR HIV SERODISCORDANT COUPLES

Women with HIV infection may wish to become pregnant even though their male sexual partner does not have HIV. Conversely, HIV uninfected women may have an infected partner. In both of these circumstances, consultation with HIV specialists experienced in management of reproductive options is critical to minimize the likelihood of HIV transmission to the uninfected individual. The guidelines below are adapted from the latest revision of the Perinatal Guidelines (http://aidsinfo.nih.gov/Guidelines/HTML/3/perinatal-guidelines/0).

Table 7.2. Recommendations for HIV Serodiscordant Couples

Panel's Recommendations
• For Serodiscordant couples who want to conceive, expert consultation is recommended so that approaches can be tailored to specific needs, which may vary from couple to couple **(AIII)**. It is important to recognize that treatment of the infected partner may not be fully protective against sexual transmission of HIV.
• Partners should be screened and treated for genital tract infections before attempting to conceive **(AII)**.
• For HIV-Infected females with HIV-uninfected male partners, the safest conception option is artificial insemination, including the option of self-insemination with a partner's sperm during the peri-ovulatory period **(AIII)**.
• For HIV-infected men with HIV-uninfected female partners, the use of sperm preparation techniques coupled with either intrauterine insemination or *in vitro* fertilization should be considered if using donor sperm from an HIV-uninfected male is unacceptable **(AII)**.
• For Serodiscordant couples who want to conceive, initiation of antiretroviral therapy (ART) for the HIV-infected partner is recommended **(AI** for CD4 T-Lymphocyte (CD4-cell) count ≤ 550 cells/mm^3, **BIII** for CD4-cell count >550 cells/mm^3). If therapy is initiated, maximal viral suppression is recommended before conception is attempted **(AIII)**.
• Periconception administration of antiretroviral pre-exposure prophylaxis (PrEP) for HIV-uninfected partners may offer an additional tool to reduce the risk of sexual transmission **(CIII)**. The utility of PrEP of the uninfected partner when the infected partner is receiving ART has not been studied.

Rating of Recommendations: A = Strong; B = Moderate; C = Optional

Rating of Evidence: I = One or more randomized trials with clinical outcomes and/or validated laboratory endpoints; II = One or more well-designed, nonrandomized trials or observational cohort studies with long-term clinical outcomes; III = Expert opinion

Reproduced from: Recommendations for Use of Antiretroviral Drugs in Pregnant HIV-1-Infected Women for Maternal Health and Interventions to Reduce Perinatal HIV Transmission in the United States. Aidsinfo.nih.gov.

The risk of transmission is greatly reduced (but not eliminated) when the infected partner is receiving suppressive antiretroviral therapy (N Engl J Med 2011; 365:493-505). There is emerging experience using pre-exposure prophylaxis to further reduce the risk; one group reports using the following procedure with no transmissions to date (AIDS 2011;25:2005-8):

1. Male partner has been successfully treated with undetectable HIV-RNA in plasma (<50 copies/ml) without the need of HIV-RNA testing in semen.

2. No report of current symptoms of genital infections and no unprotected sex with other partners.

3. LH-test in the urine is used to determine the optimal time of conception (36 h after LH-peak).

4. Administration of PrEP with tenofovir/emtricitabine, first dose at LH-peak and second 24 hours later.

An alternative to this strategy would be to offer PrEP to the uninfected person in the couple, and instruct them to use it daily until conception occurs. This combination of suppressive ART to the infected partner and PrEP for the uninfected person reduces the need for sperm washing and other advanced reproductive technologies, which are not available to all patients. In this rapidly evolving area of reproductive strategies for people with HIV, patients should be informed of all of their options.

INITIATION OF ANTIRETROVIRAL THERAPY IN PREGNANCY

Decisions regarding when to start treatment and what regimen to use depends on several factors, including; (1) gestational age of the pregnancy; (2) results of the laboratory testing (Table 7.3); and (3) known, suspected, or unknown effects of individual drugs on the fetus and newborn. An overview of antiretroviral therapy in pregnancy is shown in Table 7.4.

HIV-infected women in their first trimester of pregnancy who are not on antiretroviral therapy should begin antiretroviral therapy promptly, as early and sustained virologic suppression diminishes the risk of transmission to the newborn. For women already on ART who become pregnant, treatment should be continued. For pregnant women with acute HIV infection, treatment should be started immediately given the high HIV RNA levels associated with this condition. Before starting treatment, it is important to emphasize the need for adherence to medical therapy. Patients should also be instructed to have a low threshold for reporting any potential side effects early, especially those that may reduce medication compliance, so that treatment can be altered and/or symptomatic relief for the side effect can be provided.

GOALS OF THERAPY AND MONITORING

The goal of treatment is the same as for non-pregnant individuals: to ensure an undetectable HIV RNA using the most sensitive available assay. Once antiretroviral therapy is initiated, monitoring of HIV RNA is recommended at 1–2 weeks, then monthly thereafter until the HIV RNA is undetectable, then every 2 months after that. The CD4 cell count should be obtained every 3 months as for non-pregnant adults, although treatment should not be changed based solely on CD4 changes provided that virologic suppression is maintained. Laboratory monitoring for toxicity can be performed at the same time as HIV RNA testing.

A general overview of antiretroviral therapy during pregnancy and labor and to the newborn is summarized in Table 7.3.

In the case of virologic failure—i.e., inability to achieve an undetectable HIV RNA or viral rebound occurs—repeat resistance testing is indicated. Subsequent management will depend on assessment of medication adherence and the degree of resistance detected on testing, as described in Chapter 4. For women who have not achieved virologic suppression near the time of delivery, especially if the HIV RNA exceeds 1000 copies/mL, a scheduled cesarean delivery is recommended at 38 weeks gestation. In addition, an elective admission to the hospital for directly observed antiretroviral therapy might enable a greater decline in HIV RNA, further reducing risk of transmission.

Table 7.3. Clinical Scenario Summary Recommendations for Antiretroviral Drug Use by Pregnant HIV-Infected Women and Prevention of Perinatal Transmission of HIV-1 in the United States

Clinical Scenario	Recommendations
Non-pregnant HIV-infected women of childbearing potential (sexually active and not using contraception) who have indications for initiating antiretroviral therapy (ART)	Initiate combination antiretroviral (ARV) drug therapy as per adult treatment guidelines. When feasible, include one or more nucleoside reverse transcriptase inhibitors (NRTIs) with good placental passage as a component of the ARV regimen. • Exclude pregnancy and ensure access to effective contraception for sexually active women before starting treatment with efavirenz; alternative ART regimens that do not include efavirenz should be strongly considered in women who are planning to become pregnant. Emphasize need for women on efavirenz to review their regimens with their providers before discontinuing contraception.
HIV-infected women on ART who become pregnant	**Women:** • In general, in women who require treatment, ARV drugs should not be stopped during the first trimester or during pregnancy. • Continue current combination ARV regimen, assuming the regimen is tolerated and effective in successfully suppressing viremia. • Perform HIV ARV drug-resistance testing in women on therapy who have detectable viremia (that is, >500–1,000 copies/mL). • Continue the ART regimen during the intrapartum period (if oral zidovudine is part of the antepartum regimen, and a woman's viral load is >400 copies/mL, the oral zidovudine component of her regimen should be stopped while she receives zidovudine as an intravenous continuous infusion[a] during labor and other ARV agents are continued orally) and postpartum. • Schedule cesarean delivery at 38 weeks if plasma HIV RNA remains >1,000 copies/mL near the time of delivery. **Infants:** • Start zidovudine as soon as possible after birth and administer for 6 weeks.[b]

Table 7.3. Clinical Scenario Summary Recommendations for Antiretroviral Drug Use by Pregnant HIV-Infected Women and Prevention of Perinatal Transmission of HIV-1 in the United States (cont'd)

Clinical Scenario	Recommendations

HIV-infected pregnant women who are ARV naive	**Women:**
	Perform HIV ARV drug-resistance testing before initiating combination ARV drug therapy and repeat after initiating therapy if viral suppression is suboptimal (<1 log drop after 4 weeks on ARVs). If HIV is diagnosed late in pregnancy, the ARV regimen should be initiated promptly without waiting for the results of resistance testing.
	• Initiate combination ARV regimen.
	  • Delayed initiation of ARVs until after the first trimester can be considered in women with high CD4 T-lymphocyte (CD4-cell) counts and low HIV RNAlevels, but earlier initiation may be more effective in reducing perinatal transmission of HIV. Benefits of first trimester use must be weighed against potential fetal effects of first-trimester exposure.
	  • Avoid initiation of efavirenz or other potentially teratogenic drugs in the first trimester and drugs with known adverse potential for mother throughout the pregnancy.
	  • When feasible, include one or more NRTIs with good placental passage (zidovudine, lamivudine, emtricitabine, tenofovir, or abacavir) in the ARV regimen.
	  • Use nevirapine as a component of the ARV regimen only in women who have CD4-cell counts ≤250 cells/mm^3. Because of the increased risk of severe hepatic toxicity, use nevirapine in women with CD4-cell counts >250 cells/mm^3 only if the benefit clearly outweighs the risk.
	• Continue the combination regimen intrapartum. Continuous infusion zidovudine[a] should be administered to HIV-infected women with HIV RNA >400 copies/mL (or unknown HIV RNA) near delivery, regardless of antepartum regimen or mode of delivery. If oral zidovudine is part of the antepartum regimen, and a woman's viral load is >400 copies/mL, the oral zidovudine component of her regimen should be stopped while she receives zidovudine as an intravenous continuous infusion[a] during labor while other ARV agents are continued orally and postpartum.
	• Schedule cesarean delivery at 38 weeks if plasma HIV RNA remains >1,000 copies/mL near the time of delivery.
	• Evaluate need for continuing the combination regimen postpartum. Following delivery, considerations for continuation of the mother's ARV regimen are the same as in other non-pregnant individuals. If treatment is to be stopped and the regimen includes a drug with a long half-life, such as a non-nucleoside reverse transcriptase inhibitor. [NNRTI]), continue NRTIs for at least 7 days after stopping NNRTI.
	
	Infants:
	• Start zidovudine as soon as possible after birth and administer for 6 weeks.[b]

Table 7.3. Clinical Scenario Summary Recommendations for Antiretroviral Drug Use by Pregnant HIV-Infected Women and Prevention of Perinatal Transmission of HIV-1 in the United States (cont'd)

Clinical Scenario	Recommendations
HIV-infected pregnant women who are ARV experienced but not currently receiving ARV drugs	**Women:** • Obtain full ARV drug history, including prior resistance testing, and evaluate need for ART for maternal health. • Test for HIV ARV drug resistance before reinitiating ARV prophylaxis or therapy and retest after initiating combination ARV regimen if viral suppression is suboptimal (<1 log drop after 4 weeks on ARVs). If HIV is diagnosed late in pregnancy, the ARV regimen should be initiated promptly without waiting for the results of resistance testing. • Initiate a combination ARV regimen (that is, at least three drugs), with the regimen chosen based on results of resistance testing and history of prior therapy. • Delayed initiation of ARVs until after the first trimester can be considered in women with high CD4-cell counts and low HIV RNA levels, but earlier initiation of prophylaxis may be more effective in reducing perinatal transmission of HIV. Benefits of first trimester use must be weighed against potential fetal effects of first-trimester exposure. • Avoid initiation of efavirenz or other potentially teratogenic drugs in the first trimester and drugs with known adverse potential for the mother throughout the pregnancy. • When feasible, include one or more NRTIs with good transplacental passage (zidovudine, lamivudine, emtricitabine, tenofovir, or abacavir) as a component of the ARV regimen. • Use nevirapine as a component of therapy in women who have CD4-cell counts >250 cells/mm^3 only if the benefit clearly outweighs the risk because of the drug's association with an increased risk of severe hepatic toxicity. • Continue the combination regimen intrapartum. Continuous infusion zidovudine[a] should be administered to HIV-infected women with HIV RNA >400 copies/mL (or unknown HIV RNA) near delivery, regardless of antepartum regimen or mode of delivery. If oral zidovudine is part of the antepartum regimen, and a woman's viral load is >400 copies/mL, the oral zidovudine component of her regimen should be stopped while she receives zidovudine as an intravenous continuous infusion[a] during labor while other ARV agents are continued orally. • Evaluate need for continuing the combination regimen postpartum. Following delivery, considerations for continuation of the mother's ARV regimen are the same as in other non-pregnant adults. If treatment is to be stopped and the regimen includes a drug with a long half-life, such as NNRTIs, continue NRTIs for at least 7 days after stopping NNRTIs. • Schedule cesarean delivery at 38 weeks if plasma HIV RNA remains >1,000 copies/mL near the time of delivery.

Table 7.3. Clinical Scenario Summary Recommendations for Antiretroviral Drug Use by Pregnant HIV-Infected Women and Prevention of Perinatal Transmission of HIV-1 in the United States (cont'd)

Clinical Scenario	Recommendations
	Infants: • Start zidovudine as soon as possible after birth and administer for 6 weeks.[b]
HIV-infected women who have received no ARV before labor	**Women:** Give zidovudine as continuous infusion[a] during labor. **Infants:** Infants born to HIV-infected women who have not received antepartum ARV drugs should receive prophylaxis with a combination ARV drug regimen started as close to the time of birth as possible. Zidovudine[b] given for 6 weeks combined with three doses of nevirapine in the first week of life (at birth, 48 hours later, and 96 hours after the second dose) has been shown to be effective in a randomized controlled trial and less toxic than a three-drug regimen with nelfinavir and lamivudine for 2 weeks and 6 weeks of zidovudine. The two-drug regimen is preferred because of lower toxicity and because nelfinavir powder is no longer available in the United States. • Evaluate need for initiation of maternal therapy postpartum.
Infants born to HIV-infected women who have received no ARV before or during labor	• Infants born to HIV-infected women who have not received antepartum ARV drugs should receive prophylaxis with a combination ARV drug regimen started as close to the time of birth as possible. Zidovudine[b] given for 6 weeks combined with three doses of nevirapine in the first week of life (at birth, 48 hours later, and 96 hours after the second dose) has been shown to be effective in a randomized controlled trial and less toxic than a three-drug regimen with nelfinavir and lamivudine for 2 weeks and 6 weeks of zidovudine. The two-drug regimen is preferred because of lower toxicity and because nelfinavir powder is no longer available in the United States. • Evaluate need for initiation of maternal therapy postpartum.

Key to Abbreviations: ARV = antiretroviral; ART = antiretroviral therapy; IV = intravenously; NRTI = nucleoside reverse transcriptase inhibitor; NNRTI = non-nucleoside reverse transcriptase inhibitor

[a] Zidovudine continuous infusion: 2 mg/kg zidovudine IV over 1 hour, followed by continuous infusion of 1 mg/kg/hour until delivery.

[b] Zidovudine dosing for infants varies by gestational age: ≥35 weeks' gestation at birth is 4 mg/kg/dose orally twice daily; for infants <35 weeks of gestation at birth is 1.5 mg/kg/dose intravenously or 2.0 mg/kg/dose orally, every 12 hours, advancing to every 8 hours at 2 weeks of age if ≥30 weeks of gestation at birth or at 4 weeks of age if <30 weeks' gestation at birth.

Reproduced from: Recommendations for Use of Antiretroviral Drugs in Pregnant HIV-1-Infected Women for Maternal Health and Interventions to Reduce Perinatal HIV Transmission in the United States. Aidsinfo.nih.gov.

MANAGEMENT OF HIV-INFECTED PREGNANT WOMEN CURRENTLY RECEIVING ANTIRETROVIRAL THERAPY

Women currently receiving a <u>suppressive</u> antiretroviral regimen at the onset of pregnancy should continue the successful regimen, even in the first trimester. Discontinuation of therapy will lead to virologic rebound, potentially increasing the risk of disease progression, viral resistance, and vertical transmission. In general, the same suppressive regimen should be continued unless the regimen includes agents that might have an adverse effect on fetal or maternal outcomes. EFV should be avoided during pregnancy (especially in the first trimester) because of reports of malformations in monkeys and case reports of fetal open neural tube defects in infants exposed early in pregnancy (Arch Intern Med 2002;162:355). Because the risk of neural tube defects is restricted to the first 5 to 6 weeks of pregnancy and pregnancy is rarely recognized before 4 to 6 weeks of pregnancy, and unnecessary antiretroviral drug changes during pregnancy may be associated with loss of viral control and increased risk of perinatal transmission, efavirenz can be continued in pregnant women receiving an efavirenz-based regimen who present for antenatal care in the first trimester, provided the regimen produces virologic suppression. By contrast, women who are trying to conceive or who are sexually active without using effective or consistent contraception should not receive EFV-containing regimens. Regimens containing stavudine and didanosine should not be used during pregnancy due to an increased risk of lactic acidosis and hepatic steatosis in women on these agents; even using these drugs singly should be done with caution.

Women receiving a <u>non-suppressive</u> antiretroviral regimen at the onset of pregnancy should undergo assessment for virologic failure as described in Chapter 3. Selection of the optimal regimen is based on medication adherence, results of resistance testing, and understanding the known and unknown safety issues associated with antiretroviral agents in pregnancy.

In general, if antiretroviral therapy is given solely for prevention of perinatal HIV transmission—sometimes termed ART prophylaxis—the continuation of therapy after delivery is currently considered optional, much as treatment in non-pregnant patients with CD4 cell counts > 500. Based on current treatment guidelines for non-pregnant adults, this option would be limited to asymptomatic pregnant women with a CD4 cell count > 500 cells/mm^3 in whom treatment would be recommended provided the patient is willing to continue therapy. Depending on the pretreatment CD4 cell count and tolerability of the regimen, some women may elect to continue treatment given the possible benefits of early therapy and the documented risks of treatment interruption (N Engl J Med 2006; 355:2283–2296). During pregnancy, if treatment must be stopped for severe toxicity or pregnancy-induced hyperemesis, all drugs should generally be stopped at the same time and then reinitiated together. The exception to this practice is for NNRTI-based treatment; if possible, the NRTI backbone should be continued for 7 days after stopping the NRTI to avoid selecting for NNRTI resistance.

OTHER MANAGEMENT AND MONITORING MEASURES

A. **Other Management Considerations.** Pregnant HIV-infected women should be instructed to discontinue cigarettes, illicit drugs, and unprotected sex, and to avoid breastfeeding. Prophylaxis against opportunistic infections is indicated as for nonpregnant HIV-infected women (Chapter 5). Because of concern over antiretroviral therapy and an increase in pregnancy-induced hyperglycemia, standard glucose-loading tests should be performed earlier in pregnancy than typical, and then repeated in the third trimester.

B. **Fetal Monitoring.** Specific adverse obstetrical outcomes have not been ascribed to antiretroviral therapy. Nevertheless, many providers monitor fetal anatomy, growth, and well-being with regular frequency using ultrasound, non-stress testing, and biophysical profiles. Specifically, first trimester ultrasound is recommended to confirm gestational age and to guide the timing of scheduled cesarean delivery (recommended at 38 weeks gestation for women who have not achieved virologic suppression). For patients not seen until later in gestation, second trimester ultrasound can be used to assess fetal anatomy and determine gestational age. Second trimester ultrasound assessment of fetal anatomy is also recommended for women receiving combination antiretroviral therapy during the first trimester, especially if the regimen included EFV. Third trimester ultrasound assessment of fetal growth and well-being should also be considered for woman receiving a combination drug regimen for which there is limited experience with use in pregnancy. The need for non-stress testing and other assessments is based on ultrasound findings and the presence of maternal comorbidities.

POSTPARTUM MANAGEMENT

Children born to HIV-infected women need to be assessed for the possibility of HIV infection and for short- and long-term toxicities due to in-utero exposure to antiretroviral agents. Exposure to antiretroviral agents should become a part of the child's permanent medical record. Further arrangements are needed for long-term care of the woman, including primary and HIV-specialty care appointments, made prior to hospital discharge, and family planning counseling. Mental health status and the possibility of postpartum depression also need to be assessed, and appropriate supports need to be put into place. The importance of adherence to antiretroviral therapy postpartum should be stressed at every patient visit. Case management services best assure adequate support and compliance with healthcare needs.

Table 7.4. Antiretroviral Drug Use in Pregnant HIV-Infected Women: Pharmacokinetic and Toxicity Data in Human Pregnancy and Recommendations for Use in Pregnancy

ARV Drug Generic Name (Abbreviation) Trade Name	Formulation	Dosing Recommendations[a]	Recommendations for Use in Pregnancy	PKs in Pregnancy[b]	Concerns in Pregnancy
NRTIs			NRTIs are recommended for use as part of combination regimens, usually including two NRTIs with either an NNRTI or one or more PIs. Use of single or dual NRTIs alone is not recommended for treatment of HIV infection.		See text for discussion of potential maternal and infant mitochondrial toxicity.
Preferred Agents					
Lamivudine (3TC) Epivir	Epivir 150-, 300-mg tablets or 10-mg/mL oral solution Combivir 3TC 150 mg + ZDV 300 mg Epzicom 3TC 300 mg + ABC 600 mg	Epivir 150 mg BID or 300 mg once daily Take without regard to meals. Combivir 1 tablet BID Epzicom 1 tablet once daily	Because of extensive experience with 3TC in combination in pregnancy with ZDV, 3TC plus ZDV is a recommended dual-NRTI backbone for pregnant women.	PK not significantly altered in pregnancy; no change in dose indicated.[1] High placental transfer to fetus.	No evidence of human teratogenicity (can rule out 1.5-fold increase in overall birth defects).[2] Well tolerated; short-term safety demonstrated for mothers and infants. If hepatitis B coinfected, possible hepatitis B flare if drug stopped postpartum; see Special Situations: Hepatitis B Virus Coinfection.

Table 7.4. Antiretroviral Drug Use in Pregnant HIV-Infected Women: Pharmacokinetic and Toxicity Data in Human Pregnancy and Recommendations for Use in Pregnancy (cont'd)

ARV Drug Generic Name (Abbreviation) Trade Name	Formulation	Dosing Recommendations[a]	Recommendations for Use in Pregnancy	PKs in Pregnancy[b]	Concerns in Pregnancy
Preferred Agents, continued					
	<u>Trizivir</u>[c] 3TC 150 mg + ZDV 300 mg + ABC 300 mg	<u>Trizivir</u> 1 tablet BID			
Zidovudine (AZT, ZDV) Retrovir	<u>Retrovir</u> 100-mg capsules, 300-mg tablets, 10-mg/mL IV solution, 10-mg/ mL oral solution	<u>Retrovir</u> 300 mg BID or 200 mg TID Take without regard to meals.	Because of extensive experience with ZDV in combination in pregnancy with 3TC, ZDV plus 3TC is a recommended dual-NRTI backbone for pregnant women.	PK not significantly altered in pregnancy; no change in dose indicated.[3] High placental transfer to fetus.	No evidence of human teratogenicity (can rule out 1.5-fold increase in overall birth defects).[2] Well tolerated; short-term safety demonstrated for mothers and infants.
	<u>Combivir</u> ZDV 300 mg + 3TC 150 mg	<u>Combivir</u> 1 tablet BID			
	<u>Trizivir</u>[c] ZDV 300 mg + 3TC 150 mg + ABC 300 mg	<u>Trizivir</u> 1 tablet BID			

Alternative Agents				
Abacavir (ABC) Ziagen	<u>Ziagen</u> 300-mg tablets or 20-mg/mL oral solution <u>Epzicom</u> ABC 600 mg + 3TC 300 mg <u>Trizivir</u>[c] ABC 300 mg + ZDV 300 mg + 3TC 150 mg	<u>Ziagen</u> 300 mg BID or 600 mg once daily Take without regard to meals. <u>Epzicom</u> 1 tablet once daily <u>Trizivir</u> 1 tablet BID	Alternative NRTI for dual-NRTI backbone of combination regimens. See footnote regarding use in triple-NRTI regimen.[c]	PK not significantly altered in pregnancy; no change in dose indicated.[4] High placental transfer to fetus.	No evidence of human teratogenicity (can rule out 2-fold increase in overall birth defects).[2] Hypersensitivity reactions occur in ~5%–8% of non-pregnant individuals; a much smaller percentage are fatal and are usually associated with re-challenge. Rate in pregnancy unknown. Testing for HLA-B*5701 identifies patients at risk of reactions[5, 6] and should be done and documented as negative before starting ABC. Patients should be educated regarding symptoms of hypersensitivity reaction.

Table 7.4. Antiretroviral Drug Use in Pregnant HIV-Infected Women: Pharmacokinetic and Toxicity Data in Human Pregnancy and Recommendations for Use in Pregnancy (cont'd)

ARV Drug Generic Name (Abbreviation) Trade Name	Formulation	Dosing Recommendations[a]	Recommendations for Use in Pregnancy	PKs in Pregnancy[b]	Concerns in Pregnancy
Alternative Agents, continued					
Emtricitabine (FTC) Emtriva	Emtriva 200-mg capsule or 10-mg/mL oral solution	Emtriva 200-mg capsule once daily or 240-mg oral solution (24-mL) once daily. Take without regard to meals.	Alternative NRTI for dual-NRTI backbone of combination regimens.	PK study shows slightly lower levels in third trimester, compared with postpartum.[7] No clear need to increase dose. High placental transfer to fetus. No	No evidence of human teratogenicity (can rule out 2-fold increase in overall birth defects).[2] If hepatitis B coinfected, possible hepatitis B flareif drug stopped postpartum; see Special Situations: Hepatitis B Virus Coinfection.
	Truvada FTC 200 mg + TDF 300 mg	Truvada 1 tablet once daily		clear need to increase dose. High placental transfer to fetus.	
	Atripla FTC 200 mg + EFV[d] 600 mg + TDF 300 mg	Atripla 1 tablet at or before bedtime. Take on an empty stomach to reduce side effects.			

Tenofovir Disoproxil Fumarate (TDF) Viread	Viread 300-mg tablet	Viread 1 tablet once daily Take without regard to meals.	Alternative NRTI for dual-NRTI backbone of combination regimens. TDF would be a preferred NRTI in combination with 3TC or FTC in women with chronic HBV infection. Because of potential for renal toxicity, renal funct on should be monitored.	AUC lower in third trimester than postpartum but trough levels adequate.[8] High placental transfer to fetus.[9, 10-13]	No evidence of human teratogenicity (can rule out 2-fold increase in overall birth defects).[2] Studies in monkeys at doses approximately 2-fold higher than that for human therapeutic use show decreased fetal growth and reduction in fetal bone porosity within 2 months of starting maternal therapy.[14] Clinical studies in humans (particularly children) show bone demineralization with chronic use; clinical significance unknown.[15, 16]
	Truvada TDF 300 mg + FTC 200 mg	Truvada 1 tablet once daily			
	Atripla TDF 300 mg + EFV[d] 600 mg + FTC 200 mg	Atripla 1 tablet at or before bedtime Take on an empty stomach to reduce side effects.			

Table 7.4. Antiretroviral Drug Use in Pregnant HIV-Infected Women: Pharmacokinetic and Toxicity Data in Human Pregnancy and Recommendations for Use in Pregnancy (cont'd)

ARV Drug Generic Name (Abbreviation) Trade Name	Formulation	Dosing Recommendations[a]	Recommendations for Use in Pregnancy	PKs in Pregnancy[b]	Concerns in Pregnancy
Alternative Agents, continued					
					If hepatitis B coinfected, possible hepatitis B flare if drug stopped postpartum; see Special Situations: Hepatitis B Virus Coinfection.
Use in Special Circumstances					
Didanosine (ddl) Videx EC, generic didanosine (dose same as Videx EC)	Videx EC 125-, 200-, 250-, 400-mg capsules Buffered tablets (non-EC) no longer available Videx 10-mg/mL oral solution	**Body weight ≥60kg:** 400 mg once daily, with TDF, 250 mg once daily **Body weight <60kg:** 250 mg once daily, with TDF, 200 mg once daily Take 1/2 hour before or 2 hours after a meal. Preferred dosing with oral solution is BID	Because of the need to administer on empty stomach and potential toxicity, ddl should be used only in special circumstances where preferred or alternative NRTIs cannot be used. ddl should not be used with d4T.	PK not significantly altered in pregnancy; no change in dose indicated.[17] Moderate placental transfer to fetus.	In the APR, an increased rate of birth defects with ddl compared to general population was noted after both first trimester (19/409, 4.6%, 95% CI, 2.8–7.2) and later exposure (20/460, 4.3%, 95% CI 2.7–6.6). This difference may have been due to maternal characteristics such as older age or more advanced disease among women using ddl.

				(total daily dose divided into 2 doses).
				No specific pattern of defects was noted and clinical relevance is uncertain. Lactic acidosis, sometimes fatal, has been reported in pregnant women receiving ddI and d4T together.[19,20]
Stavudine (d4T) Zerit	Zerit 15-, 20-, 30-, 40-mg capsules or 1-mg/mL oral solution	**Body weight ≥60 kg:** 40 mg BID **Body weight <60 kg:** 30 mg BID Take without regard to meals. WHO recommends 30-mg BID dosing regardless of body weight.	Because of potential toxicities, d4T should be used only in special circumstances where preferred or alternative NRTIs cannot be used. d4T should not be used with ddI or ZDV.	PKs not significantly altered in pregnancy; no change in dose indicated.[18] High placental transfer.
				No evidence of human teratogenicity (can rule out 2-fold increase in overall birth defects).[2] Lactic acidosis, sometimes fatal, has been reported in pregnant women receiving ddI and d4T together.[19,20]
NNRTIs			NNRTIs are recommended for use in combination regimens with 2 NRTI drugs.	Hypersensitivity reactions, including hepatic toxicity, and rash more common in women; unclear if increased in pregnancy.

Table 7.4. Antiretroviral Drug Use in Pregnant HIV-Infected Women: Pharmacokinetic and Toxicity Data in Human Pregnancy and Recommendations for Use in Pregnancy (cont'd)

ARV Drug Generic Name (Abbreviation) Trade Name	Formulation	Dosing Recommendations[a]	Recommendations for Use in Pregnancy	PKs in Pregnancy[b]	Concerns in Pregnancy
Preferred Agents					
Nevirapine (NVP) Viramune	200-mg tablets or 50-mg/5-mL oral suspension	200 mg once daily for 14 days (lead-in period); thereafter, 200 mg BID. Take without regard to meals. Repeat lead-in period if therapy is discontinued for >7 days. In patients who develop mild-to-moderate rash without constitutional symptoms during lead-in, continue lead-in dosing until rash resolves, but ≤28 days total.	NVP should be initiated in pregnant women with CD4 T-lymphocyte (CD4-cell) counts >250 cells/mm³ only if benefit clearly outweighs risk because of the increased risk of potentially life-threatening hepatotoxicity in women with high CD4-cell counts. Elevated transaminase levels at baseline also may increase the risk of NVP toxicity. Women who become pregnant while taking NVP-containing regimens and are tolerating them well can continue therapy, regardless of CD4-cell count.	PK not significantly altered in pregnancy; no change in dose indicated.[21-23] High placental transfer to fetus.	No evidence of human teratogenicity (can rule out 2-fold increase in overall birth defects).[2] Increased risk of symptomatic, often rash-associated, and potentially fatal liver toxicity among women with CD4-cell counts >250/mm3 when first initiating therapy;[24,25] unclear if pregnancy increases risk.

Use in Special Circumstances			
Efavirenz[d] (EFV) Sustiva	50-, 200-mg capsules or 600-mg tablets	600 mg once daily at or before bedtime

Take on an empty stomach to reduce side effects. | Non-pregnant women of childbearing potential should undergo pregnancy testing before initiation of EFV and counseling about the potential risk to the fetus and desirability of avoiding pregnancy while on EFV-containing regimens. Alternate ARV regimens that do not include EFV should be strongly considered in women who 1) are planning to become pregnant or 2) are sexually active and not using effective contraception, assuming these alternative regimens are acceptable to the provider and are not thought to compromise the health of the woman. Because the risk of neural tube defects is restricted to the first 5–6 weeks of pregnancy and pregnancy is rarely recognized before 4–6 weeks of pregnancy, and unnecessary ARV drug changes during pregnancy may be associated with loss | AUC decreased during third trimester, compared with postpartum, but nearly all third-trimester subjects exceeded target exposure and no change in dose is indicated.[26] Moderate placental transfer to fetus. | FDA Pregnancy Class D; significant malformations (anencephaly, anophthalmia, cleft palate) were observed in 3 of 20 infants (15%) born to cynomolgus monkeys receiving EFV during the first trimester at a dose resulting in plasma levels comparable to systemic human therapeutic exposure. There are 4 retrospective case reports and 1 prospective case report of neural tube defects in humans with first-trimester exposure and 1 prospective case of anophthalmia with facial clefts;[2, 27, 28] relative risk unclear. |
| | **Atripla** EFV[d] 600 mg + FTC 200 mg + TDF 300 mg | **Atripla** 1 tablet once daily at or before bedtime | | | |

Table 7.4. Antiretroviral Drug Use in Pregnant HIV-Infected Women: Pharmacokinetic and Toxicity Data in Human Pregnancy and Recommendations for Use in Pregnancy (cont'd)

ARV Drug Generic Name (Abbreviation) Trade Name	Formulation	Dosing Recommendations[a]	Recommendations for Use in Pregnancy	PKs in Pregnancy[b]	Concerns in Pregnancy
Use in Special Circumstances, continued					
			of viral control and increased risk of perinatal transmission, EFV may be continued in pregnant women receiving an EFV-based regimen who present for antenatal care in the first trimester, provided there is virologic suppression on the regimen (see HIV-Infected Pregnant Women Who are Currently Receiving Antiretroviral Treatment).		
Insufficient Data to Recommend Use					
Etravirine (ETR) Intelence	100-, 200-mg tablets	200 mg BID Take following a meal.	Safety and PK data in pregnancy are insufficient to recommend use during pregnancy.	Limited PK data in pregnancy; in 4 pregnant women, drug levels and AUC	Limited experience in human pregnancy. Only 23 first-trimester exposures have been reported to APR. No evidence of teratogenicity in rats and rabbits.

Rilpivirine (RPV) Endurant	25-mg tablets _Complera_ RPV 25 mg + TDF 300 mg + FTC 200 mg	25 mg once daily with a meal. _Complera_ 1 tablet once daily	Safety and PK data in pregnancy are insufficient to recommend use during pregnancy.	similar to those in non-pregnant adults, suggesting no dose modification needed.[29] No PK studies in human pregnancy, placental transfer rate unknown.	No published experience in human pregnancy. No evidence of teratogenicity in rats or rabbits.
PIs			PIs are recommended for use in combination regimens with 2 NRTI drugs.		Hyperglycemia, new onset or exacerbation of diabetes mellitus, and diabetic ketoacidosis reported with PI use; unclear if pregnancy increases risk. Conflicting data regarding preterm delivery in women receiving PIs (see text).

Table 7.4. Antiretroviral Drug Use in Pregnant HIV-Infected Women: Pharmacokinetic and Toxicity Data in Human Pregnancy and Recommendations for Use in Pregnancy (cont'd)

ARV Drug Generic Name (Abbreviation) Trade Name	Formulation	Dosing Recommendations[a]	Recommendations for Use in Pregnancy	PKs in Pregnancy[b]	Concerns in Pregnancy
Preferred Agents					
Atazanavir (ATV) Reyataz (combined with low-dose RTV boosting)	100-, 150-, 200-, 300-mg capsules	ATV 300 mg + RTV 100 mg once daily. <u>Second and third trimester:</u> Some experts recommend increased dose (ATV 400 mg + RTV 100 mg once daily) in all pregnant women in the second and third trimesters. ATV package insert recommends increased dose (ATV 400 mg + RTV 100 mg once daily) in the following situations: - With TDF or H₂-receptor antagonist (not both; use of both with ATV not recommended) in	Preferred PI for use in regimens in pregnancy. Should give as low-dose RTV-boosted regimen, may use once-daily dosing. Several studies have shown decreased ATV plasma concentrations with standard dosing during pregnancy.[10,30,31] Use of an increased dose during the second and third trimesters resulted in plasma concentrations equivalent to those in non-pregnant adults on standard dosing.[32] Although some experts recommend increased ATV dosing in all women during the second and third trimesters, the package insert recommends increased ATV dosing only for ARV-	Two of three intensive PK studies of ATV with RTV boosting during pregnancy and the PK study described in the recently approved product label suggest that standard dosing in pregnancy results in decreased plasma concentrations, compared with non-pregnant adults.[10,13,30,31]	No evidence of human teratogenicity (can rule out 2-fold increase in overall birth defects).[2] Theoretical concern regarding increased indirect bilirubin levels causing significant exacerbation in physiologic hyperbilirubinemia in neonates has not been observed in clinical trials to date.[10,13,30,31,33]

	ARV-experienced patients - With EFV[c] in ARV-naive patients (Concurrent use of ATV with EFV in ARV-experienced patients is not recommended because of decreased ATV levels.) Take with food.	experienced pregnant women in the second and third trimesters also receiving either TDF or an H2-receptor antagonist or ARV-naive pregnant women receiving EFV. ATV should not be used in patients receiving both TDF and H_2 receptor antagonists or in ARV-experienced patients also taking EFV.	ATV concentrations further reduced ~25% with concomitant TDF use.[10, 13] Low placental transfer to fetus.[10, 30]	No evidence of human teratogenicity (can rule out 2-fold increase in overall birth defects).[2] Well tolerated; short-term safety demonstrated in Phase I/II studies.
Lopinavir + Ritonavir (LPV/r) Kaletra	Tablets: (LPV 200 mg + RTV 50 mg) or (LPV 100 mg + RTV 25 mg) Oral solution: Each 5 mL contains LPV 400 mg + RTV 100 mg Oral solution contains 42% alcohol and therefore may not be optimal for use in pregnancy.	LPV/r 400 mg/ 100 mg BID Second and third trimester: Some experts recommend increased dose (LPV/r 600 mg/150 mg BID) in second and third trimesters. With EFV[d] or NVP[d] PI-naive or PI-experienced patients): LPV/r 500 mg/ 125 mg tablets BID	PK studies suggest dose should be increased to 600 mg/150 mg BID in second and third trimesters, especially in PI-experienced patients. If standard dosing is used, monitor virologic response and LPV drug levels, if available. Once-daily LPV/r dosing is not recommended during pregnancy because there are no data to address whether drug levels are adequate with such administration	AUC decreased in second and third trimesters with standard dosing.[34-36] AUC with dose of LPV/r 600 mg/150 mg twice daily in third trimester in U.S. women resulted in AUC similar to that in nonpregnant adults taking	

Table 7.4. Antiretroviral Drug Use in Pregnant HIV-Infected Women: Pharmacokinetic and Toxicity Data in Human Pregnancy and Recommendations for Use in Pregnancy (cont'd)

ARV Drug Generic Name (Abbreviation) Trade Name	Formulation	Dosing Recommendations[a]	Recommendations for Use in Pregnancy	PKs in Pregnancy[b]	Concerns in Pregnancy
Preferred Agents, continued					
	therefore may not be optimal for use in pregnancy.	(Use a combination of two LPV/r 200 mg/ 50 mg tablets + one LPV/r 100 mg/ 25 mg tablet to make a total dose of LPV/r 500 mg/125 mg) or LPV/r 533 mg/133 mg oral solution (6.5mL) BID. Tablets: Take without regard to meals. Oral solution: Take with food. Not used in pregnancy: Adult dosage of LPV/r 800 mg/200 mg once daily is not recommended for use in pregnancy.		LPV/r 400 mg/100 mg dose twice daily.[30] Low placental transfer to fetus.	

Ritonavir (RTV) Norvir When used as lowdose booster with other PIs	100-mg capsules 100-mg tablets 80-mg/mL oral solution Oral solution contains 43% alcohol and therefore may not be optimal for use in pregnancy.	As PK booster for other PIs: 100–400 mg per day in 1–2 divided doses (Refer to other PIs for specific dosing recommendations.) Tablets: Take with food. Capsule and oral solution: Take with food if possible, which may improve tolerability.	Should only be used in combination with second PI as low-dose RTV "boost" to increase levels of second PI because of low drug levels in pregnant women when used as a sole PI and poor tolerance when given as full dose.	Phase I/II study in pregnancy showed lower levels during pregnancy compared with postpartum.[37] Minimal placental transfer to fetus.	No evidence of human teratogenicity (can rule out 2-fold increase in overall birth defects).[2] Limited experience at full dose in human pregnancy; should be used as low-dose RTV boosting with other PIs.
Alternative Agents					
Darunavir (DRV) Prezista (must be combined with low-dose RTV boosting)	75-, 150-, 400-, 600- and 800 mg tablets	ARV-naive patients: (DRV 800 mg + RTV 100 mg) once daily ARV-experienced patients: (DRV 800 mg + RTV 100 mg) once daily if no DRV resistance mutations (DRV 600 mg + RTV 100 mg) BID if any DRV resistance mutations	Safety and PK data in pregnancy are limited. DRV may be considered when preferred and alternative agents cannot be used. Must give as low-dose RTV-boosted regimen.	In PK study of women in the third trimester and postpartum, third-trimester DRV average plasma concentrations were decreased by 23%–28% with once- and twice-daily dosing and	Insufficient data to assess for teratogenicity in humans. No evidence of teratogenicity in mice, rats, or rabbits but low bioavailability limited exposure. Limited experience in human pregnancy.

Table 7.4. Antiretroviral Drug Use in Pregnant HIV-Infected Women: Pharmacokinetic and Toxicity Data in Human Pregnancy and Recommendations for Use in Pregnancy (cont'd)

ARV Drug Generic Name (Abbreviation) Trade Name	Formulation	Dosing Recommendations[a]	Recommendations for Use in Pregnancy	PKs in Pregnancy[b]	Concerns in Pregnancy
Alternative Agents, continued					
		Some experts recommend use of only twice-daily dosing (DRV 600 mg + RTV 100 mg BID) during pregnancy. Unboosted DRV is **not** recommended. Take with food.		third-trimester DRV trough concentrations were low, especially with once-daily dosing.[38] Some experts recommend use of only twice-daily dosing during pregnancy and investigation of use of an increased twice-daily dose is under way. Low placental transfer to fetus.[38]	

| **Saquinavir** (SQV) Invirase (available as capsules and tablets. SQV must be combined with low-dose RTV boosting.) | 500-mg tablets or 200-mg capsules | (SQV 1000 mg + RTV 100 mg) BID Unboosted SQV is **not** recommended. Take with meals or within 2 hours after a meal. | PK data on SQV capsules and the tablet formulation in pregnancy are limited. RTV-boosted SQV capsules or SQV tablets are alternative PIs for combination regimens in pregnancy and are alternative initial ARV recommendations for non-pregnant adults. Must give as low-dose RTV-boosted regimen. | Limited PK data on capsules and the 500-mg tablet formulation suggest that 1000-mg SQV capsules/ 100 mg RTV given twice daily achieves adequate SQV drug levels in pregnant women.[39] Minimal placental transfer to fetus. | Insufficient data to assess for teratogenicity in humans. No evidence of teratogenicity in rats or rabbits but low bioavailability limited exposure. Well tolerated; short-term safety demonstrated for mothers and infants for SQV in combination with low-dose RTV. Baseline ECG recommended before starting because PR and/or QT interval prolongations have been observed and drug is contraindicated in patients with pre-existing cardiac conduction system disease. |

Table 7.4. Antiretroviral Drug Use in Pregnant HIV-Infected Women: Pharmacokinetic and Toxicity Data in Human Pregnancy and Recommendations for Use in Pregnancy (cont'd)

ARV Drug Generic Name (Abbreviation) Trade Name	Formulation	Dosing Recommendations[a]	Recommendations for Use in Pregnancy	PKs in Pregnancy[b]	Concerns in Pregnancy
Use in Special Circumstances					
Indinavir (IDV) Crixivan (combined with low-dose RTV boosting)	100-, 200-, 400- mg capsules	With RTV: (IDV 800 mg + RTV 100–200 mg) BID Take without regard to meals. Not used in pregnancy: Adult dosage of IDV (without RTV) 800 mg every 8 hours is not recommended for use in pregnancy.	Because of twice-daily dosing, pill burden, and potential for renal stones, IDV should only be used when preferred and alternative agents cannot be used. Must give as low-dose RTV-boosted regimen.	Two studies including 18 women receiving IDV 800 mg TID showed markedly lower levels during pregnancy compared with postpartum, although suppression of HIV RNA levels was seen. [40,41] In a study of RTV-boosted IDV (400 mg IDV/100 mg RTV twice daily), 82% of	No evidence of human teratogenicity (can rule out 2-fold increase in overall birth defects). [2] Theoretical concern regarding increased indirect bilirubin levels, which may exacerbate physiologic hyperbilirubinemia in neonates, but minimal placental passage. Use of unboosted IDV during pregnancy is not recommended.

| **Nefinavir** (NFV) Viracept | 250-, 625-mg tablets 50-mg/g oral powder | 1250 mg BID Take with food. Not used in pregnancy: Adult dosage of NFV 750 mg TID is not recommended for use in pregnancy. | Given PK data and extensive experience with use in pregnancy, NFV might be considered in special circumstances for prophylaxis of transmission in women in whom therapy would not otherwise be indicated when alternative agents are not tolerated. In clinical trials of initial therapy in non-pregnant adults, NFV-based regimens had a lower rate of viral response compared with LPV/r-or EFV-based regimens but similar viral response to ATV-or NVP-based regimens. | Adequate drug levels are achieved in pregnant women with NFV 1250 mg given twice daily, although levels are variable in late pregnancy.[22,43,44] In a study of women in their second and third trimesters dosed at 1250 mg twice daily, women in the third trimester had lower concentration of NFV than those women met the target trough level.[42] Minimal placental transfer to fetus. | No evidence of human teratogenicity (can rule out 2-fold increase in overall birth defects).[2] Well tolerated; short-term safety demonstrated for mothers and infants. |

Table 7.4. Antiretroviral Drug Use in Pregnant HIV-Infected Women: Pharmacokinetic and Toxicity Data in Human Pregnancy and Recommendations for Use in Pregnancy (cont'd)

ARV Drug Generic Name (Abbreviation) Trade Name	Formulation	Dosing Recommendations[a]	Recommendations for Use in Pregnancy	PKs in Pregnancy[b]	Concerns in Pregnancy
Use in Special Circumstances, continued					
				in the second trimester.[44] In a study of the new 625-mg tablet formulation dosed at 1250 mg twice daily, lower AUC and peak levels were observed during the third trimester than postpartum.[45] Minimal to low placental transfer to fetus.	

Insufficient Data to Recommend Use

Fosamprenavir (FPV) Lexiva (a prodrug of amprenavir) (recommended to be combined with low-dose RTV boosting)	700-mg tablet 50-mg/mL oral suspension	ARV-naive patients: • FPV 1400 mg BID or • (FPV 1400 mg + RTV 100–200 mg) once daily or • (FPV 700 mg + RTV 100 mg) BID PI-experienced patients (once-daily dosing not recommended): • (FPV 700 mg + RTV 100 mg) BID With EFV: • (FPV 700 mg + RTV 100 mg) BID or • (FPV 1400 mg + RTV 300 mg) once daily Tablet: Take without regard to meals (if not boosted with RTV tablet). Suspension: Take without food. FPV with RTV tablet: Take with meals.	Safety and PK data in pregnancy are insufficient to recommend routine use during pregnancy in ARV-naive patients. Recommended to be given as low-dose RTV-boosted regimen.	With RTV boosting, AUC is reduced during the third trimester. However, exposure is greater during the third trimester with boosting than in non-pregnant adults without boosting and trough concentrations achieved during the third trimester were adequate for patients without PI resistance mutations.[46] Low placental transfer to fetus.	Insufficient data to assess for teratogenicity in humans. Increased fetal loss in rabbits but no increase in defects in rats and rabbits. Limited experience in human pregnancy.

Table 7.4. Antiretroviral Drug Use in Pregnant HIV-Infected Women: Pharmacokinetic and Toxicity Data in Human Pregnancy and Recommendations for Use in Pregnancy (cont'd)

ARV Drug Generic Name (Abbreviation) Trade Name	Formulation	Dosing Recommendations[a]	Recommendations for Use in Pregnancy	PKs in Pregnancy[b]	Concerns in Pregnancy
Insufficient Data to Recommend Use, continued					
Tipranavir (TPV) Aptivus (must be combined with low-dose RTV boosting)	250-mg capsules or 100-mg/mL oral solution	(TPV 500 mg + RTV 200 mg) BID Unboosted TPV is **not** recommended. TPV taken with RTV tablets: Take with meals. TPV taken with RTV capsules or solution: Take without regard to meals.	Safety and PK data in pregnancy are insufficient to recommend routine use during pregnancy in ARV-naive patients. Must give as lowdose RTV-boosted regimen.	Limited PK studies in human pregnancy. Moderate placental transfer to fetus reported in one patient.[47]	Insufficient data to assess for teratogenicity in humans. No teratogenicity in rats or rabbits. Limited experience in human pregnancy.
Entry Inhibitors					
Insufficient Data to Recommend Use					
Enfuvirtide (T20) Fuzeon	• Injectable—supplied as lyophilized powder • Each vial contains 108 mg of T20; reconstitute	90 mg (1mL) SQ BID	Safety and PK data in pregnancy are insufficient to recommend use during pregnancy in ARV-naive patients.	Limited PK studies in human pregnancy. No placental transfer to fetus, based on very limited data.[47, 48]	Insufficient data to assess for teratogenicity in humans. No evidence of teratogenicity in rats or rabbits. Minimal data in human pregnancy.[47, 49]

	with 1.1 mL of sterile water for injection for delivery of approximately 90 mg/1 mL.				Insufficient data to assess for teratogenicity in humans. No evidence of teratogenicity in rats or rabbits. Limited experience in human pregnancy.
Maraviroc (MVC) Selzentry	150, 300-mg tablets	• **150 mg BID** when given with strong CYP3A inhibitors (with or without CYP3A inducers) including PIs (except: TPV/r) • **300 mg BID** when given with NRTIs, NVP, RAL, T-20, TPV/r, and other drugs that are not strong CYP3A inhibitors or inducers • **500 mg BID** when given with CYP3A inducers, including EFV, ETR (without a CYP3A inhibitor) Take without regard to meals.	Safety and PK data in pregnancy are insufficient to recommend use during pregnancy in ARV-naive patients.	No PK studies in human pregnancy. Unknown placental transfer rate to fetus.	

Table 7.4. Antiretroviral Drug Use in Pregnant HIV-Infected Women: Pharmacokinetic and Toxicity Data in Human Pregnancy and Recommendations for Use in Pregnancy (cont'd)

ARV Drug Generic Name (Abbreviation) Trade Name	Formulation	Dosing Recommendations[a]	Recommendations for Use in Pregnancy	PKs in Pregnancy[b]	Concerns in Pregnancy
Integrase Inhibitors					
Use in Special Circumstances					
Raltegravir (RAL) Isentress	400-mg tablets	400 mg BID <u>With rifampin:</u> 800 mg BID Take without regard to meals.	Safety and PK data in pregnancy are limited; can be considered for use in special circumstances when preferred and alternative agents cannot be used.	During third trimester, RAL PK showed extensive variability but RAL exposure was not consistently altered compared with postpartum and historical data. The standard dose appears appropriate during pregnancy.[50] Variable but high placental transfer to fetus.[50, 51]	Insufficient data to assess for teratogenicity in humans. Increased skeletal variants in rats, no increase in defects in rabbits. Limited experience in human pregnancy.

Table 7.4. Antiretroviral Drug Use in Pregnant HIV-Infected Women: Pharmacokinetic and Toxicity Data in Human Pregnancy and Recommendations for Use in Pregnancy (cont'd)

Key to Abbreviations: APR = Antiretroviral Pregnancy Registry, ARV = antiretroviral, AUC = area under the curve, BID = twice daily, CI = confidence interval, CYP = cytochrome P, EC = enteric coated, ECG = electrocardiogram, FDA = Food and Drug Administration, HBV = hepatitis B virus, IV = intravenous, NNRTI = non-nucleoside reverse transcriptase inhibitor, NRTI = nucleoside/nucleotide reverse transcriptase inhibitor, PI = protease inhibitor, PK = pharmacokinetic, PPI = proton pump inhibitor, SQ = subcutaneous injection, TID = three times daily, WHO = World Health Organization

^a Dosage should be adjusted in renal or hepatic insufficiency (see *Adult Guidelines, Appendix B, Table 7*).

^b Placental transfer categories—Mean or median cord blood/maternal delivery plasma drug ratio:

        High: >0.6

        Moderate: 0.3–0.6

        Low: 0.1–0.3

        Minimal: <0.1

^c Triple-NRTI regimens including abacavir have been less potent virologically compared with PI-based combination ARV drug regimens. Triple-NRTI regimens should be used only when an NNRTI- or PI-based combination regimen cannot be used, such as because of significant drug interactions.

^d See Teratogenicity for discussion of efavirenz and risks in pregnancy.

Reproduced from: Recommendations for Use of Antiretroviral Drugs in Pregnant HIV-1-Infected Women for Maternal Health and Interventions to Reduce Perinatal HIV Transmission in the United States. Aidsinfo.nih.gov.

1. Moodley J, Moodley D, Pillay K, et al. Pharmacokinetics and antiretroviral activity of lamivudine alone or when coadministered with zidovudine in human immunodeficiency virus type 1-infected pregnant women and their offspring. J Infect Dis. Nov 1998;178(5):1327-1333. Available at http://www.ncbi.nlm.nih.gov/pubmed/9780252.

2. Antiretroviral Pregnancy Registry Steering Committee. Antiretroviral pregnancy registry international interim report for 1 Jan 1989 - 31 January 2012. Wilmington, NC: Registry Coordinating Center; 2012. Available at http://www.APRegistry.com.

3. O'Sullivan MJ, Boyer PJ, Scott GB, et al. The pharmacokinetics and safety of zidovudine in the third trimester of pregnancy for women infected with human immunodeficiency virus and their infants: phase I acquired immunodeficiency syndrome clinical trials group study (protocol 082). Zidovudine

Collaborative Working Group. Am J Obstet Gynecol. 1993;168(5):1510-1516. Available at http://www.ncbi.nlm.nih.gov/entrez/query.fcgi?cmd=Retrieve&db=pubmed&dopt=Abstract&list_uids=8098905.

4. Best BM, Mirochnick M, Capparelli EV, et al. Impact of pregnancy on abacavir pharmacokinetics. AIDS. Feb 28 2006;20(4):553-560. Available at http://www.ncbi.nlm.nih.gov/pubmed/16470119.

5. Mallal S, Phillips E, Carosi G, et al. HLA-B*5701 screening for hypersensitivity to abacavir. N Engl J Med. Feb 7 2008;358(6):568-579. Available at http://www.ncbi.nlm.nih.gov/pubmed/18256392.

6. Saag M, Balu R, Phillips E, et al. High sensitivity of human leukocyte antigen-b*5701 as a marker for immunologically confirmed abacavir hypersensitivity in white and black patients. Clin Infect Dis. Apr 1 2008;46(7):1111-1118. Available at http://www.ncbi.nlm.nih.gov/pubmed/18444831.

7. Best BM, Stek AM, Mirochnick M, et al. Lopinavir tablet pharmacokinetics with an increased dose during pregnancy. J Acquir Immune Defic Syndr. Aug 2010;54(4):381-388. Available at http://www.ncbi.nlm.nih.gov/pubmed/20632458.

8. Burchett SK, Best B, Mirochnick M, et al. Tenofovir pharmacokinetics during pregnancy, at delivery and postpartum. Paper presented at: 14th Conference on Retroviruses and Opportunistic Infections (CROI); February 25-28, 2007; Los Angeles, CA. Abstract 738b.

9. Hirt D, Urien S, Ekouevi DK, et al. Population pharmacokinetics of tenofovir in HIV-1-infected pregnant women and their neonates (ANRS 12109). Clin Pharmacol Ther. Feb 2009;85(2):182-189. Available at http://www.ncbi.nlm.nih.gov/pubmed/18987623.

10. Mirochnick M, Best BM, Stek AM, et al. Atazanavir pharmacokinetics with and without tenofovir during pregnancy. J Acquir Immune Defic Syndr. Apr 15 2011;56(5):412-419. Available at http://www.ncbi.nlm.nih.gov/pubmed/21283017.

11. Mirochnick M, Kunwenda N, Joao E, et al. Tenofovir disoproxil fumarate (TDF) pharmacokinetics (PK) with increased doses in HIV-1 infected pregnant women and their newborns (HPTN 057). Paper presented at: 11th International Workshop on Clinical Pharmacology of HIV Therapy; April 7-9, 2010; Sorrento, Italy. Abstract 3.

12. Flynn PM, Mirochnick M, Shapiro DE, et al. Pharmacokinetics and safety of single-dose tenofovir disoproxil fumarate and emtricitabine in HIV-1-infected pregnant women and their infants. Antimicrob Agents Chemother. Dec 2011;55(12):5914-5922. Available at http://www.ncbi.nlm.nih.gov/pubmed/21896911.

13. Mirochnick M, Kafulafula G, et al. The pharmacokinetics (PK) of tenofovir disoproxil fumarate (TDF) after administration to HIV-1 infected pregnant women and their newborns. Paper presented at: 16th Conference on Retroviruses and Opportunistic Infections (CROI); February 8-11, 2009; Montreal, Canada. Abstract 940.

14. Tarantal AF, Castillo A, Ekert JE, Bischofberger N, Martin RB. Fetal and maternal outcome after administration of tenofovir to gravid rhesus monkeys (Macaca mulatta). J Acquir Immune Defic Syndr. Mar 1 2002;29(3):207-220. Available at http://www.ncbi.nlm.nih.gov/pubmed/11873070.

15. Gafni RI, Hazra R, Reynolds JC, et al. Tenofovir disoproxil fumarate and an optimized background regimen of antiretroviral agents as salvage therapy: impact on bone mineral density in HIV-infected children. Pediatrics. Sep 2006;118(3):e711-718. Available at http://www.ncbi.nlm.nih.gov/pubmed/16923923.

16. Schooley RT, Ruane P, Myers RA, et al. Tenofovir DF in antiretroviral-experienced patients: results from a 48-week, randomized, double-blind study. AIDS. Jun 14 2002;16(9):1257-1263. Available at http://www.ncbi.nlm.nih.gov/pubmed/12045491.

17. Wang Y, Livingston E, Patil S, et al. Pharmacokinetics of didanosine in antepartum and postpartum human immunodeficiency virus-infected pregnant women and their neonates: an AIDS clinical trials group study. J Infect Dis. 1999;180(5):1536-1541. Available at http://www.ncbi.nlm.nih.gov/entrez/query.fcgi?cmd=Retrieve&db=Retrieve&dopt=Abstract&list_uids=10515813.

18. Wade NA, Unadkat JD, Huang S, et al. Pharmacokinetics and safety of stavudine in HIV-infected pregnant women and their infants: Pediatric AIDS Clinical Trials Group protocol 332. J Infect Dis. Dec 15 2004;190(12):2167-2174. Available at http://www.ncbi.nlm.nih.gov/pubmed/15551216.

19. Bristol-Myers Squibb Company. Healthcare provider important drug warning letter. January 5, 2001. Available at http://www.bms.com.

20. Sarner L, Fakoya A. Acute onset lactic acidosis and pancreatitis in the third trimester of pregnancy in HIV-1 positive women taking antiretroviral medication. Sex Transm Infect. Feb 2002 78(1):58-59. Available at http://www.ncbi.nlm.nih.gov/pubmed/11872862.

21. Capparelli EV, Aweeka F, Hitti J, et al. Chronic administration of nevirapine during pregnancy: impact of pregnancy on pharmacokinetics. HIV Med. Apr 2008;9(4):214-220. Available at http://www.ncbi.nlm.nih.gov/pubmed/18366444.

22. Aweeka F, Lizak P, Frenkel L, et al. Steady-state nevirapine pharmacokinetics during 2nd and 3rd trimester pregnancy and postpartum: PACTG 1022. Paper presented at: 11th Conference on Retroviruses and Opportunistic Infections (CROI); February 8-11, 2004; San Francisco, CA. Abstract 932.

23. Mirochnick M, Siminski S, Fenton T, Luco M, Sullivan JL. Nevirapine pharmacokinetics in pregnant women and in their infants after in utero exposure. Pediatr Infect Dis J. Aug 2001;20(8):803-805. Available at http://www.ncbi.nlm.nih.gov/pubmed/11734746.

24. Baylor MS, Johann-Liang R. Hepatotoxicity associated with nevirapine use. J Acquir Immune Defic Syndr. 2004;35(5):538-539. Available at http://www.ncbi.nlm.nih.gov/entrez/query.fcgi?cmd=Retrieve&db=pubmed&dopt=Abstract&list_uids=15021321.

25. Dieterich DT, Robinson PA, Love J, Stern JO. Drug-induced liver injury associated with the use of nonnucleoside reverse-transcriptase inhibitors. Clin Infect Dis. 2004;38 (Suppl 2):S80-89. Available at http://www.ncbi.nlm.nih.gov/entrez/query.fcgi?cmd=Retrieve&db=pubmed&dopt=Abstract&list_uids=14986279.

26. Cressey TR, Stek A, Capparelli E, et al. Efavirenz pharmacokinetics during the third trimester of pregnancy and postpartum. J Acquir Immune Defic Syndr. Mar 1 2012;59(3):245-252. Available at http://www.ncbi.nlm.nih.gov/pubmed/22083071.

27. De Santis M, Carducci B, De Santis L, Cavaliere AF, Straface G. Periconceptional exposure to efavirenz and neural tube defects. Arch Intern Med. Feb 11 2002;162(3):355. Available at http://www.ncbi.nlm.nih.gov/pubmed/11822930.

28. Fundaro C, Genovese O, Rendeli C, Tamburrini E, Salvaggio E. Myelomeningocele in a child with intrauterine exposure to efavirenz. AIDS. Jan 25 2002;16(2):299-300. Available at http://www.ncbi.nlm.nih.gov/pubmed/11807320.

29. Izurieta P, Kakuda TN, Feys C, Witek J. Safety and pharmacokinetics of etravirine in pregnant HIV-1-infected women. HIV Med. Apr 2011;12(4):257-258. Available at http://www.ncbi.nlm.nih.gov/pubmed/21371239.

30. Ripamonti D, Cattaneo D, Maggiolo F, et a. Atazanavir plus low-dose ritonavir in pregnancy: pharmacokinetics and placental transfer. AIDS. Nov 30 2007;21(18):2409-2415. Available at http://www.ncbi.nlm.nih.gov/pubmed/13025877.

31. Conradie F, Zorrilla C, Josipovic D, et al. Safety and exposure of once-daily ritonavir-boosted atazanavir in HIV-infected pregnant women. HIV Med. Oct 2011;12(9):570-579. Available at http://www.ncbi.nlm.nih.gov/pubmed/21569187

32. Mirochnick M, Stek A, Capparelli EV, et al. Pharmacokinetics of increased dose atazanavir with and without tenofovir during pregnancy. Paper presented at: 12th International Workshop on Clinical Pharmacology of HIV Therapy; April 13-16, 2011; Miami, FL.

33. Natha M, Hay P, Taylor G, et al. Atazanavir use in pregnancy: a report of 33 cases. Paper presented at: 14th Conference on Retroviruses and Opportunistic Infections (CROI); February 25-28, 2007; Los Angeles, CA. Abstract 750.

34. Cressey TR, Jourdain G, Rawangban B, et al. Pharmacokinetics and virologic response of zidovudine/lopinavir/ritonavir initiated during the third trimester of pregnancy. AIDS. Sep 10 201C;24(14):2193-2200. Available at http://www.ncbi.nlm.nih.gov/pubmed/20625263.

35. Stek AM, Mirochnick M, Capparelli E, et al. Reduced lopinavir exposure during pregnancy. AIDS. Oct 3 2006;20(15):1931-1939. Available at http://www.ncbi.nlm.nih.gov/pubmed/16988514.

36. Lambert JS, Else LJ, Jackson V, et al. Therapeutic drug monitoring of lopinavir/ritonavir in pregnancy. HIV Med. Mar 2011;12(3):166-173. Available at http://www.ncbi.nlm.nih.gov/pubmed/20726906.

37. Scott GB, Rodman JH, Scott WA, et al. for the PACTG 354 Protocol Team. Pharmacokinetic and virologic response to ritonavir (RTV) in combination with zidovudine (XDV) and lamivudine (3TC) in HIV-1 infected pregnant women and their infants. Paper presented at: 9th Conference on Retroviruses and Opportunistic Infections (CROI); February 24-28, 2002; Seattle, WA. Abstract 794-W. Available at http://www.retroconference.org/2002/.

38. Capparelli EV, Best BM, Stek A, et al. Pharmacokinetics of darunavir once or twice daily during pregnancy and postpartum. Paper presented at: 3rd International Workshop on HIV Pediatrics; July 15-16, 2011; Rome, Italy.

39. van der Lugt J, Colbers A, Molto J, et al. The pharmacokinetics, safety and efficacy of boosted saquinavir tablets in HIV type-1-infected pregnant women. Antivir Ther. 2009;14(3):443-450. Available at http://www.ncbi.nlm.nih.gov/pubmed/19474478.

40. Unadkat JD, Wara DW, Hughes MD, et al. Pharmacokinetics and safety of indinavir in human immunodeficiency virus-infected pregnant women. Antimicrob Agents Chemother. Feb 2007;51(2):783-786. Available at http://www.ncbi.nlm.nih.gov/pubmed/17158945.

41. Hayashi S, Beckerman K, Homma M, Kosel BW, Aweeka FT. Pharmacokinetics of indinavir in HIV-positive pregnant women. AIDS. May 26 2000;14(8):1061-1062. Available at http://www.ncbi.nlm.nih.gov/pubmed/10853990.

42. Ghosn J, De Montgolfier I, Cornelie C, et al. Antiretroviral therapy with a twice-daily regimen containing 400 milligrams of indinavir and 100 milligrams of ritonavir in human immunodeficiency virus type 1-infected women during pregnancy. Antimicrob Agents Chemother. Apr 2008;52(4):1542-1544. Available at http://www.ncbi.nlm.nih.gov/pubmed/18250187.

43. Bryson YJ, Mirochnick M, Stek A, et al. Pharmacokinetics and safety of nelfinavir when used in combination with zidovudine and lamivudine in HIV-infected pregnant women: Pediatric AIDS Clinical Trials Group (PACTG) Protocol 353. HIV Clin Trials. Mar-Apr 2008;9(2):115-125. Available at http://www.ncbi.nlm.nih.gov/pubmed/18474496.

44. Villani P, Floridia M, Pirillo MF, et al. Pharmacokinetics of nelfinavir in HIV-1-infected pregnant and nonpregnant women. Br J Clin Pharmacol. Sep 2006;62(3):309-315. Available at http://www.ncbi.nlm.nih.gov/pubmed/16934047.

45. Read JS, Best BM, Stek AM, et al. Pharmacokinetics of new 625 mg nelfinavir formulation during pregnancy and postpartum. HIV Med. Nov 2008;9(10):875-882. Available at http://www.ncbi.nlm.nih.gov/pubmed/18795962.

46. Capparelli EV, Stek A, Best B, et al. Boosted fosamprenavir pharmacokinetics during Pregnancy. Paper presented at: 17th Conference on Retroviruses and Opportunistic Infections (CROI); February 16-19, 2010; San Francisco, CA. Abstract 908.

47. Weizsaecker K, Kurowski M, Hoffmeister B, Schurmann D, Feiterna-Sperling C. Pharmacokinetic profile in late pregnancy and cord blood concentration of tipranavir and enfuvirtide. Int J STD AIDS. May 2011;22(5):294-295. Available at http://www.ncbi.nlm.nih.gov/pubmed/21571982.

48. Brennan-Benson P, Pakianathan M, Rice P, et al. Enfuvirtide prevents vertical transmission of multidrug-resistant HIV-1 in pregnancy but does not cross the placenta. AIDS. Jan 9 2006;20(2):297-299. Available at http://www.ncbi.nlm.nih.gov/pubmed/16511429.

49. Meyohas MC, Lacombe K, Carbonne B, Morand-Joubert L, Girard PM. Enfuvirtide prescription at the end of pregnancy to a multi-treated HIV-infected woman with virological breakthrough. AIDS. Sep 24 2004;18(14):1966-1968. Available at http://www.ncbi.nlm.nih.gov/pubmed/15335987.

50. Best BM, Capparelli EV, Stek A, et al. Raltegravir pharmacokinetics during pregnancy. Paper presented at: 50th Interscience Conference on Antimicrobial Agents and Chemotherapy (ICAAC); September 12-15, 2010; Boston, MA.

51. McKeown DA, Rosenvinge M, Donaghy S, et al. High neonatal concentrations of raltegravir following transplacental transfer in HIV-1 positive pregnant women. AIDS. Sep 24 2010;24(15):2416-2418. Available at http://www.ncbi.nlm.nih.gov/pubmed/20827058.

REFERENCES AND SUGGESTED READINGS

Antiretroviral Pregnancy Registry Steering Committee. Antiretroviral pregnancy registry international interim report for 1 Jan 1989 - 31 January 2012. Wilmington, NC: Registry Coordinating Center; 2012. Available at http://www.APRegistry.com.

Aweeka F, Lizak P, Frenkel L, et al. Steady state nevirapine pharmacokinetics during 2nd and 3rd trimester pregnancy and postpartum: PACTG 1022. Paper presented at: 11th Conference on Retroviruses and Opportunistic Infections (CROI); February 8-11, 2004; San Francisco, CA. Abstract 932.

Baylor MS, Johann-Liang R. Hepatotoxicity associated with nevirapine use. J Acquir Immune Defic Syndr. 2004;35(5):538 539. Available at http://www.ncbi.nlm.nih.gov/entrez/query.fcgi?cmd=Retrieve&db=pubmed&dopt=Abstract&list_uids=15021321.

Best BM, Capparelli EV, Stek A, et al. Raltegravir pharmacokinetics during pregnancy. Paper presented at: 50th Interscience Conference on Antimicrobial Agents and Chemotherapy (ICAAC); September 12-15, 2010; Boston, MA.

Best BM, Mirochnick M, Capparelli EV, et al. Impact of pregnancy on abacavir pharmacokinetics. AIDS. Feb 28 2006;20(4):553-560. Available at http://www.ncbi.nlm.nih.gov/pubmed/16470119.

Best BM, Stek AM, Mirochnick M, et al. Lopinavir tablet pharmacokinetics with an increased dose during pregnancy. J Acquir Immune Defic Syndr. Aug 2010;54(4):381-388. Available at http://www.ncbi.nlm.nih.gov/pubmed/20632458.

Brennan-Benson P, Pakianathan M, Rice P, et al. Enfuvirtide prevents vertical transmission of multidrug-resistant HIV-1 in pregnancy but does not cross the placenta. AIDS. Jan 9 2006;20(2):297-299. Available at http://www.ncbi.nlm.nih.gov/pubmed/16511429.

Bristol-Myers Squibb Company. Healthcare provider important drug warning letter. January 5, 2001. Available at http://www.bms.com.

Bryson YJ, Mirochnick M, Stek A, et al. Pharmacokinetics and safety of nelfinavir when used in combination with zidovudine and lamivudine in HIV-infected pregnant women: Pediatric AIDS Clinical Trials Group (PACTG) Protocol 353. HIV Clin Trials. Mar-Apr 2008;9(2):115-125. Available at http://www.ncbi.nlm.nih.gov/pubmed/18474496.

Burchett SK, Best B, Mirochnick M, et al. Tenofovir pharmacokinetics during pregnancy, at delivery and postpartum. Paper presented at: 14th Conference on Retroviruses and Opportunistic Infections (CROI); February 25-28, 2007; Los Angeles, CA. Abstract 738b.

Capparelli EV, Aweeka F, Hitti J, et al. Chronic administration of nevirapine during pregnancy: impact of pregnancy on pharmacokinetics. HIV Med. Apr 2008;9(4):214-220. Available at http://www.ncbi.nlm.nih.gov/pubmed/18366444.

Capparelli EV, Best BM, Stek A, et al. Pharmacokinetics of darunavir once or twice daily during pregnancy and postpartum. Paper presented at: 3rd International Workshop on HIV Pediatrics; July 15-16, 2011; Rome, Italy.

Capparelli EV, Stek A, Best B, et al. Boosted fosamprenavir pharmacokinetics during Pregnancy. Paper presented at: 17th Conference on Retroviruses and Opportunistic Infections (CROI); February 16-19, 2010; San Francisco, CA. Abstract 908.

Conradie F, Zorrilla C, Josipovic D, et al. Safety and exposure of once-daily ritonavir-boosted atazanavir in HIV-infected pregnant women. HIV Med. Oct 2011;12(9):570-579. Available at http://www.ncbi.nlm.nih.gov/pubmed/21569187

Cressey TR, Jourdain G, Rawangban B, et al. Pharmacokinetics and virologic response of zidovudine/lopinavir/ritonavir initiated during the third trimester of pregnancy. AIDS. Sep 10 2010;24(14):2193-2200. Available at http://www.ncbi.nlm.nih.gov/pubmed/20625263.

Cressey TR, Stek A, Capparelli E, et al. Efavirenz pharmacokinetics during the third trimester of pregnancy and postpartum. J Acquir Immune Defic Syndr. Mar 1 2012;59(3):245-252. Available at http://www.ncbi.nlm.nih.gov/pubmed/22083071.

De Santis M, Carducci B, De Santis L, Cavaliere AF, Straface G. Periconceptional exposure to efavirenz and neural tube defects. Arch Intern Med. Feb 11 2002;162(3):355. Available at http://www.ncbi.nlm.nih.gov/pubmed/11822930.

Dieterich DT, Robinson PA, Love J, Stern JO. Drug-induced liver injury associated with the use of nonnucleoside reverse-transcriptase inhibitors. Clin Infect Dis. 2004;38 (Suppl 2):S80-89. Available at http://www.ncbi.nlm.nih.gov/entrez/query.fcg i?cmd=Retrieve&db=pubmed&dopt=Abstract&l ist_uids=14986279.

Flynn PM, Mirochnick M, Shapiro DE, et al. Pharmacokinetics and safety of single-dose tenofovir disoproxil fumarate and emtricitabine in HIV-1-infected pregnant women and their infants. Antimicrob Agents Chemother. Dec 2011;55(12):5914-5922. Available at http://www.ncbi.nlm.nih.gov/pubmed/21896911.

Fundaro C, Genovese O, Rendeli C, Tamburrini E, Salvaggio E. Myelomeningocele in a child with intrauterine exposure to efavirenz. AIDS. Jan 25 2002;16(2):299-300. Available at http://www.ncbi.nlm.nih.gov/pubmed/11807320.

Gafni RI, Hazra R, Reynolds JC, et al. Tenofovir disoproxil fumarate and an optimized background regimen of antiretroviral agents as salvage therapy: impact on bone mineral density in HIV-infected children. Pediatrics. Sep 2006;118(3):e711-718. Available at http://www.ncbi.nlm.nih.gov/pubmed/16923923.

Ghosn J, De Montgolfier I, Cornelie C, et al. Antiretroviral therapy with a twice-daily regimen containing 400 milligrams of indinavir and 100 milligrams of ritonavir in human immunodeficiency virus type 1-infected women during pregnancy. Antimicrob Agents Chemother. Apr 2008;52(4):1542-1544. Available at http://www.ncbi.nlm.nih.gov/pubmed/18250187.

Hayashi S, Beckerman K, Homma M, Kosel BW, Aweeka FT. Pharmacokinetics of indinavir in HIV-positive pregnant women. AIDS. May 26 2000;14(8):1061-1062. Available at http://www.ncbi.nlm.nih.gov/pubmed/10853990.

Hirt D, Urien S, Ekouevi DK, et al. Population pharmacokinetics of tenofovir in HIV-1-infected pregnant women and their neonates (ANRS 12109). Clin Pharmacol Ther. Feb 2009;85(2):182-189. Available at http://www.ncbi.nlm.nih.gov/pubmed/18987623.

Izurieta P, Kakuda TN, Feys C, Witek J. Safety and pharmacokinetics of etravirine in pregnant HIV-1-infected women. HIV Med. Apr 2011;12(4):257-258. Available at http://www.ncbi.nlm.nih.gov/pubmed/21371239.

Lambert JS, Else LJ, Jackson V, et al. Therapeutic drug monitoring of lopinavir/ritonavir in pregnancy. HIV Med. Mar 2011;12(3):166-173. Available at http://www.ncbi.nlm.nih.gov/pubmed/20726906.

Mallal S, Phillips E, Carosi G, et al. HLA-B*5701 screening for hypersensitivity to abacavir. N Engl J Med. Feb 7 2008;358(6):568-579. Available at http://www.ncbi.nlm.nih.gov/pubmed/18256392.

McKeown DA, Rosenvinge M, Donaghy S, et al. High neonatal concentrations of raltegravir following transplacental transfer in HIV-1 positive pregnant women. AIDS. Sep 24 2010;24(15):2416-2418. Available at http://www.ncbi.nlm.nih.gov/pubmed/20827058.

Meyohas MC, Lacombe K, Carbonne B, Morand-Joubert L, Girard PM. Enfuvirtide prescription at the end of pregnancy to a multi-treated HIV-infected woman with virological breakthrough. AIDS. Sep 24 2004;18(14):1966-1968. Available at http://www.ncbi.nlm.nih.gov/pubmed/15353987.

Mirochnick M, Best BM, Stek AM, et al. Atazanavir pharmacokinetics with and without tenofovir during pregnancy. J Acquir Immune Defic Syndr. Apr 15 2011;56(5):412-419. Available at http://www.ncbi.nlm.nih.gov/pubmed/21283017.

Mirochnick M, Kafulafula G, et al. The pharmacokinetics (PK) of tenofovir disoproxil fumarate (TDF) after administration to HIV-1 infected pregnant women and their newborns. Paper presented at: 16th Conference on Retroviruses and Opportunistic Infections (CROI); February 8-11, 2009; Montreal, Canada. Abstract 940.

Mirochnick M, Kunwenda N, Joao E, et al. Tenofovir disoproxil fumarate (TDF) pharmacokinetics (PK) with increased doses in HIV-1 infected pregnant women and their newborns (HPTN 057). Paper presented at: 11th International Workshop on Clinical Pharmacology of HIV Therapy; April 7-9, 2010; Sorrento, Italy. Abstract 3.

Mirochnick M, Siminski S, Fenton T, Lugo M, Sullivan JL. Nevirapine pharmacokinetics in pregnant women and in their infants after in utero exposure. Pediatr Infect Dis J. Aug 2001;20(8):803-805. Available at http://www.ncbi.nlm.nih.gov/pubmed/11734746.

Mirochnick M, Stek A, Capparelli EV, et al. Pharmacokinetics of increased dose atazanavir with and without tenofovir during pregnancy. Paper presented at: 12th International Workshop on Clinical Pharmacology of HIV Therapy; April 13-16, 2011; Miami, FL.

Moodley J, Moodley D, Pillay K, et al. Pharmacokinetics and antiretroviral activity of lamivudine alone or when coadministered with zidovudine in human immunodeficiency virus type 1-infected pregnant women and their offspring. J Infect Dis. Nov 1998;178(5):1327-1333. Available at http://www.ncbi.nlm.nih.gov/pubmed/9780252.

Natha M, Hay P, Taylor G, et al. Atazanavir use in pregnancy: a report of 33 cases. Paper presented at: 14th Conference on Retroviruses and Opportunistic Infections (CROI); February 25-28, 2007; Los Angeles, CA. Abstract 750.

O'Sullivan MJ, Boyer PJ, Scott GB, et al. The pharmacokinetics and safety of zidovudine in the third trimester of pregnancy for women infected with human immunodeficiency virus and their infants: phase I acquired immunodeficiency syndrome clinical trials group study (protocol 082). Zidovudine Collaborative Working Group. Am J Obstet Gynecol. 1993;168(5):1510-1516. Available at http://www.ncbi.nlm.nih.gov/entrez/query.fcgi?cmd=Retrieve&db=pubmed&dopt=Abstract&list_uids=8098905.

Read JS, Best BM, Stek AM, et al. Pharmacokinetics of new 625 mg nelfinavir formulation during pregnancy and postpartum. HIV Med. Nov 2008;9(10):875-882. Available at http://www.ncbi.nlm.nih.gov/pubmed/18795962.

Ripamonti D, Cattaneo D, Maggiolo F, et al. Atazanavir plus low-dose ritonavir in pregnancy: pharmacokinetics and placental transfer. AIDS. Nov 30 2007;21(18):2409-2415. Available at http://www.ncbi.nlm.nih.gov/pubmed/18025877.

Saag M, Balu R, Phillips E, et al. High sensitivity of human leukocyte antigen-b*5701 as a marker for immunologically confirmed abacavir hypersensitivity in white and black patients. Clin Infect Dis. Apr 1 2008;46(7):1111-1118. Available at http://www.ncbi.nlm.nih.gov/pubmed/18444831.

Sarner L, Fakoya A. Acute onset lactic acidosis and pancreatitis in the third trimester of pregnancy in HIV 1 positive women taking antiretroviral medication. Sex Transm Infect. Feb 2002;78(1):58-59. Available at http://www.ncbi.nlm.nih.gov/pubmed/11872862.

Schooley RT, Ruane P, Myers RA, et al. Tenofovir DF in antiretroviral-experienced patients: results from a 48-week, randomized, double-blind study. AIDS. Jun 14 2002;16(9):1257-1263. Available at http://www.ncbi.nlm.nih.gov/pubmed/12045491.

Scott GB, Rodman JH, Scott WA, et al. for the PACTG 354 Protocol Team. Pharmacokinetic and virologic response to ritonavir (RTV) in combination with zidovudine (XDV) and lamivudine (3TC) in HIV-1 infected pregnant women and their infants. Paper presented at: 9th Conference on Retroviruses and Opportunistic Infections (CROI); February 24-28, 2002; Seattle, WA. Abstract 794-W. Available at http://www.retroconference.org/2002/.

Stek AM, Mirochnick M, Capparelli E, et al. Reduced lopinavir exposure during pregnancy. AIDS. Oct 3 2006;20(15):1931-1939. Available at http://www.ncbi.nlm.nih.gov/pubmed/16988514.

Tarantal AF, Castillo A, Ekert JE, Bischofberger N, Martin RB. Fetal and maternal outcome after administration of tenofovir to gravid rhesus monkeys (Macaca mulatta). J Acquir Immune Defic Syndr. Mar 1 2002;29(3):207-220. Available at http://www.ncbi.nlm.nih.gov/pubmed/11873070.

Unadkat JD, Wara DW, Hughes MD, et al. Pharmacokinetics and safety of indinavir in human immunodeficiency virus-infected pregnant women. Antimicrob Agents Chemother. Feb 2007;51(2):783-786. Available at http://www.ncbi.nlm.nih.gov/pubmed/17158945.

van der Lugt J, Colbers A, Molto J, et al. The pharmacokinetics, safety and efficacy of boosted saquinavir tablets in HIV type-1-infected pregnant women. Antivir Ther. 2009;14(3):443-450. Available at http://www.ncbi.nlm.nih.gov/pubmed/19474478.

Villani P, Floridia M, Pirillo MF, et al. Pharmacokinetics of nelfinavir in HIV-1-infected pregnant and nonpregnant women. Br J Clin Pharmacol. Sep 2006;62(3):309-315. Available at http://www.ncbi.nlm.nih.gov/pubmed/16934047.

Wade NA, Unadkat JD, Huang S, et al. Pharmacokinetics and safety of stavudine in HIV-infected pregnant women and their infants: Pediatric AIDS Clinical Trials Group protocol 332. J Infect Dis. Dec 15 2004;190(12):2167-2174. Available at http://www.ncbi.nlm.nih.gov/pubmed/15551216.

Wang Y, Livingston E, Patil S, et al. Pharmacokinetics of didanosine in antepartum and postpartum human immunodeficiency virus–infected pregnant women and their neonates: an AIDS clinical trials group study. J Infect Dis. 1999;180(5):1536-1541. Available at http://www.ncbi.nlm.nih.gov/entrez/query.fcgi?cmd=Retrieve&db=pubmed&dopt=Abstract&list_uids=10515813.

Weizsaecker K, Kurowski M, Hoffmeister B, Schurmann D, Feiterna-Sperling C. Pharmacokinetic profile in late pregnancy and cord blood concentration of tipranavir and enfuvirtide. Int J STD AIDS. May 2011;22(5):294-295. Available at http://www.ncbi.nlm.nih.gov/pubmed/21571982.

Chapter 8

Post-Exposure and Pre-Exposure Prophylaxis

OCCUPATIONAL POST-EXPOSURE PROPHYLAXIS (PEP)

The CDC estimates > 600,000 significant exposures to blood-borne pathogens occur yearly. Of 56 confirmed cases of HIV acquisition in healthcare workers, more than 90% involved percutaneous exposure, with the remaining cases due to mucous membrane/non-intact skin exposure. Estimates of HIV seroconversion rates after percutaneous and mucous membrane exposure to HIV-infected blood are 0.3% and 0.09%, respectively; lower rates of transmission occur after nonintact skin exposure, and no transmission has thus far been reported to occur through intact skin. (By comparison, the risks of seroconversion after percutaneous exposure to Hepatitis B and Hepatitis C viruses are 30% and 3%, respectively.) Risk factors for increased risk of HIV transmission after percutaneous exposure include deep injury (odds ratio 16.1), visible blood on device (odds ratio 5.2), source patient is terminally ill (odds ratio 6.4), or needle was in source patient's artery/vein (odds ratio 5.1); ZDV prophylaxis reduces the risk of transmission (odds ratio 0.2). All guidelines suggest PEP should be administered as soon as possible after exposure, but there is no absolute window (e.g., within 1–2 weeks) after which PEP should be withheld following serious exposure.

National guidelines for occupational post-exposure prophylaxis were updated in 2013 (Infect Control Hosp Epidemiology 2013;34:875-892). They are available on line free of charge http://www.jstor.org/stable/10.1086/672271. These guidelines replace a 2005 version with several substantial changes, including: 1) All PEP regimens should consist of three antiviral drugs; 2) the preferred PEP regimen is TDF/FTC plus raltegravir, with several alternative choices listed; 3) if a newer fourth-generation combination HIV p24 antigen–HIV antibody test is utilized for follow-up HIV testing of exposed HCP, HIV testing may be concluded 4 months after exposure.

The content in this chapter is adapted from both these updated guidelines and those issued by New York State (http://www.hivguidelines.org/clinical-guidelines/post-exposure-prophylaxis/hiv-prophylaxis-following-occupational-exposure/). Additional information can be found at the National Clinicians' Post-exposure Prophylaxis Hotline (http://www.nccc.ucsf.edu/about_nccc/pepline/ or 888-448-4911). Occupationally acquired HIV infections and PEP failures should be reported to the CDC at 404-639-2050.

Table 8.1. Estimated Per-Act Probability of Acquiring HIV from an Infected Source, by Exposure Act[1]

Type of Exposure	Risk per 10,000 Exposures
Parenteral	
Blood Transfusion	9,000[2]
Needle-sharing during injection drug use	67[3]
Percutaneous (needle-stick)	30[4]

Table 8.1. Estimated Per-Act Probability of Acquiring HIV from an Infected Source, by Exposure Act[1] (cont'd)

Type of Exposure	Risk per 10,000 Exposures
Sexual	
Receptive anal intercourse	50[5, 6]
Receptive penile-vaginal intercourse	10[5, 6, 7]
Insertive anal intercourse	6.5[5, 6]
Insertive penile-vaginal intercourse	5[5, 6]
Receptive oral intercourse	Low[5, 9]
Insertive oral intercourse	Low[5, 9]
Other[8]	
Biting	Negligible[10]
Spitting	negligible
Throwing body fluids (including semen or saliva)	negligible
Sharing sex toys	negligible

1. Factors that increase the risk of HIV transmission include sexually transmitted infections, early and late-stage HIV infection, and a high level of HIV in the blood. Factors that reduce the risk of HIV transmission include condom use, male circumcision, and use of antiretrovirals.
2. Donegan E, Stuart M, Niland JC, et al. Infection with human immunodeficiency virus type 1 (HIV-1) among recipients of antibody-positive blood donations. *Ann Intern Med* 1990;113(10):733–739.
3. Kaplan EH, Heimer R. A model-based estimate of HIV infectivity via needle sharing. *J Acquir Immune Defic Syndr* 1992;5(11):1116–1118.
4. Bell DM. Occupational risk of human immunodeficiency virus infection in healthcare workers: an overview. *Am J Med* 1997;102(5B):9–15.
5. Varghese B, Maher JE, Peterman TA, Branson BM, Steketee RW. Reducing the risk of sexual HIV transmission: quantifying the per-act risk for HIV on the basis of choice of partner, sex act, and condom use. *Sex Transm Dis* 2002;29(1):38–43.
6. European Study Group on Heterosexual Transmission of HIV. Comparison of female to male and male to female transmission of HIV in 563 stable couples. *BMJ* 1992;304(6830):809–813.
7. Leynaert B, Downs AM, de Vincenzi I; European Study Group on Heterosexual Transmission of HIV. Heterosexual transmission of HIV: variability of infectivity throughout the course of infection. *Am J Epidemiol* 1998;148(1):88–96.
8. HIV transmission through these exposure routes is technically possible but extremely unlikely and not well documented.
9. HIV transmission through oral sex has been documented, but rare. Accurate estimates of risk are not available.
10. Pretty LA, Anderson GS, Sweet DJ. Human bites and the risk of human immunodeficiency virus transmission. *Am J Forensic Med Pathol* 1999;20(3):232–239.

Data from: *MMWR Recomm Rep* 54 (RR–2): 1–20.

Further Reading

Cohen MS, Chen YQ, McCauley M, et al; HPTN 052 Study Team. Prevention of HIV-1 Infection with early antiretroviral therapy. *N Engl J Med* 2011;365(6):493–505.

Weller SC, Davis-Beaty K. *Condom effectiveness in reducing heterosexual HIV transmission (Review)*. The Cochrane Collaboration. Wiley and Sons, 2011.

General recommendations for management include:

- Initiate PEP as soon as possible after exposure and continue PEP for 4 weeks if HIV infection in the source patient cannot be excluded
- Seek expert consultation for a wide range of situations, in particular when the source patient has viral resistance or the exposed individual may be pregnant (see Table 8.2)
- Offer pregnancy testing to all women of childbearing age not known to be pregnant
- Advise exposed persons to seek medical evaluation for any acute illness during follow-up
- Perform HIV-antibody testing and HIV RNA testing for any illness compatible with an acute retroviral syndrome (e.g., pharyngitis, fever, rash, myalgia, fatigue, malaise, lymphadenopathy)

Table 8.2. Situations for Which Expert Consultation for Human Immunodeficiency Virus (HIV) Postexposure Prophylaxis (PEP) Is Recommended

Delayed (i.e., later than 72 hours) exposure report
- Interval after which benefits from PEP are undefined

Unknown source (e.g., needle in sharps disposal container or laundry)
- Use of PEP to be decided on a case-by-case basis
- Consider severity of exposure and epidemiologic likelihood of HIV exposure
- Do not test needles or other sharp instruments for HIV

Known or suspected pregnancy in the exposed person
- Provision of PEP should not be delayed while awaiting expert consultation

Breast-feeding in the exposed person
- Provision of PEP should not be delayed while awaiting expert consultation

Known or suspected resistance of the source virus to antiretroviral agents
- If source person's virus is known or suspected to be resistant to 1 or more of the drugs considered for PEP, selection of drugs to which the source person's virus is unlikely to be resistant is recommended
- Do not delay initiation of PEP while awaiting any results of resistance testing of the source person's virus

Toxicity of the initial PEP regimen
- Symptoms (e.g., gastrointestinal symptoms and others) are often manageable without changing PEP regimen by prescribing antimotility or antiemetic agents
- Counseling and support for management of side effects is very important, as symptoms are often exacerbated by anxiety

Serious medical illness in the exposed person
- Significant underlying illness (e.g., renal disease) or an exposed provider already taking multiple medications may increase the risk of drug toxicity and drug-drug interactions

Expert consultation can be made with local experts or by calling the National Clinicians' Post-Exposure Prophylaxis Hotline (PEPline) at 888-448-4911.

- Perform HIV-antibody testing for at least 6 months post-exposure (at baseline, 6 weeks, 3 months, and 6 months)

- Advise exposed persons to use precautions to prevent secondary transmission during follow-up, especially during the first 6–12 weeks, when most HIV-infected patients will seroconvert. Precautions include sexual abstinence or use of condoms, refrain from donating blood, plasma, organs, tissue or semen, and discontinuation of breast-feeding after high-risk exposures

- Evaluate exposed persons taking PEP within 72 hours after exposure, and monitor for drug toxicity for at least 2 weeks. Approximately 50% will experience nausea, malaise, headache, or anorexia, and about one-third will discontinue PEP due to drug toxicity. Lab monitoring

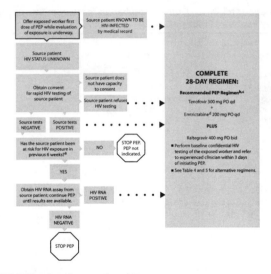

Figure 8.1. PEP Following Occupational Exposure

a   Depending on the test used, the window period may be shorter than 6 weeks. Clinicians should contact appropriate laboratory authorities to determine the window period for the test that is being used.

b   If the source is known to be HIV-infected, information about his/her viral load, ART medication history, and history of antiretroviral drug resistance should be obtained when possible to assist in selection of a PEP regimen.[9]
    Initiation of the first dose of PEP should not be delayed while awaiting this information and/or results of resistance testing. When this information becomes available, the PEP regimen may be changed if needed in consultation with an experienced provider.

Reproduced from: New York State Department of Health AIDS Institute, 2013.

should include (at a minimum) a CBC, serum creatinine, liver function tests, serum glucose (if receiving a protease inhibitor to detect hyperglycemia), and monitoring for HBV and HCV. Serious adverse events should be reported to the FDA's MedWatch Program

- If available, employees with workplace exposure should follow up in their designated occupational health sites according to employer policies. This will help retain rights and/ or benefits defined by the job in case of infection

Table 8.3A. Follow-Up of Healthcare Personnel (HCP) Exposed to Known or Suspected Human Immunodeficiency Virus (HIV)-Positive Sources

Counseling (at the time of exposure and at follow-up appointments). Exposed HCP should be advised to use precautions (e.g., use of barrier contraception and avoidance of blood or tissue donations, pregnancy, and, if possible, breastfeeding) to prevent secondary transmission, especially during the first 6-12 weeks after exposure.

For exposures for which postexposure prophylaxis (PEP) is prescribed, HCP should be informed regarding the following:

- Possible drug toxicities (e.g., rash and hypersensitivity reactions that could imitate acute HIV seroconversion and the need for monitoring)
- Possible drug interactions
- The need for adherence to PEP regimens

Early reevaluation after exposure. Regardless of whether a healthcare provider is taking PEP, reevaluation of exposed HCP within 72 hours after exposure is strongly recommended, as additional information about the exposure or source person may be available.

Follow-up testing and appointments. Follow-up testing at a minimum should include the following:

- HIV testing at baseline and at 6 weeks, 12 weeks, and 6 months after exposure; alternatively, if the clinician is certain that a fourth-generation combination HIV p24 antigen-HIV antibody test is being utilized, then HIV testing could be performed at baseline, 6 weeks after exposure, and 4 months after exposure
- Complete blood counts and renal and hepatic function tests (at baseline and 2 weeks after exposure; further testing may be indicated if abnormalities are detected)

HIV testing results should preferably be given to the exposed healthcare provider at face-to-face appointments.

Reproduced from: Updated U.S. Public Health Service Guidelines for the Management of Occupational Exposures to HIV and Recommendations for Postexposure Prophylaxis/CDC.

Table 8.3B. Human Immunodeficiency Virus (HIV) Postexposure Prophylaxis (PEP) Regimens

Preferred HIV PEP Regimen
Raltegravir (Isentress; RAL) 400 mg PO twice daily
Plus
Truvada, 1 PO once daily
(Tenofovir DF [Viread; TDF] 300 mg + emtricitabine [Emtriva; FTC] 200 mg)

Table 8.3B. Human Immunodeficiency Virus (HIV) Postexposure Prophylaxis (PEP) Regimens (cont'd)

Alternative Regimens
(May combine 1 drug or drug pair from the left column with 1 pair of nucleoside/nucleotide reverse-transcriptase inhibitors from the right column; prescribers unfamiliar with these agents/ regimens should consult physicians familiar with the agents and their toxicities)[a]

Raltegravir (Isentress; RAL)	Tenofovir DF (Viread; TDF) + emtricitabine (Emtriva; FTC); available as Truvada
Darunavir (Prezista; DRV) + ritonavir (Norvir; RTV)	
Etravirine (Intelence; ETR)	Tenofovir DF (Viread; TDF) + lamivudine (Epivir; 3TC)
Rilpivirine (Edurant; RPV)	Zidovudine (Retrovir; ZDV; AZT) + lamivudine (Epivir; 3TC); available as Combivir
Atazanavir (Reyataz; ATV) + ritonavir (Norvir; RTV)	
Lopinavir/ritonavir (Kaletra; LPV/RTV)	Zidovudine (Retrovir; ZDV; AZT) + emtricitabine (Emtriva; FTC)

The following alternative is a complete fixed-dose combination regimen, and no additional antiretrovirals are needed: Stribild (elvitegravir, cobicistat, tenofovir DF, emtricitabine)

Alternative Antiretroviral Agents for Use as PEP Only with Expert Consultation
Abacavir (Ziagen; ABC)
Efavirenz (Sustiva; EFV)
Enfuvirtide (Fuzeon; T20)
Fosamprenavir (Lexiva; FOSAPV)
Maraviroc (Selzentry; MVC)
Saquinavir (Invirase; SQV)
Stavudine (Zerit; d4T)

Antiretroviral Agents Generally Not Recommended for Use as PEP
Didanosine (Videx EC; ddI)
Nelfinavir (Viracept; NFV)
Tipranavir (Aptivus; TPV)

Antiretroviral Agents Contraindicated as PEP
Nevirapine (Viramune; NVP)

Note: For consultation or assistance with HIV PEP, contact the National Clinicians' Post-Exposure Prophylaxis Hotline at telephone number 888-448-4911 or visit its website at http://www.nccc.ucsf.edu/ about_ccc/pepline/. DF, disoproxil fumarate; PO, per os.
[a] The alternatives regimens are listed in order of preference; however, other alternatives may be reasonable based on patient and clinician preference.

Data from: Updated U.S. Public Health Service Guidelines for the Management of Occupational Exposures to HIV and Recommendations for Postexposure Prophylaxis/CDC.

NONOCCUPATIONAL POST-EXPOSURE PROPHYLAXIS (NPEP)

In January, 2005, the US Department of Health and Human Services issued recommendations for antiretroviral PEP after sexual, injection-drug use, and other nonoccupational exposures to HIV (MMWR 2005;54[RR-2]:1–28). These guidelines are currently undergoing revision, and as a result we suggest that the same antiviral regimens listed in the 2013 guidelines for occupational PEP be used in this context as well.

An interim resource for non-occupational PEP management is the New York State State Department of Health AIDS Institute, which updated its non-occupational PEP guidelines in 2013 (http://www.hivguidelines.org/clinical-guidelines/post-exposure-prophylaxis/hiv-prophylaxis-following-non-occupational-exposure/#table1). These are used to frame the discussion below.

A. **Evaluation.** The evaluation of a person seeking nonoccupational PEP should include Evaluation: Risk assessment and initiation of nPEP should occur in clinical settings that can provide the following:

- Assessment of HIV risk following exposure
- HIV and STI testing and treatment
- Prevention and risk-reduction counseling
- Clinicians with expertise in the use of ART
- Timely access to care and initiation of nPEP

If all of these services are not available, clinicians should assess the exposure and initiate nPEP when indicated according to the criteria and recommendations in these guidelines. The patient should then be referred for follow-up care to a clinician who has experience in the use of antiretroviral agents and who can provide ongoing prevention counseling.

Treating clinicians who do not have access to experienced HIV clinicians should call the National Clinicians' Consultation Center PEPline at 1-888-448-4911 to review the case.

Patients who present for nPEP should be evaluated as soon as possible in order to initiate therapy, if indicated, within recommended timeframes (preferably < 72 hours).

When an HIV exposure occurs, the events and the subsequent interventions should be clearly documented in order to facilitate determination of the effectiveness of nPEP.

B. **Use of Antiretroviral Therapy.** As noted above, the same preferred and alternative regimens used for occupational PEP should be used for non-occupational PEP (see Table 8.4). The duration of therapy is 28 days.

C. **Follow-up Testing.** The updated New York State non-occupational PEP guidelines are summarized in Table 8.5 below. Note that the duration of follow-up is limited to 12 weeks; the expert panel no longer recommends the 6-month follow-up visit because such delayed seroconversion has not been reported since 1990, presumably due to the far greater sensitivity of current HIV antibody testing.

Table 8.4. Consideration of nPEP According to the Type of Risk Exposure

Types of Exposures for Which nPEP Should Be Recommended (higher-risk exposures)	• Receptive and insertive vaginal or anal intercourse[a] • Needle sharing[a] • Injuries with exposure to blood or other potentially infected fluids from a source known to be HIV-infected or HIV status is unknown (including needlesticks with a hollow-bore needle, human bites, accidents)
Lower-Risk Exposures That Require Case-by-Case Evaluation for nPEP (lower-risk exposures: assess for factors that increase risk before recommending initiation of nPEP)	• Oral-vaginal contact (receptive and insertive) • Oral-anal contact (receptive and insertive) • Receptive penile-oral contact with or without ejaculation • Insertive penile-oral contact with or without ejaculation
	Factors that increase risk: • Source person is known to be HIV-infected with high viral load • An oral mucosa that is not intact (e.g., oral lesions, gingivitis, wounds) • Blood exposure — it is important to note that blood exposure can be minimal and therefore not recognized by the exposed person. If the exposed person reports frank blood exposure, PEP would be indicated • Presence of genital ulcer disease or other STIs
Types of Exposures That Do Not Warrant nPEP (no risk)	• Kissing[b] • Oral-to-oral contact without mucosal damage (mouth-to-mouth resuscitation) • Human bites not involving blood • Exposure to solid-bore needles or sharps not in recent contact with blood[c] • Mutual masturbation without skin breakdown or blood exposure

[a] With a source known to be HIV-infected or HIV status is unknown.

[b] There is no risk associated with close-mouthed kissing. There is a remote risk associated with open-mouthed kissing if there are sores or bleeding gums and blood is exchanged.

[c] Examples of solid-bore needles include tattoo needles and lancets used by diabetics to measure blood-sugar levels.

Reproduced from: New York State Department of Health AIDS Institute, 2013.

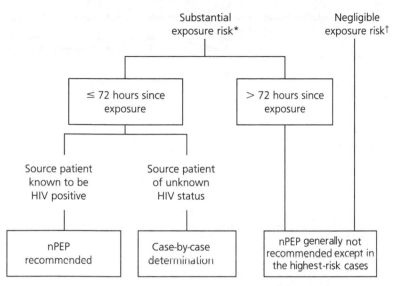

Figure 8.2. Evaluation and Treatment of Possible Nonoccupational HIV Exposures

nPEP = nonoccupational post-exposure prophylaxis

* Substantial risk for HIV exposure = exposure of vagina, rectum, eye, mouth, or other mucous membrane, nonintact skin, or percutaneous contact with blood, semen, vaginal secretions, rectal secretions, breast milk, or any body fluid that is visibly contaminated with blood when the source is know to be HIV-infected

† Negligible risk for HIV exposure = exposure of vagina, rectum, eye, mouth, or other mucous membrane, intact or nonintact skin, or percutaneous contact with urine, nasal secretions, saliva, sweat, or tears if not visibly contaminated with blood regardless of the known or suspected HIV status of the source

Reproduced from: Centers for Disease Control and Prevention, MMWR January 21, 2005 / 54(RR02);1–20.

Table 8.5. Monitoring Recommendations After Initiation of PEP Regimens Following Non-occupational Exposures

	Baseline	Week 1	Week 2	Week 3	Week 4	Week 12
Clinic Visit	√	√ Or by telephone	√ Or by telephone	√ Or by telephone	√	
Pregnancy Test	√					
Serum liver enzymes, BUN, creatinine, CBCᵃ	√		√		√	

Table 8.5. Monitoring Recommendations After Initiation of PEP Regimens Following Non-occupational Exposures (cont'd)

	Baseline	Week 1	Week 2	Week 3	Week 4	Week 12
HIV test[b]	√				√	√
STI Screening *(for exposures unrelated to sexual assault)*[b]: **GC/CT NAAT (based on site of exposure) RPR** See *HIV Prophylaxis for Victims of Sexual Assault* for recommendations in cases of sexual assault.	√		√ (consider)			
Hepatitis B and C[b]	For post-exposure management for hepatitis B and C, see Section IX: *Non-Occupational Exposures to Hepatitis B and C*					

[a] CBC should be obtained for all exposed persons at baseline. Follow-up CBC is indicated only for those receiving a zidovudine-containing regimen.
[b] Recommended even if PEP is declined.

Reproduced from: New York State Department of Health AIDS Institute, 2013.

PRE-EXPOSURE PROPHYLAXIS

Pre-Exposure prophylaxis (PrEP) refers to the practice of giving high-risk HIV uninfected individuals antiretroviral therapy to prevent them from becoming infected. PrEP has been shown to be effective in high men who have sex with men (MSM), heterosexual men and women, and injection drug users.

The first study demonstrating that PrEP is effective was the iPrEx study, which included nearly 2500 HIV-negative MSM in South America, the U.S., Thailand, and South Africa and randomized them in a double-blinded fashion to receive once-daily oral TDF/FTC or placebo (N Engl J Med 2010; 363:2587–2599). Those receiving active PrEP had a 44% reduction in the risk of acquiring HIV, with the efficacy much better in those with good medication adherence. No major toxicity was seen in the TDF/FTC group. Subsequently, additional studies conducted in sub-Saharan Africa among heterosexual men and women have also shown PrEP to be effective provided medication adherence is adequate. Studies that have failed to demonstrate the efficacy of PrEP have invariably shown very low rates of pill taking by the participants.

Based on the results of these studies, the CDC issued an interim guidance on the use of PrEP in clinical practice, initially for MSM and subsequently for heterosexuals and injection drug users. Note that in the United States, these recommendations apply only to high risk individuals; the incidence of HIV among heterosexuals at "community risk" in the United States is too low to warrant PrEP. Similarly, MSM and injection drug users who are at low risk for HIV would not be candidates for PrEP.

The full reports are available at http://www.cdc.gov/mmwr/preview/mmwrhtml/mm6003a1.htm?s_cid=mm6003a1_w and http://www.cdc.gov/mmwr/preview/mmwrhtml/mm6131a2.htm?s_cid=mm6131a2_e and http://www.cdc.gov/mmwr/preview/mmwrhtml/mm6223a2.htm.

Before initiating PrEP

Determine eligibility
- Document negative HIV antibody test(s) immediately before starting PrEP medication.
- Test for acute HIV infection if patient has symptoms consistent with acute HIV infection.
- Confirm that patient is at substantial, ongoing, high risk for acquiring HIV infection.
- Confirm that calculated creatinine clearance is ≥ 60 mL per minute (via Cockcroft–Gault formula).

Other recommended actions
- Screen for hepatitis B infection; vaccinate against hepatitis B if susceptible, or treat if active infection exists, regardless of decision about prescribing PrEP.
- Screen and treat as needed for STIs.

Beginning PrEP medication regimen

- Prescribe 1 tablet of Truvada* (TDF [300 mg] plus FTC [200 mg]) daily.
- In general, prescribe no more than a 90-day supply, renewable only after HIV testing confirms that patient remains HIV-uninfected.
- If active hepatitis B infection is diagnosed, consider using TDF/FTC for both treatment of active hepatitis B infection and HIV prevention.
- Provide risk-reduction and PrEP medication adherence counseling and condoms.

Follow-up while PrEP medication is being taken

- Every 2–3 months, perform an HIV antibody test; document negative result.
- Evaluate and support PrEP medication adherence at each follow-up visit, more often if inconsistent adherence is identified.
- Every 2–3 months, assess risk behaviors and provide risk-reduction counseling and condoms. Assess STI symptoms and, if present, test and treat for STI as needed.
- Every 6 months, test for STI even if patient is asymptomatic, and treat as needed.
- 3 months after initiation, then yearly while on PrEP medication, check blood urea nitrogen and serum creatinine.

On discontinuing PrEP (at patient request, for safety concerns, or if HIV infection is acquired)

- Perform HIV test(s) to confirm whether HIV infection has occurred.
- If HIV positive, order and document results of resistance testing and establish linkage to HIV care.
- If HIV negative, establish linkage to risk-reduction support services as indicated.
- If active hepatitis B is diagnosed at initiation of PrEP, consider appropriate medication for continued treatment of hepatitis B.

Abbreviations: HIV = human immunodeficiency virus; STI = sexually transmitted infection; TDF = tenofovir disoproxil fumarate; FTC = emtricitabine.

Chapter 9

Antiretroviral, Anti-HBV, and Anti-HCV Drug Summaries

David W. Kubiak, PharmD, BCPS
Demary Torres, PharmD

This section contains prescribing information pertinent to the clinical use of antiretroviral agents in adults, as compiled from a variety of sources, including MICROMEDEX®, Micromedex 2.0 Up to Date on-line version 21.2®, Department of Health and Human Services Guidelines for the use of antiretroviral agents in HIV-1-infected adults and adolescents (www.aidsinfo.nih.gov/guidelines/), March 27, 2013, manufacturers' product information, among others. The information provided is not exhaustive, and the reader is referred to other drug information references and the manufacturer's product literature for further information. Clinical use of the information provided and any consequences that may arise from its use are the responsibilities of the prescribing physician. The authors, editors, and publisher do not warrant or guarantee the information contained in this section, and do not assume and expressly disclaim any liability for errors or omissions or any consequences that may occur from such. **The use of any drug should be preceded by careful review of the package insert, which provides indications and dosing approved by the U.S. Food and Drug Administration. This information can be obtained on the website provided at the end of the reference list for each drug summary.**

Drugs are listed alphabetically by generic name; trade names follow in parentheses. To search by trade name, consult the index. Each drug summary contains the following information:

Usual Dose. Represents the usual dose to treat HIV infection in adult patients with normal hepatic and renal function. Additional information can be found in the manufacturer's package insert and product literature.

Bioavailability. Refers to the percentage of the dose reaching the systemic circulation from the site of administration (PO or IM). For PO antibiotics, bioavailability refers to the percentage of dose adsorbed from the GI tract.

Excreted Unchanged. Refers to the percentage of drug excreted unchanged, and provides an indirect measure of drug concentration in the urine/feces.

Serum Half-Life (normal/ESRD). The serum half-life ($T_{1/2}$) is the time (in hours) in which serum concentration falls by 50%. Serum half-life is useful in determining dosing interval. If the half-life of drugs eliminated by the kidneys is prolonged in end-stage renal disease (ESRD), then the total daily dose is reduced in proportion to the degree of renal dysfunction. If the half-life in ESRD is similar to the normal half-life, then the total daily dose does not change.

Plasma Protein Binding. Expressed as the percentage of drug reversibly bound to serum albumin. It is the unbound (free) portion of a drug that equilibrates with tissues and imparts antiviral activity. Plasma protein binding is not typically a factor in antimicrobial effectiveness unless binding exceeds 95%. Decreases in serum albumin (nephrotic syndrome, liver disease) or competition for protein binding from other drugs or endogenously produced substances (uremia, hyperbilirubinemia) will increase the percentage of free drug available for antimicrobial activity, and may require a decrease in dosage. Increases in serum binding proteins (trauma, surgery, critical illness) will decrease the percentage of free drug available for antimicrobial activity, and may require an increase in dosage.

Volume of Distribution (V_d). Represents the apparent volume into which the drug is distributed, and is calculated as the amount of drug in the body divided by the serum concentration (in liters/kilogram). V_d is related to total body water distribution (V_d H_2O = 0.7 L/kg). Hydrophilic (water soluble) drugs are restricted to extracellular fluid and have a $V_d \leq 0.7$ L/kg. In contrast, hydrophobic (highly lipid soluble) drugs penetrate most fluids/tissues of the body and have a large V_d. Drugs that are concentrated in certain tissues (e.g., liver) can have a V_d greatly exceeding total body water. V_d is affected by organ profusion, membrane diffusion/permeability, lipid solubility, protein binding, and state of equilibrium between body compartments. For hydrophilic drugs, increases in V_d may occur with burns, heart failure, dialysis, sepsis, cirrhosis, or mechanical ventilation; decreases in V_d may occur with trauma, hemorrhage, pancreatitis (early), or GI fluid losses. Increases in V_d may require an increase in total daily drug dose for antimicrobial effectiveness; decreases in V_d may require a decrease in drug dose. In addition to drug distribution, V_d reflects binding avidity to cholesterol membranes and concentration within organ tissues (e.g., liver).

Mode of Elimination. Refers to the primary route of inactivation/excretion of the drug, which impacts dosing adjustments in renal/hepatic failure.

Dosage Adjustments. Each grid provides dosing adjustments based on renal and hepatic function. Antimicrobial dosing for hemodialysis (HD)/peritoneal dialysis (PD) patients is the same as indicated for patients with a CrCl < 10 mL/min. Some antimicrobial agents require a supplemental dose immediately after hemodialysis (post-HD)/peritoneal dialysis (post-PD), following the supplemental dose, antimicrobial dosing should once again resume as indicated for a CrCl < 10 mL/min. "No change" indicates no change from the usual dose. "Avoid" indicates the drug should be avoided in the setting described. "None" indicates no supplemental dose is required. "No information" indicates there are insufficient data from which to make a dosing recommendation. Dosing recommendations are based on data, experience, or pharmacokinetic parameters. CVVH dosing recommendations represent general guidelines, since antibiotic removal is dependent on area/type of filter, ultrafiltration rates, and sieving coefficients; replacement dosing should be individualized and guided by serum levels, if possible. Creatinine clearance (CrCl) is used to gauge the degree of renal insufficiency, and can be estimated by the following calculation: CrCl (mL/min) = [(140 – age) × weight (kg)] / [72 × serum creatinine (mg/dL)]. The calculated value is multiplied by 0.85 for females. It is important to recognize that due to age-dependent decline in renal function, elderly patients with "normal" serum creatinines may have low CrCls requiring dosage adjustments. (For example, a 70-year-old, 50-kg female with a serum creatinine of 1.2 mg/dL has an estimated CrCl of 34 mL/min.) "Antiretroviral Dosage Adjustment" grids indicate recommended dosage adjustments when protease inhibitors (PIs) and non-nucleoside reverse transcriptase inhibitor (NNRTIs) are combined or used in conjunction with rifampin or rifabutin. These grids were compiled, in part, from "Guidelines for the Use of Antiretroviral Agents in HIV-Infected Adults and Adolescents," Panel on Clinical Practices for Treatment of HIV Infection, Department of Health and Human Services, www.aidsinfo.nih.gov/guidelines/. March 27, 2013.

Drug Interactions. Refers to common/important drug interactions, as compiled from various sources. If a specific drug interaction is well-documented, then other drugs from the same drug class (e.g., atorvastatin) may also be listed, based on theoretical considerations. Drug interactions may occur as a consequence of altered absorption (e.g., metal ion chelation of tetracycline), altered distribution (e.g., sulfonamide displacement of barbiturates from serum albumin), altered metabolism (e.g., rifampin–induced hepatic P-450 metabolism of theophylline/warfarin; chloramphenicol inhibition of phenytoin metabolism), or altered excretion (e.g., probenecid competition with penicillin for active transport in the kidney).

Adverse Side Effects. Common/important side effects are indicated.

Allergic Potential. Described as low or high. Refers to the likelihood of a hypersensitivity reaction to a particular antimicrobial.

Safety in Pregnancy. Designated by the U.S. Food and Drug Administration's (USFDA) use-in-pregnancy letter code (Table 9.1).

Antiretroviral Pregnancy Registry. To monitor maternal-fetal outcomes of pregnant women exposed to antiretroviral drugs, an Antiretroviral Pregnancy Registry has been established. Clinicians who are treating HIV-infected pregnant women are strongly encouraged to report cases of prenatal exposure to antiretroviral drugs (either administered alone or in combinations). The registry collects observational, non-experimental data regarding antiretroviral exposure during pregnancy for the purpose of assessing potential teratogenicity. Telephone: 910-251-9087 or 1-800-258-4263. Website: http://www.apregistry.com/who.htm; e-mail: registries@kendle.com

Comments. Includes various useful information for each antiretroviral agent.

Selected References. These references are classic, important, or recent. When available, the website containing the manufacturer's prescribing information/package insert is provided.

Table 9.1. USFDA Use-in-Pregnancy Letter Code

Category	Interpretation
A	**Controlled studies show no risk.** Adequate, well-controlled studies in pregnant women have not shown a risk to the fetus in any trimester of pregnancy
B	**No evidence of risk in humans.** Adequate, well-controlled studies in pregnant women have not shown increased risk of fetal abnormalities despite adverse findings in animals, or, in the absence of adequate human studies, animal studies show no fetal risk. The chance of fetal harm is remote, but remains a possibility
C	**Risk cannot be ruled out.** Adequate, well-controlled human studies are lacking, and animal studies have shown a risk to the fetus or are lacking. There is a chance of fetal harm if the drug is administered during pregnancy, but potential benefit from use of the drug may outweigh potential risk
D	**Positive evidence of risk.** Studies in humans or investigational or post-marketing data have demonstrated fetal risk. Nevertheless, potential benefit from use of the drug may outweigh potential risk. For example, the drug may be acceptable if needed in a life-threatening situation or serious disease for which safer drugs cannot be used or are ineffective
X	**Contraindicated in pregnancy.** Studies in animals or humans or investigational or post-marketing reports have demonstrated positive evidence of fetal abnormalities or risk which clearly outweigh any possible benefit to the patient

Data from: USFDA.

Abacavir (Ziagen) ABC

Drug Class: Antiretroviral NRTI (nucleoside reverse transcriptase inhibitor)
Usual Dose: HLA-B*5701 negative patients—300 mg (PO) BID
How Supplied: Oral Solution: 20 mg/mL, Oral Tablet: 300 mg
Pharmacokinetic Parameters:
Peak serum level: 3 mcg/mL
Bioavailability: 83%
Excreted unchanged (urine): 1.2%
Serum half-life (normal/ESRD): 1.5/8 hrs
Plasma protein binding: 50%
Volume of distribution (V_d): 0.86 L/kg
Primary Mode of Elimination: Hepatic
Dosage Adjustments*

CrCl 50–80 mL/min	No change
CrCl 10–50 mL/min	No change
CrCl < 10 mL/min	No change
Post-HD dose	None
Post-PD dose	None
CVVH dose	No change
Mild hepatic insufficiency	200 mg (PO) QD
Moderate or severe hepatic insufficiency	Avoid

Drug Interactions: Methadone (↑ methadone clearance with abacavir 600 mg BID); ethanol (↑ abacavir serum levels/half-life and may ↑ toxicity).
Adverse Effects: *Abacavir may cause severe hypersensitivity reactions (see comments), usually during the first 4–6 weeks of therapy, which may be fatal;* report cases of hypersensitivity syndrome to Abacavir Hypersensitivity Registry at 1-800-270-0425. Drug fever/rash, abdominal pain/diarrhea, nausea, vomiting, anorexia, insomnia, weakness, headache, ↑ SGOT/SGPT, hyperglycemia, hypertriglyceridemia, lactic acidosis with hepatic steatosis (rare, but potentially life-threatening toxicity with use of NRTIs). Potential for increased cardiovascular events, especially in patients with cardiovascular risk factors.
Allergic Potential: High (~ 5%)
Safety in Pregnancy: C
Comments: May be taken with or without foods. **HLA-B*5701 testing should precede the use of abacavir or an abacavir-containing regimen to reduce the risk of hypersensitivity reaction. Immediately and permanently discontinue if a hypersensitivity reaction occurs; never restart abacavir sulfate/lamivudine following a hypersensitivity reaction** or if hypersensitivity cannot be ruled out, which may include fever, rash, fatigue, nausea, vomiting, diarrhea, abdominal pain, anorexia, respiratory symptoms., which may include fever, rash, fatigue, nausea, vomiting, diarrhea, abdominal pain, anorexia, respiratory symptoms. Ethanol increases abacavir levels by 41%.
Cerebrospinal Fluid Penetration: 27–33%

REFERENCES:
Carr A, Workman C, Smith DE, et al. Abacavir substitution for nucleoside analogs in patients with HIV lipoatrophy. A randomized trial. JAMA 288:207–15, 2002.
Cutrell A, Brothers C, Yeo J, et al. Abacavir and the potential risk of myocardial infarction. Lancet 2008 April 1, e-pub.
Katalama C, Clotet B, Plettenberg A, et al. The role of abacavir (AVC, 1592) in antiretroviral therapy-experiences patients: results from randomized, double-blind, trial. CNA3002 European Study Team. AIDS 14:781–9, 2000.
Keating MR. Antiviral agents. Mayo Clin Proc 67:160–78, 1992.

"Usual dose" assumes normal renal/hepatic function. * For renal insufficiency, give usual dose × 1 followed by maintenance dose per CrCl. For dialysis patients, dose the same as for CrCl < 10 mL/min and give supplemental (post-HD/PD dose) immediately after dialysis. CrCl = creatinine clearance; CVVH = continuous veno-venous hemo-filtration; HD/PD = hemodialysis/peritoneal dialysis. See pp. 214–216 for explanations, pp. xi–xii for abbreviations.

Mallal S, Phillips E, Carosi G, et al. HLA-B*5701 screening for hypersensitivity to abacavir. N Engl J Med 358:568–79, 2008.

McDowell JA, Lou Y, Symonds WS, et al. Multiple-dose pharmacokinetics and pharmacodynamics of abacavir alone and in combination with zidovudine in human immunodeficiency virus-infected adults. Antimicrob Agents Chemother 44:2061–7, 2000.

Panel on Antiretroviral Guidelines for Adults and Adolescents. Guidelines for the use of antiretroviral agents in HIV-1-infected adults and adolescents. Department of Health and Human Services. March 27, 2013; 1–240. Available at **http://www.aidsinfo.nih.gov/contentfiles/lvguidelines/adultandadolescentgl.pdf**.

Staszewski S, Keiser P, Mantaner J, et al. Abacavir-lamivudine-zidovudine vs. indinavir-lamivudine-zidovudine in antiretroviral-naïve HIV-infected adults: a randomized equivalence trial. JAMA 285:1155–63, 2001.

Abacavir + Lamivudine (Epzicom)

Drug Class: Antiretroviral NRTI combination
Usual Dose: HLA-B*5701 negative patients—Epzicom tablet = abacavir 600 mg + lamivudine 300 mg. Usual dose: 1 tablet QD
How supplied: Oral Tablet: Contains 300 mg Abacavir Sulfate + 600 mg Lamivudine
Pharmacokinetic Parameters:
Peak serum level: 3/1.5 mcg/L
Bioavailability: 83/86%
Excreted unchanged (urine): 1.2/71%
Serum half-life (normal/ESRD): (1.5/8)/(5–7/20) hrs
Plasma protein binding: 50/36%
Volume of distribution (V_d): 0.86/1.3 L/kg
Primary Mode of Elimination: Hepatic/Renal
Dosage Adjustments*

CrCl < 50 mL/min	Not recommended
Post-HD dose	Not recommended
Post-PD dose	Not recommended

CVVH dose	Not recommended
Mild hepatic insufficiency	Contraindicated
Moderate or severe hepatic insufficiency	Contraindicated

Drug Interactions: Methadone (↑ methadone clearance with abacavir 600 mg BID); ethanol (↑ abacavir serum levels/half-life; may ↑ toxicity); didanosine, zalcitabine (↑ risk of pancreatitis); TMP-SMX (↑ lamivudine levels); zidovudine (↑ zidovudine levels).
Adverse Effects: Abacavir may cause severe hypersensitivity reactions that may be fatal (see comments), usually during the first 4–6 weeks of therapy; report cases of hypersensitivity reactions to Abacavir Hypersensitivity Registry at 1-800-270-0425. Drug fever, rash, abdominal pain, diarrhea, nausea, vomiting, anorexia, anemia, leukopenia, photophobia, depression, insomnia, weakness, headache, cough, nasal complaints, dizziness, peripheral neuropathy, myalgias, ↑ AST/ALT, hyperglycemia, hypertriglyceridemia, pancreatitis, lactic acidosis with hepatic steatosis (rare, but potentially life-threatening toxicity with the NRTIs).
Allergic Potential: High (~ 5%)/Low
Safety in Pregnancy: C
Comments: May be taken with or without food. **HLA-B*5701 testing should precede the use of abacavir or an abacavir-containing regimen to reduce the risk of hypersensitivity reaction. Immediately and permanently discontinue if a hypersensitivity reaction occurs; never restart abacavir sulfate/lamivudine following a hypersensitivity reaction** or if hypersensitivity cannot be ruled out, which may include fever, rash, fatigue, nausea, vomiting, diarrhea, abdominal pain, anorexia, respiratory symptoms. Potential cross-resistance with

---

"Usual dose" assumes normal renal/hepatic function. * For renal insufficiency, give usual dose × 1 followed by maintenance dose per CrCl. For dialysis patients, dose the same as for CrCl < 10 mL/min and give supplemental (post-HD/PD dose) immediately after dialysis. CrCl = creatinine clearance; CVVH = continuous veno-venous hemo-filtration; HD/PD = hemodialysis/peritoneal dialysis. See pp. 214–216 for explanations, pp. xi–xii for abbreviations.

didanosine. Lamivudine prevents development of ZDV resistance and restores ZDV susceptibility. For patients co-infected with HIV and HBV, monitor hepatic function closely during therapy and for several months afterward.

Cerebrospinal Fluid Penetration: 27–33/15%

REFERENCES:

Mallal S, Phillips E, Carosi G, et al. HLA-B*5701 screening for hypersensitivity to abacavir. N Engl J Med 358:568–79, 2008.

No authors listed. Two once-daily fixed-dose NRTI combination for HIV. Med Lett Drugs Ther. 47: 19–20, 2005.

Panel on Antiretroviral Guidelines for Adults and Adolescents. Guidelines for the use of antiretroviral agents in HIV-1-infected adults and adolescents. Department of Health and Human Services. March 27, 2013; 1–240. Available at **http://www. aidsinfo.nih.gov/contentfiles/lvguidelines/ adultandadolescentgl.pdf**.

Sosa N, Hill-Zabala C, Dejesus E, et al. Abacavir and lamivudine fixed-dose combination tablet once daily compared with abacavir and lamivudine twice daily in HIV-infected patients over 48 weeks. J Acquir Immune Defic Syndr 40:422–7, 2005.

Abacavir + Lamivudine + Zidovudine (Trizivir)

Drug Class: Antiretroviral NRTI combination
Usual Dose: HLA-B*5701 negative patients—Trizivir tablet = abacavir 300 mg + lamivudine 150 mg + zidovudine 300 mg. Usual dose = 1 tablet (PO) BID
How supplied: Oral Tablet: Contains 300 mg Abacavir Sulfate + 600 mg Lamivudine
Pharmacokinetic Parameters:
Peak serum level: 3/1.5/1.2 mcg/mL
Bioavailability: 86/86/64%
Excreted unchanged (urine): 1.2/90/16%
Serum half-life (normal/ESRD): [1.5/6/1.1]/8/20/2.2] hrs

Plasma protein binding: 30/36/20%
Volume of distribution (V_d): 0.86/1.3/1.6 L/kg
Primary Mode of Elimination: Hepatic/renal
Dosage Adjustments*

CrCl < 50 mL/min	Avoid
Post-HD or Post-PD	Avoid
CVVH dose	Avoid
Moderate or severe hepatic insufficiency	Not recommended

Drug Interactions: Amprenavir, atovaquone (↑ zidovudine levels); clarithromycin (↓ zidovudine levels); cidofovir (↑ zidovudine levels, flu-like symptoms); doxorubicin (neutropenia); stavudine (antagonistic to zidovudine; avoid combination); TMP-SMX (↑ lamivudine and zidovudine levels); zalcitabine (↓ lamivudine levels).
Adverse Effects: HLA-B*5701 testing should precede the use of abacavir or an abacavir-containing regimen to reduce the risk of hypersensitivity reaction. Immediately and permanently discontinue if a hypersensitivity reaction occurs; never restart abacavir sulfate/lamivudine/zidovudine following a hypersensitivity reaction or if hypersensitivity cannot be ruled out, which may include fever, rash, fatigue, nausea, vomiting, diarrhea, abdominal pain, anorexia, respiratory symptoms. Most common (> 5%): nausea, vomiting, diarrhea, anorexia, insomnia, fever/chills, headache, malaise/fatigue. Others (less common): peripheral neuropathy, myopathy, steatosis, pancreatitis. Lab abnormalities: mild hyperglycemia, anemia, LFT elevations, hypertriglyceridemia, leukopenia.
Allergic Potential: High (~ 5%)
Safety in Pregnancy: C
Comments: Avoid in patients with CrCl < 50 mL/min. May be taken with or without food. HBV hepatitis may relapse if lamivudine is discontinued.

"Usual dose" assumes normal renal/hepatic function. * For renal insufficiency, give usual dose × 1 followed by maintenance dose per CrCl. For dialysis patients, dose the same as for CrCl < 10 mL/min and give supplemental (post-HD/PD dose) immediately after dialysis. CrCl = creatinine clearance; CVVH = continuous veno-venous hemo-filtration; HD/PD = hemodialysis/peritoneal dialysis. See pp. 214–216 for explanations, pp. xi–xii for abbreviations.

REFERENCES:

Havlir DV, Lange JM. New antiretrovirals and new combinations. AIDS 12(Suppl A):S165–74, 1998.

Mallal S, Phillips E, Carosi G, et al. HLA-B*5701 screening for hypersensitivity to abacavir. N Engl J Med 358:568–79, 2008.

McDowell JA, Lou Y, Symonds WS, et al. Multiple-dose pharmacokinetics and pharmacodynamics of abacavir alone and in combination with zidovudine in human immunodeficiency virus-infected adults. Antimicrob Agents Chemother 44:2061–7, 2000.

Panel on Antiretroviral Guidelines for Adults and Adolescents. Guidelines for the use of antiretroviral agents in HIV-1-infected adults and adolescents. Department of Health and Human Services. March 27, 2013; 1–240. Available at **http://www. aidsinfo.nih.gov/contentfiles/lvguidelines/ adultandadolescentgl.pdf**.

Three new drugs for HIV infection. Med Lett Drugs Ther 40:114–6, 1998.

Weverling GJ, Lange JM, Jurriaans S, et al. Alternative multidrug regimen provides improved suppression of HIV-1 replication over triple therapy. AIDS 12:117–22, 1998.

Adefovir dipivoxil (Hepsera)

Drug Class: Anti-Hepatitis B agent (Nucleotide Reverse Transcriptase Inhibitor)
Usual Dose: 10 mg (PO) QD
How supplied: Oral Tablet: 10 mg
Pharmacokinetic Parameters:
Peak serum level: 18 ng/mL
Bioavailability: 59%
Excreted unchanged (urine): 45%
Serum half-life (normal/ESRD): 7.5/9 hrs
Plasma protein binding: 4%
Volume of distribution (V_d): 0.4 L/kg
Primary Mode of Elimination: Renal
Dosage Adjustments*

CrCl ≥ 50 mL/min	10 mg (PO) QD
CrCl 20–50 mL/min	10 mg (PO) q2d

CrCl 10–20 mL/min	10 mg (PO) q3d
Hemodialysis	10 mg (PO) q7d
Post-HD or PD dose	No information
CVVH dose	No information
Moderate or severe hepatic insufficiency	No change

Drug Interactions: No significant interaction with lamivudine, TMP-SMX, acetaminophen, ibuprofen.
Adverse Effects: Asthenia, headache, abdominal pain, nausea, flatulence, diarrhea, dyspepsia.
Allergic Potential: Low
Safety in Pregnancy: C
Comments: May be taken with or without food. Does not inhibit CP450 isoenzymes. Do not discontinue abruptly to avoid exacerbation of HBV hepatitis.
Cerebrospinal Fluid Penetration: No data

REFERENCES:

Buti M, Esteban R. Adefovir dipivoxil. Drugs of Today 39:127–35, 2003.

Cundy KC, Burditch-Crovo P, Walker RE, et al. Clinical pharmacokinetics of adefovir in human HIV-1 infected patients. Antimicrob Agents Chemother 35:2401–2405, 1995.

Davis GL. Update on the management of chronic hepatitis B. Rev Gastroenterol Disord 2: 106–15, 2002.

Hadziyannis SJ, Tassopoulos NC, Heathcote E, et al. Adefovir dipivoxil for the treatment of hepatitis B e antigen-negative chronic hepatitis B. N Engl J Med 348:800–7, 2003.

Perrillo R, Schiff E, Yoshida E, et al. Adefovir for the treatment of lamivudine-resistant hepatitis B mutants. Hepatology 32:129–34, 2000.

Peters MG, Hann Hw H, Martin P, et al. Adefovir dipivoxil alone or in combination with lamivudine in patients with lamivudine-resistant chronic hepatitis B. Gastroenterology 126:90–101, 2004.

"Usual dose" assumes normal renal/hepatic function. * For renal insufficiency, give usual dose × 1 followed by maintenance dose per CrCl. For dialysis patients, dose the same as for CrCl < 10 mL/min and give supplemental (post-HD/PD dose) immediately after dialysis. CrCl = creatinine clearance; CVVH = continuous veno-venous hemo-filtration; HD/PD = hemodialysis/peritoneal dialysis. See pp. 214–216 for explanations, pp. xi–xii for abbreviations.

Atazanavir (Reyataz) ATV

Drug Class: Antiretroviral protease inhibitor
Usual Dose: 400 mg (PO) QD; 300 mg (PO) QD when given with ritonavir 100 mg (PO) QD
How Supplied: Oral Capsule: 100 mg, 150 mg, 200 mg, 300 mg
Pharmacokinetic Parameters:
Peak serum level: 3152 ng/mL
Bioavailability: No data
Excreted unchanged (urine) (urine/feces): 7%/20%
Serum half-life (normal/ESRD): 7 hrs/no data
Plasma protein binding: 86%
Volume of distribution (V_d): No data
Primary Mode of Elimination: Hepatic
Dosage Adjustments*

CrCl < 50 mL/min	No data
Post-HD or PD dose	No data
CVVH dose	No data
Moderate hepatic insufficiency	300 mg (PO) QD
Severe hepatic insufficiency	Avoid

Antiretroviral Dosage Adjustments

Delavirdine	No information
Didanosine	Give atazanavir 2 hrs before or 1 hr after didanosine buffered formulations
Efavirenz	Do not coadminister with unboosted ATV. In treatment-naïve patients (ATV 400 mg + RTV 100 mg) once daily. Do not coadminister in treatment-experienced patients.
Indinavir	Avoid combination

Lopinavir/ ritonavir	ATV 300 mg once daily + LPV/r 400/100 mg BID
Nelfinavir	No information
Nevirapine	Do not co-administer with atazanavir +/– ritonavir
Ritonavir	Atazanavir 300 mg/d + ritonavir 100 mg/d as single daily dose with food
Saquinavir	↑ saquinavir (soft-gel) levels; no information
Rifampin	Avoid combination
Rifabutin	150 mg q2d or 3x/week
Etravirine	Do not co-administer with atazanavir +/– ritonavir
Maraviroc	MVC 150 mg BID with ATV +/– RTV
Raltegravir	No change

Drug Interactions: Antacids or buffered medications (↓ atazanavir levels; give atazanavir 2 hours before or 1 hour after); H$_2$-receptor blockers (↓ atazanavir levels. In <u>treatment-naïve</u> patients taking an H$_2$-receptor antagonist, give either atazanavir 400 mg once daily with food at least 2 hours before and at least 10 hours after the H$_2$-receptor antagonist, or give atazanavir 300 mg once daily with ritonavir 100 mg once daily with food, without the need for separation from the H$_2$-receptor antagonist. In <u>treatment-experienced</u> patients, give atazanavir 300 mg once daily with ritonavir 100 mg once daily with food at least 2 hours before and at least 10 hours after the H$_2$-receptor antagonist); antiarrhythmics (↑ amiodarone, systemic lidocaine, quinidine levels; prolongs PR interval; monitor antiarrhythmic levels); antidepressants (↑ tricyclic

"Usual dose" assumes normal renal/hepatic function. * For renal insufficiency, give usual dose × 1 followed by maintenance dose per CrCl. For dialysis patients, dose the same as for CrCl < 10 mL/min and give supplemental (post-HD/PD dose) immediately after dialysis. CrCl = creatinine clearance; CVVH = continuous veno-venous hemo-filtration; HD/PD = hemodialysis/peritoneal dialysis. See pp. 214–216 for explanations, pp. xi–xii for abbreviations.

antidepressant levels; monitor levels); calcium channel blockers (↑ calcium channel blocker levels, ↑ PR interval; ↓ diltiazem dose by 50%; use with caution; consider ECG monitoring); clarithromycin (↑ clarithromycin and atazanavir levels; consider 50% dose reduction; consider alternate agent for infections not caused by MAI); cyclosporine, sirolimus, tacrolimus (↑ immunosuppressant levels; monitor levels); ethinyl estradiol, norethindrone (↑ oral contraceptive levels; use lowest effective oral contraceptive dose); lovastatin, simvastatin (↑ risk of myopathy, rhabdomyolysis; avoid combination); sildenafil (↑ sildenafil levels; do not give more than 25 mg q2h); tadalafil (max. 10 mg/72 hours); vardenafil (max. 2.5 mg/72 hours); St. John's wort (avoid combination); warfarin (↑ warfarin levels; monitor INR); rivaroxaban (↑ rivaroxaban); tenofovir (tenofovir reduces systemic exposure to atazanavir. Whenever the two are coadministered, the recommended dose of atazanavir is 300 mg once daily with ritonavir 100 mg once daily). *Drugs that should not be coadministered with atazanavir* include alfuzosin beta-blockers, cisapride, pimozide, rifampin, irinotecan, midazolam, triazolam, lovastatin, simvastatin, bepridil, some ergot derivatives, indinavir, proton pump inhibitors, St. John's wort.

Adverse Effects: Reversible, asymptomatic ↑ in indirect (unconjugated) bilirubin may occur. Asymptomatic, dose-dependent ↑ PR interval (~ 24 msec). Use with caution with drugs that ↑ PR interval (e.g., beta-blockers, verapamil, digoxin). May ↑ risk of hyperglycemia/diabetes. May ↑ risk of bleeding in hemophilia (types A + B). Rare cases of Stevens-Johnson syndrome, erythema multiforme, and toxic skin eruptions, including drug rash, eosinophilia and systemic symptoms (DRESS) syndrome, that have been reported.

Allergic Potential: Low

Cerebrospinal Fluid Penetration: Intermediate
Safety in Pregnancy: B
Comments: Monitor LFTs in patients with HBV, HCV. Take 400 mg (two 200-mg capsules) once daily with food.
Cerebrospinal Fluid Penetration: Intermediate

REFERENCES:

Colonno RJ, Thiry A, Limoli K, Parkin N. Activities of atazanavir (BMS-232632) against a large panel of Human Immunodeficiency Virus Type 1 clinical isolates resistant to one or more approved protease inhibitors. *Antimicrob Agents Chemother* 47: 1324–33, 2003.

Haas DW, Zala C, Schrader S, et al. Therapy with atazanavir plus saquinavir in patients failing highly active antiretroviral therapy: a randomized comparative pilot trial. *AIDS* 17: 1339–1349, 2003.

Havlir DV, O'Marro SD. Atazanavir: new option for treatment of HIV infection. *Clin Infect Dis* 38: 1599–604, 2004.

Jemsek JG, Arathoon E, Arlotti M, et al. Body fat and other metabolic effects of atazanavir and efavirenz, each administered in combination with zidovudine plus lamivudine, in antiretroviral-naïve HIV-infected patients. *Clin Infect Dis* 42:273–80, 2006.

Panel on Antiretroviral Guidelines for Adults and Adolescents. Guidelines for the use of antiretroviral agents in HIV-1-infected adults and adolescents. Department of Health and Human Services. March 27, 2013; 1–240. Available at **http://www.aidsinfo.nih.gov/contentfiles/lvguidelines/adultandadolescentgl.pdf**.

Piliero PJ. Atazanavir: a novel HIV-1 protease inhibitor. Expert Opin Investig Drugs 11:1295–301, 2002.

Sanne I, Piliero P, Squires K, et al. Results of a phase 2 clinical trial at 48 weeks (AI424–007): a dose-ranging, safety, and efficacy comparative trial of atazanavir at three doses in combination with didanosine and stavudine in antiretroviral-naïve subjects. *J Acquir Immune Defic Syndr* 32:18–29, 2003.

Wang F, Ross J. Atazanavir: a novel azapeptide inhibitor of HIV-1 protease. *Formulary* 38:691–702, 2003.

"Usual dose" assumes normal renal/hepatic function. * For renal insufficiency, give usual dose × 1 followed by maintenance dose per CrCl. For dialysis patients, dose the same as for CrCl < 10 mL/min and give supplemental (post-HD/PD dose) immediately after dialysis. CrCl = creatinine clearance; CVVH = continuous veno-venous hemo-filtration; HD/PD = hemodialysis/peritoneal dialysis. See pp. 214–216 for explanations, pp. xi–xii for abbreviations.

Boceprevir (Victrelis)

Drug Class: Anti-Hepatitis C agent (NS3/4A protease inhibitor)
Usual Dose: 800 mg (PO) TID with food
How Supplied: Oral Capsule: 200 MG
Pharmacokinetic Parameters:
Peak serum level: 1723 nanograms/mL
Bioavailability: not studied
Excreted unchanged: 8% (feces) 3% (urine)
Serum half-life (normal/ESRD): 3.4 hrs / no data
Plasma protein binding: 75%
Volume of distribution (Vd): 772 L
Primary mode of Elimination: feces
Dosage Adjustments*

CrCl 50–80 mL/min	No change
CrCl 30–49 mL/min	No change
CrCl < 30 mL/min	No change
ESRD	No change
Post-HD dose	No change
Post-PD dose	No data
CVVH dose	No data
Mild – moderate hepatic insufficiency	No change
Severe hepatic insufficiency	No change

Antiretroviral Dosage Adjustments: Limited data in co-administration with HIV ARVs. Raltegravir based HAART may be feasible.
Drug Interactions: Boceprevir is a strong inhibitor of CYP3A4/5 and p-glycoprotein (P-gp). Drugs metabolized primarily by CYP3A4/5 and p-glycoprotein (P-gp) may have increased exposure when administered with boceprevir. Boceprevir does not induce or inhibit: CYP1A2, CYP2A6, CYP2B6, CYP2C8, CYP2C9, CYP2C19, CYP2D6 or CYP2E1. Boceprevir is primarily metabolized by aldo-ketoreductase (AKR) and partly by CYP3A4/5 and P-gp. Boceprevir may affect the plasma concentrations of the following co-administered drugs: ↑ antiarrhythmics, ↑ digoxin, ↑ or ↓ warfarin, ↑ trazodone, ↑ desipramine, ↑ clarithromycin, ↑ carbamazepine (↓ boceprevir), ↑ or ↓ Phenobarbital (↓ boceprevir), ↑ or ↓ phenytoin (↓ boceprevir), ↓ escitalopram, ↑ desipramine, ↑ antifungals [trazodone, ketoconazole, itraconazole, posaconazole, voriconazole (↑ boceprevir)], ↑ colchicine, ↑ rifabutin (↓ boceprevir), ↑ rifampin (↓ boceprevir), ↑ alprazolam, ↑ midazolam, ↑ calcium channel blockers, ↔ dexamethasone (↓ boceprevir), ↑ fluticasone, ↑ budesonide, ↑ bosentan, ↔ efavirenz (↓ boceprevir), ↓ or ↑ ritonivir (↓ boceprevir), ↑ atorvastatin, ↓ ethinyl estradiol, ↑drospirenone, ↑ cyclosporine, ↑ sirolimus, ↑ tacolimus, ↑ salmeterol, ↓ or ↑ methadone, ↓ or ↑ buprenorphine, ↑ PDE5 inhibitors (sildenafil max 25mg q48H, tadalafil max 10mg q72h, vardenafil max 2.5mg q72h)
Adverse Effects: Most common adverse reactions (> 35% of all patients in clinical trials): fatigue, anemia, nausea, headache and dysgeusia. Other adverse events reported in clinical trials: alopecia 22–27%, decreased appetite 25–26%, xeroderma 18–22%, diarrhea 25%, nausea 43–46%, dysgeusia 35–44%, vomiting 15–20%, xerostomia 11–15%, anemia 45–50%, thrombocytopenia <1–4%, neutropenia 14–25%, arthralgia 19–23%, asthenia 15–21%, insomnia 30–34%, fatigue 55–58%, shivering 33–34%,
Allergic Potential: low
Safety in Pregnancy: B (X when administered with ribavirin)

"Usual dose" assumes normal renal/hepatic function. * For renal insufficiency, give usual dose × 1 followed by maintenance dose per CrCl. For dialysis patients, dose the same as for CrCl < 10 mL/min and give supplemental (post-HD/PD dose) immediately after dialysis. CrCl = creatinine clearance; CVVH = continuous veno-venous hemo-filtration; HD/PD = hemodialysis/peritoneal dialysis. See pp. 214–216 for explanations, pp. xi–xii for abbreviations.

Comments: Must be taken with 7–9 hours apart with a meal or light snack. Must not be used as monotherapy for HCV and must only be used in combination with peginterferon alfa and ribavirin. Boceprevir only has clinically significant activity against HCV genotype 1 and should not be used to treat patients infected with other HCV genotypes. The safety and efficacy of boceprevir not been studied in patients with decompensated cirrhosis, patients with an organ transplant, who are co-infected with HIV, or HBV. Clinical data on boceprevir use in the pediatric or pregnant populations have not been established.

Cerebrospinal Fluid Penetration: no data

Alias: SCH 503034

REFERENCES:

Product Information: VICTRELIS® oral capsules, boceprevir oral capsules. Merck & Co, Inc, Whitehouse Station, NJ, 2011.

Bacon BR, Gordon SC, Lawitz E, et al: Boceprevir for previously treated chronic HCV genotype 1 infection. N Engl J Med 2011; 364(13):1207–1217.

Poordad F, McCone J Jr, Bacon BR, et al: Boceprevir for untreated chronic HCV genotype 1 infection. N Engl J Med 2011; 364(13):1195–1206.

Kwo PY, Lawitz EJ, McCone J, et al. Efficacy of boceprevir, an NS3 protease inhibitor, in combination with peginterferon alfa-2b and ribavirin in treatment-naive patients with genotype 1 hepatitis C infection (SPRINT-1): an open-label, randomised, multicentre phase 2 trial. Lancet. Aug 28 2010;376(9742):705–716.

Foote BS, Spooner LM, Belliveau PP. Boceprevir: a protease inhibitor for the treatment of chronic hepatitis C. Ann Pharmacother. Sep 2011;45(9): 1085–1093.

C Kasserra, E Hughes, M Treitel, et al. Clinical Pharmacology of BOC: Metabolism, Excretion, and Drug-Drug Interactions. 18th Conference on Retroviruses and Opportunistic Infections (CROI 2011). Boston. February 27–March 2, 2011. Abstract 118.

Ramanathan S, Mathias AA, German P, Kearney BP. Clinical pharmacokinetic and pharmacodynamic profile of the HIV integrase inhibitor elvitegravir. Clinical pharmacokinetics. Apr 2011;50(4):229–244.

de Kanter CT, Blonk MI, Colbers AP, Schouwenberg BJ, Burger DM. Lack of a Clinically Significant Drug-Drug Interaction in Healthy Volunteers Between the Hepatitis C Virus Protease Inhibitor Boceprevir and the HIV Integrase Inhibitor Raltegravir. Clinical infectious diseases: an official publication of the Infectious Diseases Society of America. Oct 19 2012.

Website: www.victrelis.com

Darunavir Ethanolate (Prezista) DRV

Drug Class: Antiretroviral protease inhibitor

Usual Dose: Treatment-naïve patients: 800 mg (two 400 mg tablets) of darunavir (PO) QD + 100 mg of ritonavir (PO) QD. Treatment-experienced patients: 600 mg (one 600-mg tablet) of darunavir (PO) BID plus 100 mg of ritonavir (PO) BID

How Supplied: Oral Tablet: 75 mg, 150 mg, 400 mg, 600 mg, 800 mg

Pharmacokinetic Parameters:

Peak serum level: 3578 ng/mL

Bioavailability: 37% (alone) 82% (with ritonavir)

Excreted unchanged: 41.2% (feces), 7.7% (urine)

Serum half-life (normal/ESRD): 15/15 hrs

Plasma protein binding: 95%

Volume of distribution (V_d): not studied

Primary Mode of Elimination: Fecal/renal

Dosage Adjustments*

CrCl 50–80 mL/min	No change
CrCl 10–50 mL/min	No change
CrCl < 10 mL/min	No change
Post-HD dose	No change
Post-PD dose	No change

"Usual dose" assumes normal renal/hepatic function. * For renal insufficiency, give usual dose × 1 followed by maintenance dose per CrCl. For dialysis patients, dose the same as for CrCl < 10 mL/min and give supplemental (post-HD/PD dose) immediately after dialysis. CrCl = creatinine clearance; CVVH = continuous veno-venous hemo-filtration; HD/PD = hemodialysis/peritoneal dialysis. See pp. 214–216 for explanations, pp. xi–xii for abbreviations.

CVVH dose	No change
Mild hepatic insufficiency	Not studied
Moderate or severe hepatic insufficiency	Not studied

Antiretroviral Dosage Adjustments

Efavirenz	No change
Nevirapine	No change
Didanosine	1 hour before or 1 hour after darunavir
Tenofovir	No change
Fosamprenavir	No change
Indinavir	No information
Lopinavir/ritonavir	Avoid
Saquinavir	Avoid
Rifabutin	150 mg QOD
Etravirine	No change
Maraviroc	150 mg BID
Raltegravir	No change

Drug Interactions: Alfuzosin Indinavir, ketaconazole, nevirapine, tenofovir (↑ darunavir levels); lopinavir/ritonavir, saquinavir, efavirenz (↓ darunavir levels); concomitant administration of darunavir/ritonavir with agents highly dependent on CYP3A for clearance, astemizole, cisapride, dihydroergotamine, ergonovine, ergotamine, methylergonovine, midazolam, pimozide, terfenadine, midazolam, triazolam (may ↓ darunavir levels and ↓ effectiveness); sildenafil, vardenafil, tadalafil (↑ PDE-5 inhibitors; sildenafil do not exceed 25 mg in 48 hrs, vardenafil do not exceed 2.5 mg in 72 hrs, or tadalafil do not exceed 10 mg in 72 hrs); rivaroxaban (↑ rivaroxaban); Warfarin (↑ warfrin, monitor INR).

Adverse Effects: Diarrhea, nausea, headache, nasopharyngitis.
Allergic Potential: High (see comments)
Safety in Pregnancy: C
Comments: Always take with food (increases AUC, Cmax by approximately 30%). Must be given with ritonavir to boost bioavailability. Darunavir contains a sulfonamide moiety (as do fosamprenavir and tipranavir); use with caution in patients with sulfonamide allergies. A mild-to-moderate rash occurred in 7% of patients receiving the drug in clinical trial; it did not usually require drug cessation, but severe rashes (including Stevens-Johnson syndrome) have been reported.
Cerebrospinal Fluid Penetration: No data

REFERENCES:

Clotet B, Bellos N, Moloina JM, et al. Efficacy and safety of darunavir-ritonavir at week 48 in treatment-experienced patients with HIV-1 infection in POWER 1 and 2: a pooled subgroup analysis of data from two randomised trials. *Lancet* 369:1169–78, 2007.

De Meyer SM, Spinosa-Guzman S, Vangeneugden TJ, et al. Efficacy of once-daily darunavir/ritonavir 800/100 mg in HIV-infected, treatment-experienced patients with no baseline resistance-associated mutations to darunavir. *J Acquir Immune Defic Syndr* 49(2):179–82, 2008.

De Meyer S, Azijn H, Surleraux D, et al. TMC114, a novel human immunodeficiency virus type 1 protease inhibitor active against protease inhibitor-resistant viruses, including a broad range of clinical isolates. *Antimicrob Agents Chemother* 49:2314–21, 2005.

Dominique L.N.G, Surleraux T, Abdellah Tahri T, et al. Discovery and selection of TMC114, a next generation HIV-I protease inhibitor. *J Med Chem* 48: 1813–22, 2005.

Grinsztejn, B. TMC114/r is well tolerated in 3-class-experienced patients: week 24 of POWER 1 (TMC114–C213). Tibotec Pharmaceuticals. Rio de Janerio, Brazil. Available from URL: www.tibotec.com

Katlama C. TMC114/r outperforms investigator-selected PI(s) in 3-class-experienced patients: week 24 primary

---

"Usual dose" assumes normal renal/hepatic function. * For renal insufficiency, give usual dose × 1 followed by maintenance dose per CrCl. For dialysis patients, dose the same as for CrCl < 10 mL/min and give supplemental (post-HD/PD dose) immediately after dialysis. CrCl = creatinine clearance; CVVH = continuous veno-venous hemo-filtration; HD/PD = hemodialysis/peritoneal dialysis. See pp. 214–216 for explanations, pp. xi–xii for abbreviations.

efficacy analysis of POWER 1 (TMC114–C213). Tibotec Pharmaceuticals. Rio de Janerio, Brazil. Available from URL: www.tibotec.com

Madruga JV, Berger D, McMurchie M, et al. Efficacy and safety of darunavir-ritonavir compared with that of lopinavir-ritonavir at 48 weeks in treatment-experienced, HIV-infected patients in TITAN: a randomized controlled phase III trial. *Lancet* 370:3–5, 2007.

Ortiz R, Dejesus E, Khanlou H, et al. Efficacy and safety of once-daily darunavir/ritonavir versus lopinavir/ritonavir in treatment-naive HIV-1-infected patients at week 48 (ARTMIS). *AIDS* 2008;22(12): 1389–97.

Panel on Antiretroviral Guidelines for Adults and Adolescents. Guidelines for the use of antiretroviral agents in HIV-1-infected adults and adolescents. Department of Health and Human Services. March 27, 2013; 1–240. Available at http://www.aidsinfo.nih.gov/contentfiles/lvguidelines/adultandadolescentgl.pdf.

Product Information: PREZISTA(TM) oral tablets, darunavir oral tablets. Tibotec Therapeutics, Inc, Raritan, NJ, 2006.

Sorbera LA, Castaner J, Bayes M. Darunavir. Anti-HIV agent HIV protease inhibitor. Drugs of the Future. 30:441–449, 2005.

Website: www.prezista.com

CrCl 50–80 mL/min	No change
CrCl 10–50 mL/min	No change
CrCl < 10 mL/min	No change
Post-HD dose	None
Post-PD dose	None
CVVH dose	No change
Moderate hepatic insufficiency	No information
Severe hepatic insufficiency	No information/ use caution

Antiretroviral Dosage Adjustments

Efavirenz	No information
Indinavir	Indinavir 600 mg TID
Lopinavir/ ritonavir	No information
Nelfinavir	No information (monitor for neutropenia)
Nevirapine	No information
Ritonavir	Delavirdine: no change; ritonavir: No information
Saquinavir soft-gel	Saquinavir soft-gel 800 mg TID (monitor transaminases)
Rifampin, rifabutin	Avoid combination
Statins	Not recommended

Delavirdine (Rescriptor)

Drug Class: Antiretroviral NNRTI (non-nucleoside reverse transcriptase inhibitor)
Usual Dose: 400 mg (PO) BID
How Supplied: Oral Tablet: 100 mg, 200 mg
Pharmacokinetic Parameters:
Peak serum level: 35 mcg/mL
Bioavailability: 85%
Excreted unchanged (urine): 5%
Serum half-life (normal/ESRD): 5.8 hrs/no data
Plasma protein binding: 98%
Volume of distribution (V$_d$): 0.5 L/kg
Primary Mode of Elimination: Hepatic
Dosage Adjustments*

Drug Interactions: Antiretrovirals, rifabutin, rifampin (see dose adjustment grid, above); astemizole, terfenadine, benzodiazepines, cisapride, H$_2$ blockers, proton pump inhibitors, ergot alkaloids, quinidine, statins (avoid if possible); carbamazepine, phenobarbital, phenytoin (may ↓ delavirdine levels, monitor

---

"Usual dose" assumes normal renal/hepatic function. * For renal insufficiency, give usual dose × 1 followed by maintenance dose per CrCl. For dialysis patients, dose the same as for CrCl < 10 mL/min and give supplemental (post-HD/PD dose) immediately after dialysis. CrCl = creatinine clearance; CVVH = continuous veno-venous hemo-filtration; HD/PD = hemodialysis/peritoneal dialysis. See pp. 214–216 for explanations, pp. xi–xii for abbreviations.

anticonvulsant levels); clarithromycin, dapsone, nifedipine, warfarin ($\uparrow$ interacting drug levels); sildenafil (do not exceed 25 mg in 48 hrs); tadalafil (max. 10 mg/72 hrs); vardenafil (max. 2.5 mg/72 hrs).

Adverse Effects: Drug fever/rash, Stevens-Johnson syndrome (rare), headache, nausea/vomiting, diarrhea, $\uparrow$ SGOT/SGPT.

Allergic Potential: High

Safety in Pregnancy: C

Comments: May be taken with or without food, but food decreases absorption by 20%. May disperse four 100-mg tablets in > 3 oz. water to produce slurry; 200-mg tablets should be taken as intact tablets and not used to make an oral solution. Separate dosing with ddI or antacids by 1 hour.

Cerebrospinal Fluid Penetration: 0.4%

REFERENCES:

Been-Tiktak AM, Boucher CA, Brun-Vezinet F, et al. Efficacy and safety of combination therapy with delavirdine and zidovudine: A European/Australian phase II trial. *Intern J Antimicrob Agents* 11:13–21, 1999.

Conway B. Initial therapy with protease inhibitor-sparing regimens: Evaluation of nevirapine and delavirdine. *Clin Infect Dis* 2:130–4, 2000.

Demeter LM, Shafer RW, Meehan PM, et al. Delavirdine susceptibilities and associated reverse transcriptase mutations in human immunodeficiency virus type 1 isolates from patients in a phase I/II trial of delavirdine monotherapy (ACTG260). *Antimicrob Agents Chemother* 44:794–7, 2000.

Justesen US, Klitgaard NA, Brosen K, et al. Dose-dependent pharmacokinetics of delavirdine in combination with amprenavir in healthy volunteers. *J Antimicrob Chemother* 54:206–10, 2004.

Panel on Antiretroviral Guidelines for Adults and Adolescents. Guidelines for the use of antiretroviral agents in HIV-1-infected adults and adolescents. Department of Health and Human Services. March 27, 2013; 1–240. Available at **http://www.aidsinfo.nih.gov/contentfiles/lvguidelines/adultandadolescentgl.pdf**.

Didanosine (Videx) ddI

Drug Class: Antiretroviral NRTI (nucleoside reverse transcriptase inhibitor)

Usual Dose: 400 mg QD for weight > 60 kg; 250 QD for < 60 kg

How Supplied:

Generic—Oral Capsule, Delayed Release: 125 mg, 200 mg, 250 mg, 400 mg

Videx EC—Oral Capsule, Delayed Release: 125 mg, 200 mg, 250 mg, 400 mg

Videx—Oral Tablet, Chewable: 100 mg

Videx Pediatric—Oral Powder for Suspension: 10 mg/mL

Pharmacokinetic Parameters:

Peak serum level: 29 mcg/mL
Bioavailability: 42%
Excreted unchanged (urine): 60%
Serum half-life (normal/ESRD): 1.6/4.1 hrs
Plasma protein binding: $\leq$ 5%
Volume of distribution (V_d): 1.1 L/kg

Primary Mode of Elimination: Renal

Dosage Adjustments*: > 60 kg/[< 60 kg]:

CrCl 30–59 mL/min	200 mg (PO) QD (125 mg [PO] QD)
CrCl 10–29 mL/min	125 mg (PO) QD (125 mg [PO] QD)
CrCl < 10 mL/min	125 mg (PO) QD (not recommended)
Post-HD dose	No information
Post-PD dose	100 mg (PO)
CVVH dose	150 mg (PO) QD
Moderate hepatic insufficiency	No change
Severe hepatic insufficiency	No change

"Usual dose" assumes normal renal/hepatic function. * For renal insufficiency, give usual dose × 1 followed by maintenance dose per CrCl. For dialysis patients, dose the same as for CrCl < 10 mL/min and give supplemental (post-HD/PD dose) immediately after dialysis. CrCl = creatinine clearance; CVVH = continuous veno-venous hemo-filtration; HD/PD = hemodialysis/peritoneal dialysis. See pp. 214–216 for explanations, pp. xi–xii for abbreviations.

Drug Interactions: Alcohol, lamivudine, pentamidine, valproic acid (↑ risk of pancreatitis); dapsone, fluoroquinolones, ketoconazole, itraconazole, tetracyclines (↓ absorption of interacting drug; give 2 hours after didanosine); dapsone, INH, metronidazole, nitrofurantoin, stavudine, vincristine, zalcitabine, neurotoxic drugs or history of neuropathy (↑ risk of neuropathy); dapsone (↓ dapsone absorption, which increases risk of PCP); tenofovir (if possible, avoid concomitant tenofovir due to impaired CD4 response and increased risk of virologic failure). Avoid ribavirin in HIV patients.

Adverse Effects: Headache, depression, nausea, vomiting, GI upset/abdominal pain, diarrhea, drug fever/rash, anemia, leukopenia, thrombocytopenia, hepatotoxicity/hepatic necrosis, pancreatitis (may be fatal; ↑ risk in patients on concomitant tenofovir), hypertriglyceridemia, hyperuricemia, lactic acidosis, lipoatrophy, wasting, dose-dependent (≥ 0.06 mg/kg/d) peripheral neuropathy, hyperglycemia, reports of noncirrhotic portal hypertension lactic acidosis with hepatic steatosis (rare, but potentially life-threatening toxicity with use of NRTIs; *pregnant women taking didanosine + stavudine may be at increased risk*).

Allergic Potential: Low

Safety in Pregnancy: B; should be avoided in pregnancy as it may cause fatal pancreatitis

Comments: Available as buffered powder for oral solution and enteric-coated extended-release capsules (Videx EC 400 mg PO QD). Take 30 minutes before or 2 hours after meal (food decreases serum concentrations by 49%). Avoid in patients with alcoholic cirrhosis/history of pancreatitis. Use with caution with ribavirin. Na$^+$ content = 11.5 mEq/g. Buffered tablets discontinued by US manufacturer in February 2006.

Cerebrospinal Fluid Penetration: 20%

REFERENCES:

Barreiro P, Corbaton A, Nunez M, et al. Tolerance of didanosine as enteric-coated capsules versus buffered tablets. *AIDS Patient Care STDS* 18:329–31, 2004.

Hirsch MS, D'Aquila RT. Therapy for human immunodeficiency virus infection. *N Engl J Med* 328:1686–95, 1993.

HIV Trialists' Collaborative Group. Zidovudine, didanosine, and zalcitabine in the treatment of HIV infection: Meta-analyses of the randomised evidence. *Lancet* 353:2014–2025, 1999.

Montaner JS, Reiss P, Cooper D, et al. A randomized, double-blind trial comparing combinations of nevirapine, didanosine, and zidovudine for HIV-infected patients: The INCAS trial. Italy, the Netherlands, Canada and Australia Study. *J Am Med Assoc* 279:930–937, 1998.

Negredo E, Molto J, Munoz-Moreno JA, et al. Safety and efficacy of once-daily didanosine, tenofovir and nevirapine as a simplification antiretroviral approach. *Antivir Ther* 9:335–42, 2004.

Panel on Antiretroviral Guidelines for Adults and Adolescents. Guidelines for the use of antiretroviral agents in HIV-1-infected adults and adolescents. Department of Health and Human Services. March 27, 2013; 1–240. Available at http://www.aidsinfo.nih.gov/contentfiles/lvguidelines/adultandadolescentgl.pdf.

Perry CM, Balfour JA. Didanosine: An update on its antiviral activity, pharmacokinetic properties, and therapeutic efficacy in the management of HIV disease. *Drugs* 52:928–62, 1996.

Rathbun RC, Martin ES 3rd. Didanosine therapy in patients intolerant of or failing zidovudine therapy. *Ann Pharmacother* 26:1347–51, 1992.

Dolutegravir (Tivicay)

Drug Class: HIV-1 integrase strand transfer inhibitor (INSTI)

Usual Dose: Treatment-naïve or treatment experienced-INSTI naïve: 50 mg once daily. Treatment-naïve or treatment-experienced INSTI naïve when coadministered with the following potent UGT1A/CYP3A inducers: efavirenz, fosamprenavir/ritonavir, tipranavir/

"Usual dose" assumes normal renal/hepatic function. * For renal insufficiency, give usual dose × 1 followed by maintenance dose per CrCl. For dialysis patients, dose the same as for CrCl < 10 mL/min and give supplemental (post-HD/PD dose) immediately after dialysis. CrCl = creatinine clearance; CVVH = continuous veno-venous hemo-filtration; HD/PD = hemodialysis/peritoneal dialysis. See pp. 214–216 for explanations, pp. xi–xii for abbreviations.

ritonavir, or rifampin: 50 mg twice daily. INSTI experienced with certain INSTI-associated resistance mutations or clinically suspected INSTI resistance: 50 mg twice daily. Can be taken with or without food.

How supplied: Oral tablet, 50 mg

Pharmacokinetic parameters
(50 mg once daily dose):
Peak serum level: 3.67 mcg/mL
Bioavailability: Not established
Excreted unchanged: 53% (feces), 31% (urine)
Serum half-life: 14 hours Plasma protein binding: 98.9%
Volume of Distribution: 17.4 L
Primary mode of elimination: Hepatic

Dosage Adjustments for Renal and Hepatic Insufficiency

CrCl 50-80 mL/min	No change
CrCl 10-50 mL/min	No change
CrCl < 10 mL/min	No change
Post-HD dose	No information
Post-PD dose	No information
Mild-moderate hepatic insufficiency	No change
Severe hepatic insufficiency	Do not use

Antiretroviral Dosage Adjustments: Increase dose to 50 mg twice-daily when coadministered with the following potent UGT1A/CYP3A inducers: efavirenz, fosamprenavir/ritonavir, tipranavir/ritonavir, or rifampin. Also increase to 50 mg twice daily when given to a patient with certain INSTI-inhibitor resistance mutations or suspected INSTI resistance.

Drug interactions: In vivo, dolutegravir inhibits tubular secretion of creatinine by inhibiting OCT2. Dolutegravir may increase plasma concentrations of drugs eliminated via OCT2 (dofetilide and metformin). Co-administration of dolutegravir and dofetilide should be avoided; close monitoring is recommended when starting or stopping dolutegravir and metformin together. A dose adjustment of metformin may be necessary. Dolutegravir should not be used with etravirine without coadministration of atazanavir/ritonavir, darunavir/ritonavir, or lopinavir/ritonavir. Rifampin, efavirenz, fosamprenavir/ritonavir, and tipranavir/ritonavir induce metabolism of dolutegravir, requiring a dolutegravir dose increase to 50 mg twice daily. Co-administration of dolutegravir with phenytoin, phenobarbital, carbamazepine, or St. John's wort will lower dolutegravir levels and should not be given together. Medications containing polyvalent cations (e.g., MG, Al, Fe, or Ca) decrease absorption of dolutegravir; dolutegravir should be administered 2 hours before or 6 hours after taking medications containing polyvalent cations.

Adverse effects: Hypersensitivity reactions characterized by rash, constitutional findings and sometimes organ dysfunction, including liver injury, have been reported. Discontinue dolutegravir and other suspect agents immediately if signs or symptoms of hypersensitivity reactions develop, as a delay in stopping treatment may result in a life-threatening reaction. The most common adverse reactions of moderate to severe intensity and incidence > 2% were insomnia and headache.

Allergic potential: Low

Safety in pregnancy: Category B. Experience in pregnancy is limited, and should be used during pregnancy only if clearly needed.

Cerebrospinal fluid: In 11 treatment-naïve subjects on dolutegravir 50 mg daily plus abacavir/lamivudine, the median dolutegravir concentration in CSF was 18 ng/mL (range: 4 ng/mL to 232 ng/mL) 2 to 6 hours postdose

---

"Usual dose" assumes normal renal/hepatic function. * For renal insufficiency, give usual dose × 1 followed by maintenance dose per CrCl. For dialysis patients, dose the same as for CrCl < 10 mL/min and give supplemental (post-HD/PD dose) immediately after dialysis. CrCl = creatinine clearance; CVVH = continuous veno-venous hemo-filtration; HD/PD = hemodialysis/peritoneal dialysis. See pp. 214–216 for explanations, pp. xi–xii for abbreviations.

after 2 weeks of treatment. The clinical relevance of this finding has not been established.

REFERENCES:

Cahn, P, Pozniak AL, Mingrone H, et al. Once-daily dolutegravir versus raltegravir in antiretroviral-experienced, integrase-inhibitor-naive adults with HIV: week 48 results from the randomised, double-blind, non-inferiority SAILING study. *The Lancet* 382:700–708, 2013.

Raffi F, Rachlis A, Stellbrink HJ, et al. Once-daily dolutegravir versus raltegravir in antiretroviral-naive adults with HIV-1 infection: 48 week results from the randomised, double-blind, non-inferiority SPRING-2 study, *The Lancet* 381:735–743, 2013.

Walmsley SL, Antela A, Clumeck N, et al. Dolutegravir plus Abacavir–Lamivudine for the Treatment of HIV-1 Infection. *N Engl J Med* 369:1807–1818, 2013.

Product Information. TIVICAY (dolutegravir) oral tablets. ViiV Healthcare, Middlesex, United Kingdom, 2013.

Efavirenz (Sustiva) EFV

Drug Class: Antiretroviral NNRTI (non-nucleoside reverse transcriptase inhibitor)
Usual Dose: 600 mg (PO) QD or QHS
How Supplied: Oral Capsule: 50 mg, 200 mg; Oral Tablet: 600 mg
Pharmacokinetic Parameters:
Peak serum level: 12.9 mcg/mL
Bioavailability: Increased with food
Excreted unchanged (urine): 14–34%
Serum half-life (normal/ESRD): 40–55 hrs/no data
Plasma protein binding: 99%
Volume of distribution (V_d): No data
Primary Mode of Elimination: Hepatic
Dosage Adjustments*

CrCl < 60 mL/min	No change
Post-HD or PD dose	None
CVVH dose	No change
Moderate or severe hepatic insufficiency	No information

Antiretroviral Dosage Adjustments

Delavirdine	No information
Indinavir	Indinavir 1000 mg TID
Lopinavir/ritonavir (l/r)	Consider l/r 533/133 mg BID in PI-experienced patients
Nelfinavir	No changes
Nevirapine	Do not coadminister
Ritonavir	Ritonavir 600 mg BID (500 mg BID for intolerance)
Saquinavir	Avoid use as sole PI
Rifampin	No changes
Rifabutin	Rifabutin 450–600 mg QD or 600 mg 2–3x/week if not on protease inhibitor
Etravirine	Do not coadminister
Maraviroc	600 mg BID
Raltegravir	No change

Drug Interactions: Antiretrovirals, rifabutin, rifampin (see dose adjustment grid, above); astemizole, terfenadine, cisapride, ergotamine, midazolam, triazolam (avoid); carbamazepine, phenobarbital, phenytoin (monitor anticonvulsant levels; use with caution); caspofungin (↓ caspofungin levels, may ↓ caspofungin effect); methadone, clarithromycin (↓ interacting drug levels; titrate methadone dose to effect; consider using azithromycin instead of clarithromycin).

Adverse Effects: Drug fever/rash, CNS symptoms (nightmares, dizziness, neuropsychiatric symptoms, difficulty concentrating, somnolence), ↑ SGOT/SGPT, E. multiforme/Stevens-Johnson syndrome (rare), false positive cannabinoid test.

Allergic Potential: High

"Usual dose" assumes normal renal/hepatic function. * For renal insufficiency, give usual dose × 1 followed by maintenance dose per CrCl. For dialysis patients, dose the same as for CrCl < 10 mL/min and give supplemental (post-HD/PD dose) immediately after dialysis. CrCl = creatinine clearance; CVVH = continuous veno-venous hemo-filtration; HD/PD = hemodialysis/peritoneal dialysis. See pp. 214–216 for explanations, pp. xi–xii for abbreviations.

Safety in Pregnancy: D

Comments: Rash/CNS symptoms usually resolve spontaneously over 2–4 weeks. Take at bedtime. Avoid taking after high fat meals (levels ↑ 50%). 600-mg dose available as single tablet.

Cerebrospinal Fluid Penetration: 0.26%–1.19%

REFERENCES:

Albrecht MA, Bosch RJ, Hammer SM, et al. Nelfinavir, efavirenz, or both after the failure of nucleoside treatment of HIV infection. *N Engl J Med* 345:398–407, 2001.

Gallant JE, DeJesus D, Arribas JR, et al. Tenofovir DF, emtricitabine, and efavirenz vs. zidovudine, lamivudine, and efavirenz for HIV. N Engl J Med 354:251–60, 2006.

Go JC, Cunha BA. Efavirenz. *Antibiotics for Clinicians* 5:1–8, 2001.

Haas DW, Fessel WJ, Delapenha RA, et al. Therapy with efavirenz plus indinavir in patients with extensive prior nucleoside reverse-transcriptase inhibitor experience: A randomized, double-blind, placebo-controlled trial. *J Infect Dis* 183:392–400, 2001.

la Porte CJ, de Graaff-Teulen MJ, Colbers EP, et al. Effect of efavirenz treatment on the pharmacokinetics of nelfinavir boosted by ritonavir in healthy volunteers. *Br J Clin Pharmacol* 58:632–40, 2004.

Marzolini C, Telenti A, Decosterd LA, et al. Efavirenz plasma levels can predict treatment failure and central nervous system side effects in HIV-1-infected patients. *AIDS* 15:71–5, 2001.

Negredo E, Cruz L, Paredes R, et al. Virological, immunological, and clinical impact of switching from protease inhibitors to nevirapine or to efavirenz in patients with human immunodeficiency virus infection and long-lasting viral suppression. *Clin Infect Dis* 34:504–510, 2002.

Panel on Antiretroviral Guidelines for Adults and Adolescents. Guidelines for the use of antiretroviral agents in HIV-1-infected adults and adolescents. Department of Health and Human Services. March 27, 2013; 1–240. Available at **http://www.aidsinfo.nih.gov/contentfiles/lvguidelines/adultandadolescentgl.pdf.**

Efavirenz + Emtricitabine + Tenofovir disoproxil fumarate (ATRIPLA)

Drug Class: Antiretroviral agent

Usual Dose: 1 tablet (efavirenz 600 mg/emtricitabine 200 mg/tenofovir 300 mg) (PO) QD on an empty stomach

How Supplied: Oral Tablet: Contains 600 mg Efavirenz + 200 mg Emtricitabine + 300 mg Tenofovir Disoproxil Fumarate

Pharmacokinetic Parameters:

Peak serum level: 4.0/1.8 mcg/mL/ 296 ng/mL

Bioavailability: NR/93%/25%

Excreted unchanged: < 1% unchanged and 14–30% as metabolites/86%/32%

Serum half-life (normal/ESRD): (40–55 hrs/ ~ 10 hrs on hemodialysis)/(10 hrs/extended)/ (17 hrs/no data)

Plasma protein binding: 99/< 4/< 0.7%

Volume of distribution (V_d): NR/NR/1.2 L/kg

Primary Mode of Elimination: hepatic/renal/renal

Dosage Adjustments*

CrCl 50–80 mL/min	No change
CrCl 10–50 mL/min	Avoid
CrCl < 10 mL/min	Avoid
Post-HD dose	Avoid
Post-PD dose	Avoid
CVVH dose	Avoid
Mild hepatic insufficiency	No information
Moderate or severe hepatic insufficiency	No information

"Usual dose" assumes normal renal/hepatic function. * For renal insufficiency, give usual dose × 1 followed by maintenance dose per CrCl. For dialysis patients, dose the same as for CrCl < 10 mL/min and give supplemental (post-HD/PD dose) immediately after dialysis. CrCl = creatinine clearance; CVVH = continuous veno-venous hemo-filtration; HD/PD = hemodialysis/peritoneal dialysis. See pp. 214–216 for explanations, pp. xi–xii for abbreviations.

Antiretroviral Dosage Adjustments

Fosamprenavir/ ritonavir	An additional 100 mg/day (300 mg total) of ritonavir is recommended when Atripla is administered with fosamprenavir/ ritonavir QD. No change in ritonavir dose when Atripla is administered with fosamprenavir/ritonavir BID
Atazanavir	Avoid
Indinavir	Indinavir 1000 mg TID
Lopinavir/ ritonavir	Increase lopinavir/ritonavir to 600/150 mg (3 tablets) BID
Ritonavir	No information
Saquinavir	Avoid
Didanosine	Avoid
Rifabutin	Rifabutin 450–600 mg QD or 600 mg 2–3x/week if not on protease inhibitor
Rifampin	No change

Drug Interactions: Antiretrovirals, rifabutin (see dose adjustment grid above); astemizole, cisapride, ergotamine, methylergonovine, midazolam, triazolam, St John's wort (↓ efavirenz levels), voriconazole (↓ voriconazole levels; avoid), caspofungin (↓ caspofungin levels); carbamazepine, phenytoin, phenobarbital (monitor anticonvulsant levels; use with caution; potential for ↓ efavirenz levels); statins (may ↓ statin levels); methadone, (↓ methadone levels); clarithromycin (may ↓ clarithromycin effectiveness, consider using azithromycin).
Adverse Effects: Headache, diarrhea, nausea, vomiting, GI upset, lactic acidosis, osteopenia,

rash, dizziness, fatigue, lactic acidosis with hepatic steatosis (rare but potentially life-threatening with NRTIs), relapsing type B viral hepatitis, depression, vivid dreams, renal impairment.
Allergic Potential: High
Safety in Pregnancy: D
Comments: Rash/CNS effects usually resolve in a few weeks. Take at bedtime on empty stomach. High fat meals can ↑ efavirenz by 50%. Use with caution in patients with history of seizures (↑ risk of convulsions). Potential for cross-resistance to lamivudine, zalcitabine, abacavir, and didanosine. Low affinity for DNA polymerase-gamma.
Cerebrospinal Fluid Penetration: 1%/no data/no data

REFERENCES:
Gallant JE, DeJesus E, Arribas JR, et al: Tenofovir DF, emtricitabine, and efavirenz vs. zidovudine, lamivudine, and efavirenz for HIV. N Engl J Med 354:251–260, 2006.
Izzedine H, Aymard G, Launay-Vacher V, et al. Pharmacokinetics of efavirenz in a patient on maintenance haemodialysis. AIDS 14:618–619.
Panel on Antiretroviral Guidelines for Adults and Adolescents. Guidelines for the use of antiretroviral agents in HIV-1-infected adults and adolescents. Department of Health and Human Services. March 27, 2013; 1–240. Available at **http://www. aidsinfo.nih.gov/contentfiles/lvguidelines/ adultandadolescentgl.pdf**.

Elvitegravir, Cobicistat, Emtricitabine, Tenofovir disoproxil fumarate (Stribild®)

Drug Class: HIV Combination Antiretroviral Agent
Usual Dose: 1 tablet PO QD with a meal (preferably high fat)
How supplied: oral tablet: (containing; 150 mg of elvitegravir, 150 mg of cobicistat, 200 mg of emtricitabine, and 300 mg of tenofovir disoproxil fumarate)

"Usual dose" assumes normal renal/hepatic function. * For renal insufficiency, give usual dose × 1 followed by maintenance dose per CrCl. For dialysis patients, dose the same as for CrCl < 10 mL/min and give supplemental (post-HD/PD dose) immediately after dialysis. CrCl = creatinine clearance; CVVH = continuous veno-venous hemo-filtration; HD/PD = hemodialysis/peritoneal dialysis. See pp. 214–216 for explanations, pp. xi–xii for abbreviations.

Pharmacokinetic Parameters:

Peak serum level: 1.7 mcg/mL/1.1 mcg/mL/ 1.9 mcg/mL/0.45 mcg/mL

Bioavailability: 23% to 87% increased with food (high fat meals)

Excreted unchanged: 6.7% (urine)/8.2% (urine)/extensive (urine)/extensive (urine)

Serum half-life (normal/ESRD): 12.9/3.5/10/17(hrs)/no data

Plasma protein binding: 99%/98%/4%/0.7%

Volume of distribution (Vd): not data/no data/ no data/1.2 L/kg

Primary mode of Elimination: hepatic & feces/ hepatic & feces/renal/renal

Dosage Adjustments*

CrCl > 70 mL/min	No change
CrCl 30–49 mL/min	*Not recommended
CrCl < 30 mL/min	*Not recommended
ESRD	*Not recommended
Post-HD dose	*Not recommended
Post-PD dose	*Not recommended
CVVH dose	*Not recommended
Mild – moderate hepatic insufficiency	No change
Severe hepatic insufficiency	Not studied

* The fixed dose tablet is not recommended for patients with CrCl < 70ml/min, however therapy with one or more of the individual components might be possible, please refer agent specific drug monographs.

Antiretroviral Dosage Adjustments: *Please refer to individual drug monographs*

Drug Interactions: *Co-administration of STRIBILD is contraindicated with drugs that are highly dependent on CYP3A for clearance and for which elevated plasma concentrations are associated with serious and/or life-threatening events.* antiacids (↓ elvitegravir), ↑ alfuzosin, ↑ midazolam, pimozide, triazolam, rifampin (↓ elvitegravir), ↑ simvastatin, ↑ atrovastatin, ↑ fluticasone, ↑ colchicine, Avanafil (do not coadminister), ↑ sildenafil (max 25 mg in 48 hours), ↑ tadalafil, ↑ vardenafil, ↑ beta-blockers, ↑ SSRIs, ↑ TCAs, ↑ digoxin, ↑ ↓ voriconazole, ketoconazole, itraconazole, (↑ elvitegravir), rivaroxaban (↑ rivaroxaban), Warfarin (↑ warafrin, monitor INR)

Adverse Effects: *Please refer to individual drug monographs for more complete details.*

- Most common adverse drug reactions to elvitegravir/cobicistat are ≥ 10% all grades: gastrointestinal (diarrhea and nausea) and renal (proteinunria)
- Most common adverse drug reactions to emtricitabine and tenofovir disoproxil fumarate are diarrhea, nausea, fatigue, headache, dizziness, depression, insomnia, abnormal dreams, lactic acidosis, myalgia, decreased bone mineral density and rash.

Allergic Potential: low

Safety in Pregnancy: B

Comments: Must be taken with a full meal (preferably high fat), Stribild exposure was about 87% lower when administered in the fasted state. Concomitant use with other antiretrovirals, including ritonavir, is not recommended. Avoid administering Stribild with concurrent or recent use of nephrotoxic drugs. In patients coinfected with HIV-1 and HBV, abrupt withdrawal of emtricitabine or tenofovir DF have caused severe acute exacerbations of hepatitis B virus infection. Patients who fail elvitegravir can develop cross resistance to raltegravir.

Cerebrospinal Fluid Penetration: No data

"Usual dose" assumes normal renal/hepatic function. * For renal insufficiency, give usual dose × 1 followed by maintenance dose per CrCl. For dialysis patients, dose the same as for CrCl < 10 mL/min and give supplemental (post-HD/PD dose) immediately after dialysis. CrCl = creatinine clearance; CVVH = continuous veno-venous hemo-filtration; HD/PD = hemodialysis/peritoneal dialysis. See pp. 214–216 for explanations, pp. xi–xii for abbreviations.

REFERENCES:

Product Information: STRIBILD(TM) oral tablets, elvitegravir cobicistat emtricitabine tenofovir disoproxil fumarate oral tablets. Gilead Sciences, Inc. (per manufacturer), Foster City, CA, 2012.

Sax PE, DeJesus E, Mills A, et al: Co-formulated elvitegravir, cobicistat, emtricitabine, and tenofovir versus co-formulated efavirenz, emtricitabine, and tenofovir for initial treatment of HIV-1 infection: a randomised, double-blind, phase 3 trial, analysis of results after 48 weeks. Lancet 2012; 379(9835):2439–2448.

DeJesus E, Rockstroh JK, Henry K, et al: Co-formulated elvitegravir, cobicistat, emtricitabine, and tenofovir disoproxil fumarate versus ritonavir-boosted atazanavir plus co-formulated emtricitabine and tenofovir disoproxil fumarate for initial treatment of HIV-1 infection: a randomised, double-blind, phase 3, non-inferiority trial. Lancet 2012; 379(9835):2429–2438

Ramanathan S, Mathias AA, German P, Kearney BP. Clinical pharmacokinetic and pharmacodynamic profile of the HIV integrase inhibitor elvitegravir. Clinical pharmacokinetics. Apr 2011;50(4):229–244

Website: https://www.stribild.com/

Emtricitabine (Emtriva) FTC

Drug Class: Antiretroviral NRTI (nucleoside reverse transcriptase inhibitor)
Usual Dose: 200 mg (PO) QD
How Supplied: Oral Capsule: 200 mg, Oral Solution: 10 mg/mL
Pharmacokinetic Parameters:
Peak serum level: 1.8 mcg/mL
Bioavailability: 93%
Excreted unchanged (urine): 86%
Serum half-life (normal/ESRD): 10 hrs/extended
Plasma protein binding: 4%
Primary Mode of Elimination: Renal
Dosage Adjustments*

CrCl ≥ 50 mL/min	200 mg (PO) QD
CrCl 30–49 mL/min	200 mg (PO) q2d
CrCl 15–29 mL/min	200 mg (PO) q3d
CrCl < 15 mL/min	200 mg (PO) q4d
Post-HD dose	200 mg (PO) q4d
Post-PD dose	No information
CVVH dose	No information
Moderate or severe hepatic insufficiency	No change

Drug Interactions: No significant interactions with indinavir, stavudine, zidovudine, famciclovir, tenofovir.
Adverse Effects: Headache, diarrhea, nausea, rash, lactic acidosis with hepatic steatosis (rare, but potentially life-threatening with NRIIs).
Allergic Potential: Low
Safety in Pregnancy: B
Comments: May be taken with or without food. Does not inhibit CYP450 enzymes. Mean intracellular half-life of 39 hours. Potential cross-resistance to lamivudine and zalcitabine. Low affinity for DNA polymerase-gamma.
Cerebrospinal Fluid Penetration: No data

REFERENCES:

Anderson PL. Pharmacologic perspectives for once-daily antiretroviral therapy. Ann Pharmacother 38:1924–34, 2004.

Benson CA, van der Horst C, Lamarca A, et al. A randomized study of emtricitabine and lamivudine in stable suppressed patients with HIV. AIDS 18:2269–2276, 2004.

Dando TM, Wagstaff AJ. Emtricitabine/tenofovir disoproxil fumarate. Drugs 64:2075–82, 2004.

Gallant JE, DeJesus D, Arribas JR, et al. Tenofovir DF, emtricitabine, and efavirenz vs. zidovudine, lamivudine, and efavirenz for HIV. N Engl J Med 354:251–60, 2006.

"Usual dose" assumes normal renal/hepatic function. * For renal insufficiency, give usual dose × 1 followed by maintenance dose per CrCl. For dialysis patients, dose the same as for CrCl < 10 mL/min and give supplemental (post-HD/PD dose) immediately after dialysis. CrCl = creatinine clearance; CVVH = continuous veno-venous hemo-filtration; HD/PD = hemodialysis/peritoneal dialysis. See pp. 214–216 for explanations, pp. xi–xii for abbreviations.

Lim SG, Ng TN, Kung N, et al. A double-blind placebo-controlled study of emtricitabine in chronic hepatitis B. *Arch Intern Med* 166:49–56, 2006.

Panel on Antiretroviral Guidelines for Adults and Adolescents. Guidelines for the use of antiretroviral agents in HIV-1-infected adults and adolescents. Department of Health and Human Services. March 27, 2013; 1–240. Available at **http://www.aidsinfo.nih.gov/contentfiles/lvguidelines/adultandadolescentgl.pdf**.

Saag MS. Emtricitabine, a new antiretroviral agent with activity against HIV and hepatitis B virus. *Clin Infect Dis* 42;128–31, 2006.

Emtricitabine + Rilpivirine hydrochloride + Tenofovir disoproxil fumarate (Complera®)

Drug Class: HIV Combination Antiretroviral Agent
Usual Dose: 1 tablet PO QD with a high fat meal
How supplied: oral tablet: (containing 200 mg of emtricitabine, 25 mg of rilpivirine, and 300 mg of tenofovir disoproxil fumarate)
Pharmacokinetic Parameters:
Peak serum level: 1.8 mcg/mL/NR/ 0.29 mcg/mL
Bioavailability: 93%/no data/25–39%
Excreted unchanged: 14%/25%/n/a (feces) 86%/6.1%/32% (urine)
Serum half-life (normal/ESRD): 10/50/17(hrs)/ no data
Plasma protein binding: 4%/99.7%/0.7%
Volume of distribution (Vd): not data/no data/ 1.3 L/kg
Primary mode of Elimination: renal/renal & feces/renal

Dosage Adjustments*

CrCl 50–80 mL/min	No change
CrCl 30–49 mL/min	*Not recommended
CrCl < 30 mL/min	*Not recommended
ESRD	*Not recommended
Post-HD dose	*Not recommended
Post-PD dose	*Not recommended
CVVH dose	*Not recommended
Mild – moderate hepatic insufficiency	No change
Severe hepatic insufficiency	Not studied

* The fixed dose tablet is not recommended for patients with CrCl < 50ml/min, however therapy with one or more of the individual components might be possible, please refer agent specific drug monographs.

Antiretroviral Dosage Adjustments: *Please refer to individual drug monographs*
Drug Interactions: *Please refer to individual drug monographs*
Adverse Effects: *Please refer to individual drug monographs for more complete details.*

- Most common adverse drug reactions to rilpivirine (>2%, Grades 2–4) are insomnia and headache.
- Most common adverse drug reactions to emtricitabine and tenofovir disoproxil fumarate (≥ 10%) are diarrhea, nausea, fatigue, headache, dizziness, depression, insomnia, abnormal dreams, and rash.

Allergic Potential: low
Safety in Pregnancy: B
Comments: Must be taken with a full meal (preferably high fat), rilpivirine exposure was

---

"Usual dose" assumes normal renal/hepatic function. * For renal insufficiency, give usual dose × 1 followed by maintenance dose per CrCl. For dialysis patients, dose the same as for CrCl < 10 mL/min and give supplemental (post-HD/PD dose) immediately after dialysis. CrCl = creatinine clearance; CVVH = continuous veno-venous hemo-filtration; HD/PD = hemodialysis/peritoneal dialysis. See pp. 214–216 for explanations, pp. xi–xii for abbreviations.

about 40% lower when administered in the fasted state. Use with caution in patients with severe depressive disorders as depression, dysphoria, major depression, mood altered, negative thoughts, suicide attempt, and suicidal ideation, have been reported with rilpivirine. In clinical trials patients with HIV-1 RNA > 100,000 copies/mL at therapy initiation experienced virologic failure more often than patients with HIV-1 RNA < 100,000 copies/mL at the start of therapy. Patients who experience virological failure on rilpivirine may be at risk for cross-resistance to other NNRTIs and to emtricitabine/lamivudine

Cerebrospinal Fluid Penetration: no data

REFERENCES:

Product Information: COMPLERA(TM) oral tablets, emtricitabine/rilpivirine/tenofovir disoproxil fumarate oral tablets. Gilead Sciences, Inc. (per Manufacturer), Foster City, CA, 2011.

Cohen CJ, Andrade-Villanueva J, Clotet B, et al: Rilpivirine versus efavirenz with two background nucleoside or nucleotide reverse transcriptase inhibitors in treatment-naive adults infected with HIV-1 (THRIVE): a phase 3, randomized, non-inferiority trial. Lancet 2011; 378(9787):229–237.

Molina JM, Cahn P, Grinsztejn B, et al: Rilpivirine versus efavirenz with tenofovir and emtricitabine in treatment-naive adults infected with HIV-1 (ECHO): a phase 3 randomized double-blind active-controlled trial. Lancet 2011; 378(9787):238–246.

Schrijvers R, Desimmie BA, Debyser Z. Rilpivirine: a step forward in tailored HIV treatment. Lancet. Jul 16 2011;378(9787):201–203.

Panel on Antiretroviral Guidelines for Adults and Adolescents. Guidelines for the use of antiretroviral agents in HIV-1-infected adults and adolescents. Department of Health and Human Services. March 27, 2013; 1–240. Available at **http://www. aidsinfo.nih.gov/contentfiles/lvguidelines/ adultandadolescentgl.pdf.**

Website: http://www.complera.com/

Emtricitabine + Tenofovir disoproxil fumarate (Truvada)

Drug Class: Antiretroviral NRTI (nucleoside reverse transcriptase inhibitor) + nucleotide analogue

Usual Dose: One tablet (PO) QD (each tablet contains 200 mg of emtricitabine + 300 mg of tenofovir)

How Supplied: Oral Tablet: Contains 200 mg Emtricitabine + 300 mg Tenofovir Disoproxil Fumarate

Pharmacokinetic Parameters:
Peak serum level: 1.8/0.3 mcg/L
Bioavailability: 93%/27% if fasting (39% with high fat meal)
Excreted unchanged (urine): 86/32%
Serum half-life (normal/ESRD): (10 hrs/ extended)/(17 hrs/no data)
Plasma protein binding: 4/0.7–7.2%
Volume of distribution (V_d): no data/1.3 L/kg

Primary Mode of Elimination: Renal/Renal
Dosage Adjustments*

CrCl ≥ 50 mL/min	No change
CrCl 30–49 mL/min	One capsule (PO) q2d
CrCl 15–29 mL/min	Avoid
CrCl < 15 mL/min	Avoid
Post-HD dose	Avoid
Post-PD dose	Avoid
CVVH dose	Avoid
Moderate or severe hepatic insufficiency	No change

Drug Interactions: No significant interactions with indinavir, stavudine, zidovudine, famciclovir, lamivudine, lopinavir/ritonavir, efavirenz, methadone, oral contraceptives.

"Usual dose" assumes normal renal/hepatic function. * For renal insufficiency, give usual dose × 1 followed by maintenance dose per CrCl. For dialysis patients, dose the same as for CrCl < 10 mL/min and give supplemental (post-HD/PD dose) immediately after dialysis. CrCl = creatinine clearance; CVVH = continuous veno-venous hemo-filtration; HD/PD = hemodialysis/peritoneal dialysis. See pp. 214–216 for explanations, pp. xi–xii for abbreviations.

Tenofovir ↑ didanosine levels. Tenofovir reduces systemic exposure to atazanavir; whenever the two are coadministered, the recommended dose of atazanavir is 300 mg once daily with ritonavir 100 mg once daily.

Adverse Effects: Headache, diarrhea, nausea, vomiting, GI upset, rash, lactic acidosis with hepatic steatosis (rare but potentially life-threatening with NRTIs).

Allergic Potential: Low

Safety in Pregnancy: B

Comments: May be taken with or without food. Does not inhibit CYP450 enzymes. Mean intracellular half-life with emtricitabine is 39 hours. Potential cross-resistance to lamivudine, zalcitabine, abacavir, didanosine. Low affinity for DNA polymerase-gamma. Avoid coadministration with didanosine.

Cerebrospinal Fluid Penetration: No data

REFERENCES:

Dando TM, Wagstaff AJ. Emtricitabine/tenofovir disoproxil fumarate. *Drugs* 64:2075–82, 2004.

Gallant JE, DeJesus D, Arribas JR, et al. Tenofovir DF, emtricitabine, and efavirenz vs zidovudine, lamivudine, and efavirenz for HIV. *N Engl J Med* 354:251–60, 2006.

Panel on Antiretroviral Guidelines for Adults and Adolescents. Guidelines for the use of antiretroviral agents in HIV-1-infected adults and adolescents. Department of Health and Human Services. March 27, 2013; 1–240. Available at **http://www.aidsinfo.nih.gov/contentfiles/lvguidelines/adultandadolescentgl.pdf**.

Website: www.truvada.com

Enfuvirtide (Fuzeon)
ENF (T-20)

Drug Class: Antiretroviral fusion inhibitor

Usual Dose: 90 mg (SC) BID

How Supplied: Subcutaneous Powder for Solution: 90 mg

Pharmacokinetic Parameters:
Peak serum level: 4.9 mcg/mL
Bioavailability: 84.3%
Serum half-life (normal/ESRD): 3.8 hrs/ no data
Plasma protein binding: 92%
Volume of distribution (V_d): 5.5 L

Primary Mode of Elimination: Metabolized

Dosage Adjustments*

CrCl > 35 mL/min	No change
CrCl < 35 mL/min	No data
Post-HD dose	No data
Post-PD dose	No data
CVVH dose	No data
Moderate or severe hepatic insufficiency	No data

Drug Interactions: No clinically significant interactions with other antiretrovirals. Does not inhibit CYP450 enzymes.

Adverse Effects: Local injection site reactions are common. Diarrhea, nausea, fatigue may occur. Laboratory abnormalities include mild/transient eosinophilia. Pneumonia may occur, but cause is unclear and may not be due to drug therapy. Pancreatitis, myalgia, conjunctivitis (rare).

Allergic Potential: Hypersensitivity reactions may occur, including fever, chills, hypotension, rash, ↑ serum transaminases. Do not rechallenge following a hypersensitivity reaction

Safety in Pregnancy: B

Comments: Enfuvirtide interferes with entry of HIV-1 into cells by blocking fusion of HIV-1 and CD4 cellular membranes by binding to HR1 in the gp41 subunit of the HIV-1 envelope glycoprotein. Additive/synergistic with NRTIs, NNRTIs, and PIs, and no cross resistance to

---

"Usual dose" assumes normal renal/hepatic function. * For renal insufficiency, give usual dose × 1 followed by maintenance dose per CrCl. For dialysis patients, dose the same as for CrCl < 10 mL/min and give supplemental (post-HD/PD dose) immediately after dialysis. CrCl = creatinine clearance; CVVH = continuous veno-venous hemo-filtration; HD/PD = hemodialysis/peritoneal dialysis. See pp. 214–216 for explanations, pp. xi–xii for abbreviations.

other antiretrovirals in cell culture. Compared to background regimen, enfuvirtide ↑ CD4 (71 vs. 35 cells/mm³) and ↓ HIV-1 RNA (−1.52 log₁₀ vs. −0.73 log₁₀ copies/mL) at 24 weeks. Reconstitute in 1.1 mL of sterile water. SC injection should be given into upper arm, anterior thigh, or abdomen. Rotate injection sites; do not inject into moles, scars, bruises. After reconstitution, use immediately or refrigerate and use within 24 hours (no preservatives added).

REFERENCES:

Coleman CI, Musial, BL, Ross, J. Enfuvirtide: the first fusion inhibitor for the treatment of patients with HIV-1 infection. *Formulary* 38:204–222, 2003.

Kilby JM, Lalezari JP, Eron JJ, et al. The safety, plasma pharmacokinetics, and antiviral activity of subcutaneous enfuvirtide (T-20), a peptide inhibitor of gp41-mediated virus fusion, in HIV-infected adults. *AIDS Res Hum Retroviruses* 18:685–93, 2002.

Lalezari JP, Eron JJ, Carlson M, et al. A phase II clinical study of the long-term safety and antiviral activity of enfuvirtide-based antiretroviral therapy. *AIDS* 17:691–8, 2003.

Lalezari JP, Henry K, O'Hearn M, et al. TORO 1 Study Group. Enfuvirtide, an HIV-1 fusion inhibitor, for drug-resistant HIV infection in North and South America. *N Engl J Med* 348:2175–85, 2003.

Lazzarin A, Clotet B, Cooper D, et al. TORO 2 Study Group. Efficacy of enfuvirtide in patients infected with drug-resistant HIV-1 in Europe and Australia. *N Engl J Med* 348:2186–95, 2003.

Leao J, Frezzini C, Porter S. Enfuvirtide: a new class of antiretroviral therapy for HIV infection. *Oral Dis* 10:327–9, 2004.

Leen C, Wat C, Nieforth K. Pharmacokinetics of enfuvirtide in a patient with impaired renal function. *Clin Infect Dis* 4:339–55, 2004.

Panel on Antiretroviral Guidelines for Adults and Adolescents. Guidelines for the use of antiretroviral agents in HIV-1-infected adults and adolescents. Department of Health and Human Services. March 27, 2013; 1–240. Available at **http://www.aidsinfo.nih.gov/contentfiles/lvguidelines/adultandadolescentgl.pdf.**

Entecavir (Baraclude) ETV

Drug Class: Anti-hepatitis B agent—Guanosine Nucleoside Analog

Usual Dose: nucleoside-treatment-naïve patients—0.5 mg PO once daily without food; history of hepatitis B viremia while receiving lamivudine or known lamivudine resistant mutations—1 mg PO once daily, without food

How Supplied: Oral Solution: 0.05 mg/mL; Oral Tablet: 0.5 mg, 1 mg

Pharmacokinetic Parameters:

Peak serum level: 4.2 ng/mL (0.5 mg), 8.2 ng/ml (1 mg)

Bioavailability: ~ 100%

Excreted unchanged (urine): 62–73% (urine)

Serum half-life (normal/ESRD): 128–149 hrs/ no data

Plasma protein binding: 13%

Volume of distribution (V_d): extensively distributed into tissues

Primary Mode of Elimination: renal

Dosage Adjustments*

	Treatment-naïve (0.5 mg)	Lamivudine-refractory (1 mg)
CrCl > 50 mL/min	0.5 mg QD	1 mg QD
CrCl 30–50 mL/min	0.25 mg QD or 0.5 mg q2d	0.5 mg QD or 1 mg q2d
CrCl 10–30 mL/min	0.15 mg QD or 0.5 mg q3d	0.3 mg QD or 1 mg q3d
CrCl < 10 mL/min	0.05 mg QD or 0.5 mg q7d	0.1 mg QD or 1 mg q7d
Post-HD dose†	0.05 mg QD or 0.5 mg q7d	0.1 mg QD or 1 mg q7d

"Usual dose" assumes normal renal/hepatic function. * For renal insufficiency, give usual dose × 1 followed by maintenance dose per CrCl. For dialysis patients, dose the same as for CrCl < 10 mL/min and give supplemental (post-HD/PD dose) immediately after dialysis. CrCl = creatinine clearance; CVVH = continuous veno-venous hemo-filtration; HD/PD = hemodialysis/peritoneal dialysis. See pp. 214–216 for explanations, pp. xi–xii for abbreviations.

Post-PD dose[†]	0.05 mg QD or 0.5 mg q7d	0.1 mg QD or 1 mg q7d
CVVH dose	No data	No data
Mild to moderate hepatic insufficiency	No change	No change
Severe hepatic insufficiency	Mop change	No change

[†] On dialysis days, give dose after dialysis.

Antiretroviral Dosage Adjustments: None
Drug Interactions: Since entecavir is primarily eliminated by the kidneys, coadministration of entecavir with drugs that reduce renal function or compete for active tubular secretion may increase serum concentrations of either entecavir or the coadministered drug. Coadministration of entecavir with lamivudine, adefovir dipivoxil, or tenofovir disoproxil fumarate did not result in significant drug interactions.
Adverse Effects: Rash has been reported with entecavir therapy during postmarketing surveillance. Lactic acidosis and severe hepato-megaly with steatosis have been reported, predominantly in women, with the use of nucleoside analogs alone or in combination with antiretrovirals, including entecavir. Obesity and prolonged exposure may be risk factors. GI effects: Nausea/vomiting/diarrhea/indigestion have been reported in < 1% of patients. Neurologic effects: dizziness 3%, headache 3%, insomnia < 1%, somnolence < 1%. Renal effects: hematuria 9%. Fatigue 3%.
Allergic Potential: Low—Anaphylactoid reaction has been reported with

entecavir therapy during postmarketing surveillance
Safety in Pregnancy: C
Comments: Entecavir should be taken on an empty stomach (at least 2 hours after a meal and 2 hours before the next meal). Oral solution—do not dilute or mix with water or any other liquid. HIV coinfection; entecavir is not recommended in patients who are not receiving concurrent HIV treatment (i.e., highly active antiretroviral therapy) due to the risk of HIV nucleoside reverse transcriptase inhibitor resistance. Lactic acidosis and severe hepatomegaly with steatosis, including fatalities, have been reported with nucleoside analogs; patients with obesity, female gender, prolonged nucleoside exposure, or known risk factors for liver disease may be at increased risk; suspend treatment if signs or symptoms of lactic acidosis or hepatotoxicity occur. Entecavir is potent and well tolerated and has extremely low resistance rates in nucleoside/nucleotide analogue-naïve patients.
Cerebrospinal Fluid Penetration: No data
Comments: Entecavir may select for the M184V mutation in HIV. As a result, it is contraindicated in patients with HIV who are not on suppressive ART.

REFERENCES:
Chang TT, Gish RG, deMan R, et al. A comparison of entecavir and lamivudine for HBeAg-positive chronic hepatitis B. *N Engl J Med* 354(10):1001–10, 2006.
Honkoop P, de Man RA. Entecavir: a potent new antiviral drug for hepatitis B. *Expert Opin Investig Drugs* 12(4):683–8, 2003.
Lai CL, Rosmawati M, Lao J. Entecavir is superior to lamivudine in reducing hepatitis B virus DNA in patients with chronic hepatitis B infection. *Gastroenterology* 123:1831–38, 2002.
Lai CL, Shouval D, Lok AS, et al. Entecavir versus lamivudine for patients with HBeAg-negative

----

chronic hepatitis B. *N Engl J Med* 354(10):1011–20, 2006.

Product Information: BARACLUDE® oral tablets, entecavir oral tablets, solution. Bristol-Myers Squibb, Princeton, NJ, 2008.

Sherman M, Yurdaydin C, Sollano J, et al. Entecavir for treatment of lamivudine-refractory, HBeAg-positive chronic hepatitis B. *Gastroenterology* 130(7):2039–49, 2006.

Tenney DJ, Levine SM, Rose RE, et al. Clinical emergence of entecavir-resistant hepatitis B virus requires additional substitutions in virus already resistant to lamivudine. *Antimicrob Agents Chemother* 48(9):3498–3507, 2004.

Website: www.baraclude.com

Etravirine (Intelence) ETR

Drug Class: Antiretroviral NNRTI (non-nucleoside reverse transcriptase inhibitor)
Usual Dose: 200 mg (PO) BID following a meal
How Supplied: Oral Tablet: 100 mg, 200 mg
Pharmacokinetic Parameters:
Peak serum level: 296 ng/mL
Bioavailability: unknown (food increases systemic exposure)
Excreted unchanged: 81–86% (feces); 0% (urine)
Serum half-life (normal/ESRD): 41 hrs/not studied
Plasma protein binding: 99.9%
Volume of distribution (V_d): Not studied
Primary Mode of Elimination: Fecal 93.7%/renal 1.2%
Dosage Adjustments*

CrCl 50–80 mL/min	Not studied
CrCl 10–50 mL/min	Not studied
CrCl < 10 mL/min	Not studied
Post-HD dose	No change
Post-PD dose	No change
CVVH dose	Not studied

Moderate or severe hepatic insufficiency	No change
Co-infection with Hepatitis B or C virus	No change

Antiretroviral Dosage Adjustments

Atazanavir/ritonavir	Avoid
Delavirdine	Avoid (↑ etravirine)
Efavirenz/nevirapine	Avoid (↓ etravirine)
Fosamprenavir/ritonavir	Use with caution (↑ amprenavir)
Lopinavir/ritonavir	Use with caution (↑ etravirine)
Ritonavir (600 mg BID)	Avoid (↓ etravirine)
Darunavir/ritonavir	No change
Rifabutin, Rifampin	Avoid (↓ etravirine)
Tipranavir/ritonavir	Avoid (↓ etravirine)
Saquinavir/ritonavir	No change
Maraviroc	600 mg BID
Raltegravir	No change

Drug Interactions: Etravirine is a substrate for the liver enzymes CYP3A4, CYP2C9, and CYP2C19. Coadministration with drugs that inhibit or induce these enzymes may alter the therapeutic effect or adverse reaction profile of etravirine or concomitant drug. Amiodarone, bepridil, disopyramide, flecainide, lidocaine (systemic), mexiletine, propafenone, quinidine (↓ antiarrhythmic levels); warfarin (↑ warfarin levels); carbamazepine, phenobarbital, phenytoin (↓ etravirine levels); antifungals (↑ etravirine levels)—also etravirine decreases

---

"Usual dose" assumes normal renal/hepatic function. * For renal insufficiency, give usual dose × 1 followed by maintenance dose per CrCl. For dialysis patients, dose the same as for CrCl < 10 mL/min and give supplemental (post-HD/PD dose) immediately after dialysis. CrCl = creatinine clearance; CVVH = continuous veno-venous hemo-filtration; HD/PD = hemodialysis/peritoneal dialysis. See pp. 214–216 for explanations, pp. xi–xii for abbreviations.

itraconazole and ketoconazole levels and increases voriconazole levels but has no effect on fluconazole or posaconazole levels; clarithromycin ($\uparrow$ etravirine levels, $\downarrow$ clarithromycin levels), atorvastatin ($\downarrow$ atorvastatin levels), sildenafil ($\downarrow$ sildenafil levels), tadalafil ($\downarrow$ tadalafil levels), vardenafil ($\downarrow$ vardenafil levels); etravirine has no effect on methadone levels.

Adverse Effects: Hypertension, rash, abdominal pain, nausea, diarrhea, $\uparrow$ liver enzymes AST(SGOT)/ALT(SGPT), myocardial infarction, hypersensitivity reaction.

Allergic Potential: Low (< 2%)

Safety in Pregnancy: B

Comments: Severe and potentially life-threatening skin reactions have been reported, including Stevens-Johnson syndrome, hypersensitivity reaction, and erythema multiforme. Discontinue treatment if severe rash develops. Efficacy in treatment-naïve patients has not been established. Take with meals; food increases systemic exposure by 50%.

Cerebrospinal Fluid Penetration: No data

REFERENCES:

Lazzarin A, Campbell T, Clotet B, et al. Efficacy and safety of TMC125 (etravirine) in treatment-experienced HIV-1-infected patients in DUET-2: 24-week results from a randomised, double-blind, placebo-controlled trial. *Lancet* 370: 39–48, 2007.

Madruga JV, Cahn P, Grinsztejn B, et al. Efficacy and safety of TMC125 (etravirine) in treatment-experienced HIV-1-infected patients in DUET-1: 24-week results from a randomised, double-blind, placebo-controlled trial. *Lancet* 370:29–38, 2007.

Panel on Antiretroviral Guidelines for Adults and Adolescents. Guidelines for the use of antiretroviral agents in HIV-1-infected adults and adolescents. Department of Health and Human Services.

March 27, 2013; 1–240. Available at **http://www.aidsinfo.nih.gov/contentfiles/lvguidelines/adultandadolescentgl.pdf**.

Product Information: INTELENCE™ oral tablets, etravirine oral tablets. Tibotec Therapeutics, Inc., Raritan, NJ, 2008.

Fosamprenavir (Lexiva) FPV

Drug Class: Antiretroviral protease inhibitor

Usual Dose: Treatment-naïve patients: 1400 mg BID or 1400 mg + ritonavir 100–200 mg QD or 700 mg + ritonavir 100 mg BID

Treatment-experienced patients: (once daily dosing not recommended) 700 mg + ritonavir 100 mg BID

Pharmacokinetic Parameters:

Peak serum level: 4.8 mcg/mL

Bioavailability: No data

Excreted unchanged (urine): 1%

Serum half-life (normal/ESRD): 7 hrs/no data

Plasma protein binding: 90%

Volume of distribution (V_d): 6.1 L/kg

Primary Mode of Elimination: Hepatic

Dosage Adjustments*

CrCl 50–80 mL/min	No change
CrCl 10–50 mL/min	No change
CrCl < 10 mL/min	No change
Post-HD or PD dose	No change
CVVH dose	No change
Mild-moderate hepatic insufficiency (Child-Pugh score 5–8)	700 mg (PO) BID if given without ritonavir; no data with ritonavir
Severe hepatic insufficiency (Child-Pugh score 9–12)	Avoid

"Usual dose" assumes normal renal/hepatic function. * For renal insufficiency, give usual dose × 1 followed by maintenance dose per CrCl. For dialysis patients, dose the same as for CrCl < 10 mL/min and give supplemental (post-HD/PD dose) immediately after dialysis. CrCl = creatinine clearance; CVVH = continuous veno-venous hemo-filtration; HD/PD = hemodialysis/peritoneal dialysis. See pp. 214–216 for explanations, pp. xi–xii for abbreviations.

Antiretroviral Dosage Adjustments:

Didanosine	Administer didanosine 1 hour apart
Delavirdine	Avoid combination
Efavirenz	Fosamprenavir 700 mg BID + ritonavir 100 mg BID + efavirenz; fosamprenavir 1400 mg QD + ritonavir 200 mg QD + efavirenz; no data for fosamprenavir 1400 mg BID + efavirenz
Indinavir	No information
Lopinavir/ ritonavir	Avoid
Nelfinavir	No information
Nevirapine	(FPV 700 mg + RTV 100 mg) BID NVP standard
Saquinavir	No information
Rifampin	Avoid combination
Rifabutin	Reduce usual rifabutin dose by 50% (or 75% if given with fosamprenavir plus ritonavir; max. 150 mg q2d)
Etravirine	Avoid combination
Maraviroc	150 mg BID
Raltegravir	No data

Drug Interactions: Antiretrovirals (see dose adjustment grid, above). Contraindicated with: ergot derivatives, cisapride, midazolam, triazolam, pimozide, flecainide and propafenone (if administered with ritonavir). Do not coadminister with: rifampin, lovastatin, simvastatin, St. John's wort, delavirdine. Dose reduction (of other drug): atorvastatin, rifabutin, sildenafil, vardenafil, ketoconazole, itraconazole. Concentration monitoring (of other drug): amiodarone, systemic lidocaine, quinidine, warfarin (INR), rivaroxaban ($\uparrow$ rivaroxaban), tricyclic antidepressants, cyclosporin, tacrolimus, sirolimus. H_2 blockers and proton pump inhibitors interfere with absorption. Sildenafil (do not give > 25 mg/48 hrs); tadalafil (max. 10 mg/72 hrs); vardenafil (max. 2.5 mg/72 hrs).

Adverse Effects: Rash, Stevens-Johnson syndrome (rare), GI upset, headache, depression, diarrhea, hyperglycemia (including worsening diabetes, new-onset diabetes, DKA), $\uparrow$ cholesterol/triglycerides (evaluate risk for coronary disease/pancreatitis), fat redistribution, $\uparrow$ SGOT/SGPT, possible increased bleeding in hemophilia; potential increased risk of myocardial infarction has been reported.

Allergic Potential: High. Fosamprenavir is a sulfonamide; use with caution in patients with sulfonamide allergies

Safety in Pregnancy: C

Comments: Usually given in conjunction with ritonavir. May be taken with or without food. Fosamprenavir is a prodrug that is rapidly hydrolyzed to amprenavir by gut epithelium during absorption. Amprenavir inhibits CYP3A4. Fosamprenavir contains a sulfonamide moiety (as do darunavir and tipranavir).

REFERENCES:

Becker S, Thornton L. Fosamprenavir: advancing HIV protease inhibitor treatment options. *Expert Opin Pharmacother* 5:1995–2005, 2004.

Chapman TM, Plosker GL, Perry CM. Fosamprenavir: a review of its use in the management of antiretroviral therapy-naïve patients with HIV infection. *Drugs* 64:2101–24, 2004.

Lexiva (fosamprenavir) approved. *AIDS Treat News* 31;2, 2003.

"Usual dose" assumes normal renal/hepatic function. * For renal insufficiency, give usual dose × 1 followed by maintenance dose per CrCl. For dialysis patients, dose the same as for CrCl < 10 mL/min and give supplemental (post-HD/PD dose) immediately after dialysis. CrCl = creatinine clearance; CVVH = continuous veno-venous hemo-filtration; HD/PD = hemodialysis/peritoneal dialysis. See pp. 214–216 for explanations, pp. xi–xii for abbreviations.

Panel on Antiretroviral Guidelines for Adults and Adolescents. Guidelines for the use of antiretroviral agents in HIV-1-infected adults and adolescents. Department of Health and Human Services. March 27, 2013; 1–240. Available at **http://www.aidsinfo.nih.gov/ contentfiles/lvguidelines/adultandadolescentgl.pdf**.

Rodriguez-French A, Boghossian J, Gray GE, et al. The NEAT study: a 48-week open-label study to compare the antiviral efficacy and safety of GW433908 versus nelfinavir in antiretroviral therapy-naïve HIV-1-infected patients. *J Acquir Immune Defic Syndr* 35:22–32, 2004.

Indinavir (Crixivan) IDV

Drug Class: Antiretroviral protease inhibitor
Usual Dose: 800 mg (PO) TID
How Supplied: Oral Capsule: 100 mg, 200 mg, 400 mg
Pharmacokinetic Parameters:
Peak serum level: 252 mcg/mL
Bioavailability: 65% (77% with food)
Excreted unchanged (urine): < 20%
Serum half-life (normal/ESRD): 2 hrs/no data
Plasma protein binding: 60%
Volume of distribution (V_d): No data
Primary Mode of Elimination: Hepatic
Dosage Adjustments*

CrCl 50–80 mL/min	No change
CrCl 10–50 mL/min	No change
CrCl < 10 mL/min	No change
Post-HD dose	None
Post-PD dose	None
CVVH dose	No change
Moderate hepatic insufficiency	600 mg (PO) TID
Severe hepatic insufficiency	400 mg (PO) TID

Antiretroviral Dosage Adjustments

Didanosine	Administer didanosine 1 hour apart
Delavirdine	Indinavir 600 mg TID
Efavirenz	Indinavir 1000 mg TID or IDV 800 mg + RTV 100–200 mg BID
Lopinavir/ ritonavir	Indinavir 600 mg BID
Nelfinavir	Limited data for indinavir 1200 mg BID + nelfinavir 1250 mg BID
Nevirapine	Indinavir 1000 mg TID or IDV 800 mg + RTV 100–200 mg BID
Ritonavir	Indinavir 800 mg BID + ritonavir 100–200 mg BID, or 400 mg BID of each drug
Saquinavir	No information
Rifampin	Avoid combination
Rifabutin	Indinavir 1000 mg TID; rifabutin 150 mg QD or 300 mg 2–3x/week
Etravirine	Avoid combination
Maraviroc	150 mg BID
Raltegravir	No information

Drug Interactions: Antiretrovirals, rifabutin, rifampin (see dose adjustment grid, above); astemizole, terfenadine, benzodiazepines, cisapride, ergot alkaloids, statins, St. John's wort (avoid if possible); calcium channel blockers (↑ calcium channel blocker levels); carbamazepine, phenobarbital, phenytoin (↓ indinavir levels,

---

"Usual dose" assumes normal renal/hepatic function. * For renal insufficiency, give usual dose × 1 followed by maintenance dose per CrCl. For dialysis patients, dose the same as for CrCl < 10 mL/min and give supplemental (post-HD/PD dose) immediately after dialysis. CrCl = creatinine clearance; CVVH = continuous veno-venous hemo-filtration; HD/PD = hemodialysis/peritoneal dialysis. See pp. 214–216 for explanations, pp. xi–xii for abbreviations.

↑ anticonvulsant levels; monitor); tenofovir (↓ indinavir levels, ↑ tenofovir levels); clarithromycin, erythromycin, telithromycin (↑ indinavir and macrolide levels); didanosine (administer indinavir on empty stomach 1 hour apart); ethinyl estradiol, norethindrone (↑ interacting drug levels; no dosage adjustment); grapefruit juice (↓ indinavir levels); itraconazole, ketoconazole (↑ indinavir levels); sildenafil (↑ or ↓ sildenafil levels; do not exceed 25 mg in 48 hrs), tadalafil (max. 10 mg/72 hrs), vardenafil (max 2.5 mg/72 hrs); theophylline (↓ theophylline levels); rivaroxaban (↑ rivaroxaban); Warfarin (↑ warafrin, monitor INR); fluticasone nasal spray (avoid concomitant use).

Adverse Effects: Nephrolithiasis, nausea, vomiting, diarrhea, anemia, leukopenia, headache, insomnia, hyperglycemia (including worsening diabetes, new-onset diabetes, DKA), ↑ SGOT/SGPT, ↑ indirect bilirubin (2° to drug-induced Gilbert's syndrome; inconsequential), fat redistribution, lipid abnormalities (evaluate risk of coronary disease/pancreatitis), abdominal pain, possible ↑ bleeding in hemophilia, dry skin, chelitis, paronychiae.

Allergic Potential: Low

Safety in Pregnancy: C

Comments: Renal stone formation may be prevented/minimized by adequate hydration (1–3 liters water daily); ↑ risk of nephrolithiasis with alcohol. Take 1 hour before or 2 hours after meals (may take with skim milk or low-fat meal). Separate dosing with ddI by 1 hour.

Cerebrospinal Fluid Penetration: 16%

REFERENCES:

Acosta EP, Henry K, Baken L, et al. Indinavir concentrations and antiviral effect. *Pharmacotherapy* 19:708–712, 1999.

Antinori A, Giancola MI, Griserri S, et al. Factors influencing virological response to antiretroviral drugs in cerebrospinal fluid of advanced HIV-1-infected patients. *AIDS* 16:1867–76, 2002.

Deeks SG, Smith M, Holodniy M, et al. HIV-1 protease inhibitors: A review for clinicians. *JAMA* 277:145–53, 1997.

DiCenzo R, Forrest A, Fischl MA, et al. Pharmacokinetics of indinavir and nelfinavir in treatment-naïve, human immunodeficiency virus-infected subjects. *Antimicrob Agents Chemother* 48:918–23, 2004.

Go J, Cunha BA. Indinavir: A review. *Antibiotics for Clinicians* 3:81–87, 1999.

Justesen US, Andersen AB, Klitgaard NA, et al. Pharmacokinetic interaction between rifampin and the combination of indinavir and low-dose ritonavir in HIV-infected patients. *Clin Infect Dis* 38:426–9, 2004.

Kopp JB, Falloon J, Filie A, et al. Indinavir-associated intestinal nephritis and urothelial inflammation: clinical and cytologic findings. *Clin Infect Dis* 34:1122–8, 2002.

Meraviglia P, Angeli E, Del Sorbo F, et al. Risk factors for indinavir-related renal colic in HIV patients: predicative value of indinavir dose-body mass index. *AIDS* 16:2089–93, 2002.

McDonald CK, Kuritzkes DR. Human immunodeficiency virus type 1 protease inhibitors. Arch Intern Med 157:951–9, 1997.

Panel on Antiretroviral Guidelines for Adults and Adolescents. Guidelines for the use of antiretroviral agents in HIV-1-infected adults and adolescents. Department of Health and Human Services. March 27, 2013; 1–240. Available at **http://www.aidsinfo.nih.gov/contentfiles/lvguidelines/adultandadolescentgl.pdf**.

Lamivudine (Epivir) 3TC

Drug Class: Antiretroviral NRTI (nucleoside reverse transcriptase inhibitor); antiviral (Hepatitis B Virus)

Usual Dose: 150 mg (PO) BID or 300 mg (PO) QD (HIV); 100 mg (PO) QD (HBV)

How Supplied:

Epivir A/F—Oral Solution: 10 mg/mL
Epivir HBV—Oral Solution: 5 mg/mL
Epivir—Oral Solution: 10 mg/mL

"Usual dose" assumes normal renal/hepatic function. * For renal insufficiency, give usual dose × 1 followed by maintenance dose per CrCl. For dialysis patients, dose the same as for CrCl < 10 mL/min and give supplemental (post-HD/PD dose) immediately after dialysis. CrCl = creatinine clearance; CVVH = continuous veno-venous hemo-filtration; HD/PD = hemodialysis/peritoneal dialysis. See pp. 214–216 for explanations, pp. xi–xii for abbreviations.

Generic—Oral Tablet: 150, 300 mg
Pharmacokinetic Parameters:
Peak serum level: 1.5 mcg/mL
Bioavailability: 86%
Excreted unchanged (urine): 71%
Serum half-life (normal/ESRD): 5–7/20 hrs
Plasma protein binding: 36%
Volume of distribution (V_d): 1.3 L/kg
Primary Mode of Elimination: Renal
Dosage Adjustments*

CrCl 30–50 mL/min	150 mg (PO) QD
CrCl 15–30 mL/min	100 mg (PO) QD
CrCl 5–15 mL/min	50 mg (PO) QD
CrCl < 5 mL/min	25 mg (PO) QD
Post-HD dose	No information
Post-PD dose	No information
CVVH dose	No information
Moderate hepatic insufficiency	No change
Severe hepatic insufficiency	No information

Drug Interactions: Didanosine, zalcitabine
(↑ risk of pancreatitis); TMP-SMX (↑ lamivudine
levels); zidovudine (↑ zidovudine levels).
Adverse Effects: Drug fever/rash, abdominal
pain/diarrhea, nausea, vomiting, anemia,
leukopenia, photophobia, depression, cough,
nasal complaints, headache, dizziness, peripheral
neuropathy, pancreatitis, myalgias, lactic acidosis
with hepatic steatosis (rare, but potentially life-
threatening toxicity with NRTIs).
Allergic Potential: Low
Safety in Pregnancy: C
Comments: Potential cross resistance with
didanosine. Prevents development of AZT

resistance and restores AZT susceptibility.
May be taken with or without food. Effective
against HBV, but HBV may reactivate after
lamivudine therapy is stopped. Also a
component of Combivir, Trizivir, and Epzicom.
Cerebrospinal Fluid Penetration: 15%

REFERENCES:
Benson CA, van der Horst C, Lamarca A, et al.
   A randomized study of emtricitabine and lamivudine
   in stable suppressed patients with HIV. *AIDS*
   18:2269–76, 2004.
Eron JJ, Benoit SL, Jemsek J, et al. Treatment with
   lamivudine, zidovudine, or both in HIV-positive
   patients with 200 to 500 CD4 cells per cubic
   millimeter. *N Engl J Med* 333:1662–9, 1995.
Lai CI, Chien RN. Leung NW, et al. A one-year trial of
   lamivudine for chronic hepatitis B. *N Engl J Med*
   339:61–8, 1998.
Lau GK, He ML, Fong DY, et al. Preemptive use of
   lamivudine reduces hepatitis B exacerbation after
   allogeneic hematopoietic cell transplantation.
   Hepatology 36:702–9, 2002.
Leung N. Lamivudine for chronic hepatitis B. *Expert
   Rev Anti Infect Ther* 2:173–80, 2004.
Liaw YF, Sung JY, Chow WC, et al. Lamivudine for
   patients with chronic hepatitis B and advanced liver
   disease. *N Engl J Med* 351:1521–31, 2004.
Lu Y, Wang B, Yu L, et al. Lamivudine in prevention and
   treatment of recurrent HBV after liver transplantation.
   Hepatobiliary Pancreat Dis Int 3:504–7, 2004.
Marrone A, Zampino R, D'Onofrio M, et al.
   Combined interferon plus lamivudine treatment
   in young patients with dual HBV (HbeAg
   positive) and HCV chronic infection. *J Hepatol*
   41:1064–5, 2004.
Murphy RL, Brun S, Hicks C, et al. ABT-378/ritonavir
   plus stavudine and lamivudine for the treatment
   of antiretroviral-naïve adults with HIV-1 infection:
   48-week results. *AIDS* 15:F1–9, 2001.
Panel on Antiretroviral Guidelines for Adults and
   Adolescents. Guidelines for the use of antiretroviral
   agents in HIV-1-infected adults and adolescents.
   Department of Health and Human Services.
   March 27, 2013; 1–240. Available at

"Usual dose" assumes normal renal/hepatic function. * For renal insufficiency, give usual dose × 1 followed
by maintenance dose per CrCl. For dialysis patients, dose the same as for CrCl < 10 mL/min and give supplemental (post-HD/PD dose) immediately after dialysis. CrCl = creatinine clearance; CVVH = continuous
veno-venous hemo-filtration; HD/PD = hemodialysis/peritoneal dialysis. See pp. 214–216 for explanations,
pp. xi–xii for abbreviations.

http://www.aidsinfo.nih.gov/contentfiles/
lvguidelines/adultandadolescentgl.pdf.

Perry CM, Faulds D. Lamivudine. A review of its antiviral activity, pharmacokinetic properties and therapeutic efficacy in the management of HIV infection. *Drugs* 53:657–80, 1997.

Rivkina A, Rybalov S. Chronic hepatitis B: current and future treatment options. *Pharmacotherapy* 22:721–37, 2002.

Schmilovitz-Weiss H, Ben-Ari Z, Sikuler E, et al. Lamivudine treatment for acute severe hepatitis B: a pilot study. *Liver Int* 24:547–51, 2004.

Staszewski S, Morales-Ramirez J, Trashima KT, et al. Efavirenz plus zidovudine and lamivudine, efavirenz plus indinavir, and indinavir plus zidovudine and lamivudine in the treatment of HIV-1 infection in adults. *N Engl J Med* 341:1865–1873, 1999.

Lamivudine + Zidovudine (Combivir)

Drug Class: Antiretroviral NRTIs combination
Usual Dose: Combivir tablet – 150 mg lamivudine + 300 mg zidovudine. Usual dose = 1 tablet (PO) BID
How Supplied: Oral Tablet: Contains 150 mg Lamivudine + 300 mg Zidovudine
Pharmacokinetic Parameters:
Peak serum level: 2.6/1.2 mcg/mL
Bioavailability: 82/60%
Excreted unchanged (urine): 86/64%
Serum half-life (normal/ESRD): (6/1.1)/(20/2.2) hrs
Plasma protein binding: < 36/< 38%
Volume of distribution (V_d): 1.3/1.6 L/kg
Primary Mode of Elimination: Renal
Dosage Adjustments*

CrCl 50–80 mL/min	No change
CrCl 10–50 mL/min	Avoid
CrCl < 10 mL/min	Avoid
Post-HD dose	Avoid
Post-PD dose	Avoid
CVVH dose	Avoid
Moderate hepatic insufficiency	Avoid
Severe hepatic insufficiency	Avoid

Drug Interactions: Atovaquone (↑ zidovudine levels); stavudine (antagonist to stavudine; avoid combination); ganciclovir, doxorubicin (neutropenia); tipranavir (↓ zidovudine levels); TMP-SMX (↑ lamivudine and zidovudine levels); vinca alkaloids (neutropenia).
Adverse Effects: Most common (> 5%): nausea, vomiting, diarrhea, anorexia, insomnia, fever/chills, headache, malaise/fatigue. Others (less common): peripheral neuropathy, myopathy, steatosis, pancreatitis. Lab abnormalities: mild hyperglycemia, anemia, LFT elevations, hypertriglyceridemia, leukopenia.
Allergic Potential: Low
Safety in Pregnancy: C
Cerebrospinal Fluid Penetration:
Lamivudine = 12%; zidovudine = 60%

REFERENCES:

Drugs for AIDS and associated infections. *Med Lett Drug Ther* 35:79–86, 1993.

Hirsch MS, D'Aquila RT. Therapy for human immunodeficiency virus infection. *N Engl J Med* 328:1685–95, 1993.

McLeod GX, Hammer SM. Zidovudine: Five years later. *Ann Intern Med* 117:487–510, 1992.

Panel on Antiretroviral Guidelines for Adults and Adolescents. Guidelines for the use of antiretroviral agents in HIV-1-infected adults and adolescents. Department of Health and Human Services. March 27, 2013; 1–240. Available at **http://www.aidsinfo.nih.gov/contentfiles/lvguidelines/adultandadolescentgl.pdf**.

Staszewski S, Morales-Ramirez J, Trashima KT, et al. Efavirenz plus zidovudine and lamivudine, efavirenz plus indinavir, and indinavir plus zidovudine and

---

"Usual dose" assumes normal renal/hepatic function. * For renal insufficiency, give usual dose × 1 followed by maintenance dose per CrCl. For dialysis patients, dose the same as for CrCl < 10 mL/min and give supplemental (post-HD/PD dose) immediately after dialysis. CrCl = creatinine clearance; CVVH = continuous veno-venous hemo-filtration; HD/PD = hemodialysis/peritoneal dialysis. See pp. 214–216 for explanations, pp. xi–xii for abbreviations.

lamivudine in the treatment of HIV-1 infection in adults. *N Engl J Med* 341:1865–1873, 1999.

Lopinavir + Ritonavir (Kaletra) LPV/r

Drug Class: Antiretroviral protease inhibitor combination

Usual Dose: Therapy-naïve: 400/10 mg (2 tablets or 5 mL solution) BID or 800/200 mg (4 tablets or 10 mL solution) QD. Therapy-experienced: 400/100 mg BID. New tablet formulation (lopinavir 200 mg + ritonavir 50 mg) replaces capsules (lopinavir 133.3 mg + ritonavir 33.3 mg), resulting in reduction in total number of pills from 6 capsules to 4 tablets per day. Also available as an oral solution (lopinavir 400 mg + ritonavir 100 mg per 5 mL)

How Supplied: Oral Solution: Contains 80 mg/mL Lopinavir + 20 mg/mL Ritonavir; Oral Tablet: Available as 100 mg Lopinavir + 25 mg Ritonavir, or 200 mg Lopinavir + 50 mg Ritonavir

Pharmacokinetic Parameters:
Peak serum level: 9.6/≤ 1 mcg/mL
Bioavailability: No data
Excreted unchanged (urine): 3%
Serum half-life (normal/ESRD): 5–6/5–6 hrs
Plasma protein binding: 99%
Volume of distribution (V_d): No data/0.44 L/kg
Primary Mode of Elimination: Hepatic
Dosage Adjustments*

CrCl 50–80 mL/min	No change
CrCl 10–50 mL/min	No change
CrCl < 10 mL/min	No change
Post-HD dose	None
Post-PD dose	None
CVVH dose	No change

Moderate hepatic insufficiency	No change
Severe hepatic insufficiency	Avoid

Antiretroviral Dosage Adjustments

Fosamprenavir	Avoid
Delavirdine	No information
Efavirenz	LPV/r tablets 500/125 mg‡ BID; LPV/r oral solution 533/133 mg BID
Indinavir	Indinavir 600 mg BID
Nelfinavir	Same as for efavirenz
Nevirapine	Same as for efavirenz
Rifabutin	Max. dose of rifabutin 150 mg QOD (every other day) or 3 times per week
Saquinavir	Saquinavir 1000 mg BID
Etravirine	No change
Maraviroc	150 mg BID
Raltegravir	No information

Drug Interactions: Antiretrovirals, rifabutin, (see dose adjustment grid, above); astemizole, terfenadine, benzodiazepines, cisapride, ergotamine, flecainide, pimozide, propafenone, rifampin, statins, St. John's wort (avoid if possible); tenofovir (↓ lopinavir levels, ↑ tenofovir levels). ↓ effectiveness of oral contraceptives. Insufficient data on other drug interactions listed for ritonavir alone; rivaroxaban (↑ rivaroxaban), Warfarin (↑ warafrin, monitor INR).

Adverse Effects: Diarrhea (very common), headache, nausea, vomiting, asthenia, ↑ SGOT/SGPT, hepatotoxicity, abdominal

---

"Usual dose" assumes normal renal/hepatic function. * For renal insufficiency, give usual dose × 1 followed by maintenance dose per CrCl. For dialysis patients, dose the same as for CrCl < 10 mL/min and give supplemental (post-HD/PD dose) immediately after dialysis. CrCl = creatinine clearance; CVVH = continuous veno-venous hemo-filtration; HD/PD = hemodialysis/peritoneal dialysis. See pp. 214–216 for explanations, pp. xi–xii for abbreviations.

pain, pancreatitis, paresthesias, hyperglycemia (including worsening diabetes, new-onset diabetes, DKA), ↑ cholesterol/triglycerides (evaluate risk for coronary disease, pancreatitis), ↑ CPK, ↑ uric acid, fat redistribution, possible increased bleeding in hemophilia. Oral solution contains 42.4% alcohol. May prolong PR and QT interval; use with caution in patients with underlying structural heart disease, preexisting conduction system abnormalities, ischemic heart disease, or cardiomyopathies.

Allergic Potential: Low

Safety in Pregnancy: C

Comments: Tablet formulation does not require refrigeration and may be taken with or without food. With oral solution, Lopinavir serum concentrations with moderately fatty meals are increased 54%.

REFERENCES:

Benson CA, Deeks SG, Brun SC, et al. Safety and antiviral activity at 48 weeks of lopinavir/ritonavir plus nevirapine and 2 nucleoside reverse-transcriptase inhibitors in human immunodeficiency virus type 1-infected protease inhibitor-experienced patients. *J Infect Dis* 185:599–607, 2002.

Manfredi R, Calza L, Chiodo F. First-line efavirenz versus lopinavir-ritonavir-based highly active antiretroviral therapy for naïve patients. *AIDS* 18:2331–2333, 2004.

Panel on Antiretroviral Guidelines for Adults and Adolescents. Guidelines for the use of antiretroviral agents in HIV-1-infected adults and adolescents. Department of Health and Human Services. March 27, 2013; 1–240. Available at **http://www.aidsinfo.nih.gov/contentfiles/lvguidelines/adultandadolescentgl.pdf**.

Riddler S, et al. Initial treatment for HIV infection—an embarrassment of riches. *N Engl J Med* 358(20): 2095–2106. May 15, 2008.

Walmsley S, Bernstein B, King M, et al. Lopinavir-ritonavir versus nelfinavir for the initial treatment of HIV infection. *N Engl J Med* 346:2039–46, 2002.

Website: www.kaletra.com

Maraviroc (Selzentry) MVC

Drug Class: HIV-1 chemokine receptor 5 (CCR5) antagonist

Usual Dose: 150 mg, 300 mg, or 600 mg (PO) BID, depending on concomitant medications (see below), in CCR5-tropic HIV-1 isolates. Available in 150 mg and 300 mg tablets

How Supplied: Oral Tablet: 150 mg, 300 mg

Pharmacokinetic Parameters:

Peak serum level: 266–618 mcg/mL
Bioavailability: 23–33%
Excreted unchanged: 20% (urine); 76% (feces)
Serum half-life (normal/ESRD): 14–18 hrs/not studied
Plasma protein binding: 76%
Volume of distribution (V_d): 194 L

Primary Mode of Elimination: Fecal/renal

Dosage Adjustments*

CrCl 50–80 mL/min	No change
CrCl 10–25 mL/min	Use caution
CrCl < 10 mL/min	Use caution
Post-HD dose	No information
Post-PD dose	No information
CVVH dose	No information
Mild hepatic insufficiency	No information
Moderate or severe hepatic insufficiency	No information

Antiretroviral Dosage Adjustments

Protease inhibitors (except tipranavir/ritonavir), delavirdine, ketoconazole, itraconazole, clarithromycin, nefazodone, telithromycin	150 mg (PO) BID

"Usual dose" assumes normal renal/hepatic function. * For renal insufficiency, give usual dose × 1 followed by maintenance dose per CrCl. For dialysis patients, dose the same as for CrCl < 10 mL/min and give supplemental (post-HD/PD dose) immediately after dialysis. CrCl = creatinine clearance; CVVH = continuous veno-venous hemo-filtration; HD/PD = hemodialysis/peritoneal dialysis. See pp. 214–216 for explanations, pp. xi–xii for abbreviations.

| Tipranavir/ritonavir, nevirapine, all NRTIs and enfuvirtide | 300 mg (PO) BID |
| Efavirenz, rifampin, carbamazepine, phenobarbital, phenytoin | 600 mg (PO) BID |

Drug Interactions: Maraviroc is a substrate of CYP3A and P-glycoprotein and is likely to be modulated by inhibitors and inducers of these enzymes/transporters.

Adverse Effects: Hepatotoxicity has been reported. A systemic allergic reaction (e.g., pruritic rash, eosinophilia, or elevated IgE) prior to the development of hepatotoxicity may occur. Other adverse effects: cough, infection, upper respiratory tract infection, rash, pyrexia, dizziness, abdominal pain, musculoskeletal symptoms (joint/muscle pain). Myocardial infarction/ischemia reported in < 2% in clinical trials. Orthostatic hypotension, especially in patients with severe renal insufficiency.

Allergic Potential: Low

Safety in Pregnancy: B

Comments: Indicated for treatment-experienced adult patients infected with only cellular chemokine receptor (CCR) 5-tropic HIV-1 virus detectable who have evidence of viral replication and HIV-1 strains resistant to multiple antiretroviral agents. Used in combination with other antiretroviral agents. Trofile phenotype test (performed at Monogram) is needed to confirm infection with CCR5-tropic HIV-1 (also known as "R5 virus").

Cerebrospinal Fluid Penetration: No data

REFERENCES:

Dorr P, Westby M, Dobbs S, et al. Maraviroc (UK-427, 857), a potent, orally bioavailable, and selective small-molecule inhibitor of chemokine receptor CCR5 with broad-spectrum anti-human immunodeficiency virus type 1 activity. *Antimicrob Agents Chemother* 49:4721–4732, 2005.

Gulick R. Maraviroc for previously treated patients with R5 HIV-1 infection, *N Engl J Med* 359(14):1429–41. Oct 2, 2008.

Fätkenheuer G. Subgroup analyses of maraviroc in previously treated R5 HIV-1 infection. *N Engl J Med* 359(14):1442–55. Oct 2, 2008.

Lederman MM, Penn-Nicholson A, Cho M, et al. Biology of CCR5 and its role in HIV infection and treatment. *JAMA* 296:815–826, 2006.

Panel on Antiretroviral Guidelines for Adults and Adolescents. Guidelines for the use of antiretroviral agents in HIV-1-infected adults and adolescents. Department of Health and Human Services. March 27, 2013; 1–240. Available at **http://www.aidsinfo.nih.gov/contentfiles/lvguidelines/adultandadolescentgl.pdf**.

Product Information: SELZENTRY(R) oral tablets, maraviroc oral tablets. Pfizer Labs, New York, NY, 2007.

Website: www.selzentry.com

Nelfinavir (Viracept) NFV

Drug Class: Antiretroviral protease inhibitor

Usual Dose: 1250 mg (PO) BID (two 625-mg tablets per dose) with meals, or five 250-mg tabs or 750 mg (three 250-mg tabs) (PO) TID

How Supplied: Oral Powder for Suspension: 50 mg/gm, Oral Tablet: 250 mg, 625 mg

Pharmacokinetic Parameters:
Peak serum level: 35 mcg/mL
Bioavailability: 20–80%
Excreted unchanged (urine): 1–2%
Serum half-life (normal/ESRD): 4 hrs/no data
Plasma protein binding: 98%
Volume of distribution (V_d): 5 L/kg

Primary Mode of Elimination: Hepatic

Dosage Adjustments*

CrCl 50–80 mL/min	No change
CrCl 10–50 mL/min	No change
CrCl < 10 mL/min	No change

"Usual dose" assumes normal renal/hepatic function. * For renal insufficiency, give usual dose × 1 followed by maintenance dose per CrCl. For dialysis patients, dose the same as for CrCl < 10 mL/min and give supplemental (post-HD/PD dose) immediately after dialysis. CrCl = creatinine clearance; CVVH = continuous veno-venous hemo-filtration; HD/PD = hemodialysis/peritoneal dialysis. See pp. 214–216 for explanations, pp. xi–xii for abbreviations.

Post-HD dose	None
Post-PD dose	None
CVVH dose	No change
Moderate hepatic insufficiency	No information
Severe hepatic insufficiency	No information—use caution

Antiretroviral Dosage Adjustments

Delavirdine	No information (monitor for neutropenia)
Efavirenz	No changes
Indinavir	Limited data for nelfinavir 1250 mg BID + indinavir 1200 rng BID
Lopinavir/ ritonavir	Nelfinavir 1000 mq BID or lopinavir/r 600/150 mg BID
Nevirapine	No changes
Ritonavir	No information
Saquinavir	Saquinavir 1200 mg BID
Rifampin	Avoid combination
Rifabutin	Nelfinavir 1250 mg BID; rifabutin 150 mg QD or 300 mg 2–3x/week
Etravirine	No data
Maraviroc	150 mg BID
Raltegravir	No data

Drug Interactions: Antiretrovirals, rifabutin, rifampin (see dose adjustment grid, above); amiodarone, quinidine, astemizole, terfenadine, benzodiazepines, cisapride, ergot alkaloids, statins, St. John's wort (avoid if possible); carbamazepine, phenytoin, phenobarbital (↓ nelfinavir levels, ↑ anticonvulsant levels; monitor); caspofungin (↓ caspofungin levels, may ↓ caspofungin effect); clarithromycin, erythromycin, telithromycin (↑ nelfinavir and macrolide levels); didanosine (dosing conflict with food; give nelfinavir with food 2 hours before or 1 hour after didanosine); itraconazole, voriconazole, ketoconazole (↑ nelfinavir levels); lamivudine (↑ lamivudine levels); methadone (may require ↑ methadone dose); oral contraceptives, zidovudine (↓ zidovudine levels); sildenafil (↑ or ↓ sildenafil levels; do not exceed 25 mg in 48 hrs, tadalafil (max. 10 mg/72 hrs, vardenafil (max. 2.5 mg/72 hrs); rivaroxaban (↑ rivaroxaban); Warfarin (↑ warafrin, monitor INR).

Adverse Effects: Impaired concentration, nausea, abdominal pain, secretory diarrhea, ↑ SGOT/SGPT, rash, ↑ cholesterol/triglycerides (evaluate risk for coronary disease/pancreatitis), fat redistribution, hyperglycemia (including worsening diabetes, new-onset diabetes, DKA), possible increased bleeding in hemophilia.

Allergic Potential: Low

Safety in Pregnancy: B

Comments: Take with food (absorption increased 300%). New 625-mg tablet available.

Cerebrospinal Fluid Penetration: Undetectable

REFERENCES:

Albrecht MA, Bosch RJ, Hammer SM, et al. Nelfinavir, efavirenz, or both after the failure of nucleoside treatment of HIV infection. *N Engl J Med* 345: 398–407, 2001.

Clotet B, Ruiz L, Martinez-Picado J, et al. Prevalence of HIV protease mutations on failure of nelfinavir-containing HAART: a retrospective analysis of four clinical studies and two observational cohorts. *HIV Clin Trials* 3:316–23, 2002.

Deeks SG, Smith M, Holodniy M, et al. HIV-1 protease inhibitors: A review for clinicians. *JAMA* 277: 145–53, 1997.

"Usual dose" assumes normal renal/hepatic function. * For renal insufficiency, give usual dose × 1 followed by maintenance dose per CrCl. For dialysis patients, dose the same as for CrCl < 10 mL/min and give supplemental (post-HD/PD dose) immediately after dialysis. CrCl = creatinine clearance; CVVH = continuous veno-venous hemo-filtration; HD/PD = hemodialysis/peritoneal dialysis. See pp. 214–216 for explanations, pp. xi–xii for abbreviations.

DiCenzo R, Forrest A, Fischl MA, et al. Pharmacokinetics of indinavir and nelfinavir in treatment-naïve, human immunodeficiency virus-infected subjects. *Antimicrob Agents Chemother* 48:918–23, 2004.

Go J, Cunha BA. Nelfinavir: a review. *Antibiotics for Clinicians* 4:17–23, 2000.

Kaul DR, Cinti SK, Carver PL, et al. HIV protease inhibitors: Advances in therapy and adverse reactions, including metabolic complications. *Pharmacotherapy* 19:281–98, 1999.

Panel on Antiretroviral Guidelines for Adults and Adolescents. Guidelines for the use of antiretroviral agents in HIV-1-infected adults and adolescents. Department of Health and Human Services. March 27, 2013; 1–240. Available at **http://www.aidsinfo.nih.gov/contentfiles/lvguidelines/adultandadolescentgl.pdf**.

Perry CM, Benfield P. Nelfinavir. *Drugs* 54:81–7, 1997.

Simpson KN, Luo MP, Chumney E, et al. Cost-effective of lopinavir/ritonavir versus nelfinavir as the first-line highly active antiretroviral therapy regimen for HIV infection. HIV Clin Trials 5:294–304, 2004.

Walmsley S, Bernstein B, King M, et al. Lopinavir-ritonavir versus nelfinavir for the initial treatment of HIV infection. *N Engl J Med* 346:2039–46, 2002.

Website: www.viracept.com

Nevirapine (Viramune) NVP

Drug Class: Antiretroviral NNRTI
(non-nucleoside reverse transcriptase inhibitor)
Usual Dose: 200 mg (PO) QD × 2 weeks, then 200 mg (PO) BID
How Supplied:
Viramune O/S—Oral Suspension: 50 mg/5 mL
Viramune—Oral Suspension: 50 mg/5 mL, Oral Tablet: 200 mg
Viramune XR—Oral Tablet, Extended Release: 400 mg
Generic—Oral Tablet: 200 mg
Pharmacokinetic Parameters:
Peak serum level: 0.9–3.6 mcg/mL
Bioavailability: 90%

Excreted unchanged (urine): 5%
Serum half-life (normal/ESRD): 40 hrs/no data
Plasma protein binding: 60%
Volume of distribution (V_d): 1.4 L/kg
Primary Mode of Elimination: Hepatic
Dosage Adjustments*

CrCl > 20 mL/min	No change
CrCl < 20 mL/min	No change; use caution
Post-HD dose	200 mg (PO)
Post-PD dose	None
CVVH dose	No change
Moderate hepatic insufficiency	Use caution
Severe hepatic insufficiency	Avoid

Antiretroviral Dosage Adjustments

Delavirdine	No information
Efavirenz	Avoid combination
Indinavir	Indinavir 1000 mg TID
Lopinavir/ ritonavir (l/r)	Consider l/r 600/150 mg BID in PI-experienced patients
Nelfinavir	No information
Ritonavir	No changes
Saquinavir	No information
Rifampin	Not recommended
Rifabutin	Use caution
Etravirine	Avoid combination
Maraviroc	Without PI MVC 300 mg BID with PI (except TPV/r) MVC 150 mg BID
Raltegravir	No data

"Usual dose" assumes normal renal/hepatic function. * For renal insufficiency, give usual dose × 1 followed by maintenance dose per CrCl. For dialysis patients, dose the same as for CrCl < 10 mL/min and give supplemental (post-HD/PD dose) immediately after dialysis. CrCl = creatinine clearance; CVVH = continuous veno-venous hemo-filtration; HD/PD = hemodialysis/peritoneal dialysis. See pp. 214–216 for explanations, pp. xi–xii for abbreviations.

Drug Interactions: Antiretrovirals, rifabutin, rifampin (see dose adjustment grid, above); carbamazepine, phenobarbital, phenytoin (monitor anticonvulsant levels); caspofungin ($\downarrow$ caspofungin levels, may $\downarrow$ caspofungin effect); ethinyl estradiol ($\downarrow$ ethinyl estradiol levels; use additional/alternative method); ketoconazole (avoid); voriconazole ($\uparrow$ nevirapine levels); methadone ($\downarrow$ methadone levels; titrate methadone dose to effect); tacrolimus ($\downarrow$ tacrolimus levels).

Adverse Effects: Drug fever/rash (may be severe; usually occurs within 6 weeks), Stevens-Johnson syndrome, $\uparrow$ SGOT/SGPT, *fatal hepatitis*, headache, diarrhea, leukopenia, stomatitis, peripheral neuropathy, paresthesias. Greater risk of fatal hepatitis and Stevens-Johnson syndrome when CD4 > $400/mm^3$ (males) or > $250/mm^3$ (females) (monitor patients intensely for first 18 weeks of therapy).

Allergic Potential: High
Safety in Pregnancy: B
Comments: Absorption not affected by food. Not to be used for post-exposure prophylaxis because of potential for fatal hepatitis.
Cerebrospinal Fluid Penetration: 45%

REFERENCES:
D'Aquila RT, Hughes MD, Johnson VA, et al. Nevirapine, zidovudine, and didanosine compared with zidovudine and didanosine in patients with HIV-1 infection. *Ann Intern Med* 124: 1019–30, 1996.

Hammer SM, Kessler HA, Saag MS. Issues in combination antiretroviral therapy: a review. *J Acquired Immune Defic Syndr* 7:24–37, 1994.

Havlir DV, Lange JM. New antiretrovirals and new combinations. *AIDS* 12:165–74, 1998.

Herzmann C, Karcher H. Nevirapine plus zidovudine to prevent mother-to-child transmission of HIV. *N Engl J Med* 351:2013–5, 2004.

Johnson S, Chan J, Bennett CL. Hepatotoxicity after prophylaxis with a nevirapine-containing antiretroviral regimen. *Ann Intern Med* 137:146–7, 2002.

Milinkovic A, Martinez E. Nevirapine in the treatment of HIV. *Expert Rev Anti Infect Ther* 2:367–73, 2004.

Montaner JS, Reiss P, Cooper D, et al. A randomized, double-blind trial comparing combinations of nevirapine, didanosine, and zidovudine for HIV-infected patients: the INCAS trial. Italy, the Netherlands, Canada and Australia Study. *J Am Med Assoc* 279:930–937, 1998.

Negredo E, Ribalta J, Paredes R, et al. Reversal of atherogenic lipoprotein profile in HIV-1 infected patients with lipodystrophy after replacing protease inhibitors by nevirapine. *AIDS* 16:1383–9, 2002.

Panel on Antiretroviral Guidelines for Adults and Adolescents. Guidelines for the use of antiretroviral agents in HIV-1-infected adults and adolescents. Department of Health and Human Services. March 27, 2013; 1–240. Available at **http://www.aidsinfo.nih.gov/contentfiles/lvguidelines/adultandadolescentgl.pdf**.

Weverling GJ, Lange JM, Jurriaans S, et al. Alternative multidrug regimen provides improved suppression of HIV-1 replication over triple therapy. *AIDS* 12:117–22, 1998.

Website: www.viramune.com

Raltegravir (Isentress) RAL

Drug Class: HIV-1 integrase inhibitor
Usual Dose: 400 mg (PO) BID
How Supplied: Oral Tablet: 400 mg
Pharmacokinetic Parameters:
Peak serum level: 6.5 µM
Bioavailability: ~ 32% (20–43%)
Excreted unchanged: 51% (feces); 9% (urine)
Serum half-life (normal/ESRD): 9–12 hrs/ no data
Plasma protein binding: 83%
Volume of distribution (V_d): not studied
Primary Mode of Elimination: Fecal/renal

"Usual dose" assumes normal renal/hepatic function. * For renal insufficiency, give usual dose × 1 followed by maintenance dose per CrCl. For dialysis patients, dose the same as for CrCl < 10 mL/min and give supplemental (post-HD/PD dose) immediately after dialysis. CrCl = creatinine clearance; CVVH = continuous veno-venous hemo-filtration; HD/PD = hemodialysis/peritoneal dialysis. See pp. 214–216 for explanations, pp. xi–xii for abbreviations.

Dosage Adjustments*

CrCl 50–80 mL/min	No change
CrCl 10–50 mL/min	No change
CrCl < 10 mL/min	No information
Post-HD dose	No information
Post-PD dose	No information
CVVH dose	No information
Mild/moderate hepatic insufficiency	No change
Severe hepatic insufficiency	No information

Antiretroviral Dosage Adjustments

Atazanavir	No change
Atazanavir/ritonavir	No change
Efavirenz	No change
Rifampin	Raltegravir 800 mg BID
Ritonavir	No change
Tenofovir	No change
Tipranavir/ritonavir	No change
Etravirine	No changes
Nevirapine	No data
Maraciroc	No changes

Drug Interactions: Rifampin (↓ raltegravir levels, use with caution). Omeprazole (↑ raltegravir levels, no adjustment needed). In vitro, raltegravir does not inhibit CYP1A2, CYP2B6, CYP2C8, CYP2C9, CYP2C19, CYP2D6 or CYP3A and does not induce CYP3A4. In addition, raltegravir does not inhibit P-glycoprotein-mediated transport. Raltegravir

is therefore not expected to affect the pharmacokinetics of drugs that are substrates of these enzymes or P-glycoprotein (e.g., protease inhibitors, NNRTIs, methadone, opioid analgesics, statins, azole antifungals, proton pump inhibitors, oral contraceptives, anti-erectile dysfunction agents).
Adverse Effects: Nausea, headache, diarrhea, pyrexia.
Allergic Potential: Low
Safety in Pregnancy: C
Comments: May be taken with or without food. CPK elevations, myopathy, and rhabdomyolysis have been reported—use with caution in patients at increased risk for myopathy or rhabdomyolysis, such as those receiving concomitant medications known to cause these conditions (e.g., statins). Raltegravir is indicated for treatment-naïve and treatment-experienced adult patients who have evidence of viral replication and HIV-1 strains resistant to multiple antiretroviral agents. Treatment experienced patients who switch to raltegravir must have a least two other fully active agents in their regimen.
Cerebrospinal Fluid Penetration: No data

REFERENCES:
Cooper, OA. Subgroup and resistance analyses of raltegravir for resistant HIV-1 infection. *N Engl J Med* 359(4):355–65. Jul 24, 2008.
Eron JJ, Young B, Cooper DA, et al. Switch to a raltegravir-based regimen versus continuation of a lopinavir-ritonavir-based regimen in stable HIV-infected patients with suppressed viraemia (SWITCHMRK 1 and 2): two multicentre, double-blind, randomised controlled trials. *Lancet*. Jan 30; 375(9712):396–407.
Grinsztejn B, Nguyen BY, Katlama C, et al. Safety and efficacy of the HIV-1 integrase inhibitor raltegravir (MK-0518) in treatment-experienced patients with multidrug-resistant virus: a phase II randomised controlled trial. *Lancet* 369:1261–69, 2007.

Iwamoto M, Wenning LA, Nguyen BY, et al. Effects of omeprazole on plasma levels of raltegravir. *Clin Infect Dis.* Feb 15 2009;48(4):489–492.

Iwamoto M, Wenning LA, Petry AS, et al. Safety, tolerability, and pharmacokinetics of raltegravir after single and multiple doses in healthy subjects. *Clin Pharmacol Ther* 83:293–9, 2007.

Kassahun K, McIntosh I, Cui D, et al. Metabolism and Disposition in Humans of Raltegravir (MK-0518), an Anti-AIDS Drug Targeting the HIV-1 Integrase Enzyme. *Drug Metab Dispos* Epub: 1–28, 2007.

Lennox JL, DeJesus E, Lazzarin A, et al. Safety and efficacy of raltegravir-based versus efavirenz-based combination therapy in treatment-naïve patients with HIV-1 infection: a multicentre, double-blind randomised controlled trial. *Lancet.* Sep 5 2009; 374(9692):796–806.

Markowitz M, Morales-Ramirez JO, Nguyen BY, et al. Antiretroviral activity, pharmacokinetics, and tolerability of MK-0518, a novel inhibitor of HIV-1 integrase, dosed as monotherapy for 10 days in treatment-naive HIV-1-Infected Individuals. *J Acquir Immune Defic Syndr* 43:509 15, 2006.

Palmisano L, Role of integrase inhibitors in the treatment of HIV disease. *Expert Rev Anti Infect Ther* 5:67–75, 2007.

Panel on Antiretroviral Guidelines for Adults and Adolescents. Guidelines for the use of antiretroviral agents in HIV-1-infected adults and adolescents. Department of Health and Human Services. March 27, 2013; 1–240. Available at http://www.aidsinfo.nih.gov/contentfiles/lvguidelines/adultandadolescentgl.pdf.

Product Information. ISENTRESS oral tablets, raltegravir oral tablets. Merck & Co, Inc, Whitehouse Station, NJ, 2007.

Steigbigel RT. Raltegravir with optimized background therapy for resistant HIV-1 infection. *N Engl J Med* 359(4):339–54. Jul 24, 2008.

Wenning LA, Hanley WD, Brainard DM, et al. Effect of rifampin, a potent inducer of drug-metabolizing enzymes, on the pharmacokinetics of raltegravir. *Antimicrob Agents Chemother.* Jul 2009;53(7): 2852–2856.

Rilpivirine (Edurant®) RPV

Drug Class: HIV Antiretroviral Agent (Non-Nucleoside Reverse Transcriptase Inhibitor)
Usual Dose: 25 mg (PO) QD with food (treatment-naïve)
How Supplied: Oral Tablet: 25 MG
Pharmacokinetic Parameters:
Time to peak concentration: 4–5 hours
Area Under the Curve: 2397 nanograms x hr/mL
Bioavailability: unknown
Excreted unchanged: 25% (feces) 6.1% (urine)
Serum half-life (normal/ESRD): 50 hrs / no data
Plasma protein binding: 99.7 % (primarily albumin)
Volume of distribution (Vd): not studied
Primary mode of Elimination: Feces
Dosage Adjustments*

CrCl 50–80 mL/min	No Change
CrCl 30–49 mL/min	No Change
CrCl < 30 mL/min	No Change
ESRD	No Change
Post-HD dose	No Change
Post-PD dose	No Change
CVVH dose	No Change
Mild – moderate hepatic insufficiency	No Change
Severe hepatic insufficiency	No data, use caution

Antiretroviral Dosage Adjustments: It is not recommended to co-administer rilpivirine with other NNRTIs. No dose adjustment is needed when rilpivirine is co-administered with boosted and un-boosted protease inhibitors.

"Usual dose" assumes normal renal/hepatic function. * For renal insufficiency, give usual dose × 1 followed by maintenance dose per CrCl. For dialysis patients, dose the same as for CrCl < 10 mL/min and give supplemental (post-HD/PD dose) immediately after dialysis. CrCl = creatinine clearance; CVVH = continuous veno-venous hemo-filtration; HD/PD = hemodialysis/peritoneal dialysis. See pp. 214–216 for explanations, pp. xi–xii for abbreviations.

Drug Interactions: rilpivirine is a primarily metabolized by cytochrome P450 (CYP)3A. Drugs that can induce or inhibit CYP3A can affect plasma concentrations of rilpivirine. Co-administration of rilpivirine with drugs that increase gastric pH may result in decreased plasma concentrations of rilpivirine. Drugs that may reduce rilpivirine plasma concentrations: antacids, cimetidine, famotidine, ranitidine, esomeprazole, omeprazole, pantoparazole, lansoprazole, rabeprazole, nizatidine, rifampin, rifapentine, rifabutin, phenytoin, phenobarbital, oxcarbazepine. Drugs that mau increase rilpivirine plasma concentrations: ketoconazole, itraconazole, voriconazole, posaconazole, clarithromycin, erythromycin, troleandomycin. Rilpivirine may decrease methadone concentrations.

Adverse Effects: Rash 3%, Lipodystrophy, Serum cholesterol raised, Serum triglycerides raised, nausea/vomiting <1%, elevated ALT/AST/Serum bilirubin <2%, Membranous glomerulonephritis <2%, Mesangial proliferative glomerulonephritis <2%, ↑ Serum creatinine <1%, dizziness/headache/insomnia <2%, depression and suicidal thoughts – rare, vivid dreams – rare.

Allergic Potential: low
Safety in Pregnancy: B
Comments: Must be taken with a full meal (preferably high fat), rilpivirine exposure was about 40% lower when administered in the fasted state. Use with caution in patients with severe depressive disorders as depression, dysphoria, major depression, mood altered, negative thoughts, suicide attempt, and suicidal ideation, have been reported with rilpivirine. In clinical trials patients with HIV-1 RNA > 100,000 copies/mL at therapy initiation experienced virologic failure more often than patients with HIV-1 RNA < 100,000 copies/mL at the start

of therapy. Patients who experience virological failure on rilpivirine may be at risk for cross-resistance to other NNRTIs and to emtricitabine/lamivudine

Cerebrospinal Fluid Penetration: no data
Alias: (TMC-278)

REFERENCES:
Product Information: EDURANT(R) oral tablets, rilpivirine oral tablets. Tibotec Therapeutics, Raritan, NJ, 2011.
Cohen CJ, Andrade-Villanueva J, Clotet B, et al: Rilpivirine versus efavirenz with two background nucleoside or nucleotide reverse transcriptase inhibitors in treatment-naive adults infected with HIV-1 (THRIVE): a phase 3, randomized, non-inferiority trial. Lancet 2011; 378(9787):229–237.
Molina JM, Cahn P, Grinsztejn B, et al: Rilpivirine versus efavirenz with tenofovir and emtricitabine in treatment-naive adults infected with HIV-1 (ECHO): a phase 3 randomized double-blind active-controlled trial. Lancet 2011; 378(9787):238–246.
Schrijvers R, Desimmie BA, Debyser Z. Rilpivirine: a step forward in tailored HIV treatment. Lancet. Jul 16 2011;378(9787):201–203.
Panel on Antiretroviral Guidelines for Adults and Adolescents. Guidelines for the use of antiretroviral agents in HIV-1-infected adults and adolescents. Department of Health and Human Services. March 27, 2013; 1–240. Available at **http://www.aidsinfo.nih.gov/contentfiles/lvguidelines/adultandadolescentgl.pdf**.
Website: http://www.edurant-info.com/

Ritonavir (Norvir) RTV

Drug Class: Antiretroviral protease inhibitor
Usual Dose: 600 mg (PO) BID (see comments)
How Supplied: Oral Capsule, Liquid Filled: 100 mg; Oral Solution: 80 mg/mL; Oral Tablet (heat stable) 100 mg
Pharmacokinetic Parameters:
Peak serum level: 11 mcg/mL
Bioavailability: No data
Excreted unchanged (urine): 3.5%

"Usual dose" assumes normal renal/hepatic function. * For renal insufficiency, give usual dose × 1 followed by maintenance dose per CrCl. For dialysis patients, dose the same as for CrCl < 10 mL/min and give supplemental (post-HD/PD dose) immediately after dialysis. CrCl = creatinine clearance; CVVH = continuous veno-venous hemo-filtration; HD/PD = hemodialysis/peritoneal dialysis. See pp. 214–216 for explanations, pp. xi–xii for abbreviations.

Serum half-life (normal/ESRD): 4 hrs/no data
Plasma protein binding: 99%
Volume of distribution (V_d): 0.41 L/kg
Primary Mode of Elimination: Hepatic
Dosage Adjustments*

CrCl 50–80 mL/min	No change
CrCl 10–50 mL/min	No change
CrCl < 10 mL/min	No change
Post-HD dose	None
Post-PD dose	None
CVVH dose	None
Moderate hepatic insufficiency	No change
Severe hepatic insufficiency	No change; use caution

Antiretroviral Dosage Adjustments

Atazanavir	Ritonavir 100 mg QD + atazanavir 300 mg QD with food
Delavirdine	Delavirdine: no change; ritonavir: no information
Efavirenz	Ritonavir 600 mg BID (500 mg BID for intolerance)
Indinavir	Ritonavir 100–200 mg BID + indinavir 800 mg BID, or 400 mg BID of each drug
Nelfinavir	Ritonavir 400 mg BID + nelfinavir 500–750 mg BID
Nevirapine	No changes
Saquinavir	Ritonavir 400 mg BID + saquinavir 400 mg BID

Ketoconazole	Caution; do not exceed ketoconazole 200 mg QD
Rifampin	Avoid
Rifabutin	150 mg q2d or 3x/week

Drug Interactions: Antiretrovirals, rifabutin, rifampin (see dose adjustment grid, above); alprazolam, diazepam, estazolam, flurazepam, midazolam, triazolam, zolpidem, meperidine, propoxyphene, piroxicam, quinidine, amiodarone, encainide, flecainide, propafenone, astemizole, bepridil, bupropion, cisapride, clorazepate, clozapine, pimozide, St. John's wort, terfenadine (avoid); alfentanil, fentanyl, hydrocodone, tramadol, disopyramide, lidocaine, mexiletine, erythromycin, clarithromycin, rivaroxaban (↑ rivaroxaban), Warfarin (↑ warafrin, monitor INR); dronabinol, ondansetron, metoprolol, pindolol, propranolol, timolol, amlodipine, diltiazem, felodipine, isradipine, nicardipine, nifedipine, nimodipine, nisoldipine, nitrendipine, verapamil, etoposide, paclitaxel, tamoxifen, vinblastine, vincristine, loratadine, tricyclic antidepressants, paroxetine, nefazodone, sertraline, trazodone, fluoxetine, venlafaxine, fluvoxamine, cyclosporine, tacrolimus, chlorpromazine, haloperidol, perphenazine, risperidone, thioridazine, clozapine, pimozide, methamphetamine (↑ interacting drug levels); voriconazole (↓ voriconazole levels); telithromycin (↑ ritonavir levels); codeine, hydromorphone, methadone, morphine, ketoprofen, ketorolac, naproxen, diphenoxylate, oral contraceptives, theophylline (↓ interacting drug levels); carbamazepine, phenytoin, phenobarbital, clonazepam, dexamethasone, prednisone (↓ ritonavir levels, ↑ interacting drug levels; monitor anticonvulsant levels); metronidazole (disulfiram-like reaction); tenofovir, tobacco

---

"Usual dose" assumes normal renal/hepatic function. * For renal insufficiency, give usual dose × 1 followed by maintenance dose per CrCl. For dialysis patients, dose the same as for CrCl < 10 mL/min and give supplemental (post-HD/PD dose) immediately after dialysis. CrCl = creatinine clearance; CVVH = continuous veno-venous hemo-filtration; HD/PD = hemodialysis/peritoneal dialysis. See pp. 214–216 for explanations, pp. xi–xii for abbreviations.

(↓ ritonavir levels); Avanafil (do not coadminster); sildenafil (do not exceed 25 mg in 48 hrs); tadalafil (max. 10 mg/72 hrs); vardenafil (max. 2.5 mg/72 hrs); Fluticasone and Budesonide (Inhaled) co-administration can result in adrenal insufficiency, including Cushing's syndrome.

Adverse Effects: Anorexia, anemia, leukopenia, hyperglycemia (including worsening diabetes, new-onset diabetes, DKA), ↑ cholesterol/triglycerides (evaluate risk for coronary disease/pancreatitis), fat redistribution, ↑ CPK, nausea, vomiting, diarrhea, abdominal pain, circumoral/extremity paresthesias, ↑ SGOT/SGPT, pancreatitis, taste perversion, possible increased bleeding in hemophilia.

Allergic Potential: Low

Safety in Pregnancy: B

Comments: Usually used at low dose (100–200 mg/day) as pharmacokinetic "booster" of other PIs. GI intolerance decreases over time. Take with food if possible (serum levels increase 15%, fewer GI side effects). Dose escalation regimen: day 1–2 (300 mg BID), day 3–5 (400 mg BID), day 6–13 (500 mg BID), day 14 (600 mg BID). Separate dosing from ddI by 2 hours. Refrigerate capsules (not oral solution) if temperature to exceed 78°F. Do not refrigerate oral tablets, they are heat stable. Tablets are not bioequivalent to capsules and patients may experience more GI side effects when switched to tablet formulation.

Cerebrospinal Fluid Penetration: < 10%

REFERENCES:

Cameron DW, Japour AJ, Xu Y, et al. Ritonavir and saquinavir combination therapy for the treatment of HIV infection. *AIDS* 13:213–24, 1999.

Deeks SG, Smith M, Holodniy M, et al. HIV-1 protease inhibitors: a review for clinicians. *JAMA* 277: 145–53, 1997.

Kaul DR, Cinti SK, Carver PL, et al. HIV protease inhibitors: advances in therapy and adverse reactions, including metabolic complications. *Pharmacotherapy* 19:281–98, 1999.

Lea AP, Faulds D. Ritonavir. *Drugs* 52:541–6, 1996.

McDonald CK, Kuritzkes DR. Human immunodeficiency virus type 1 protease inhibitors. *Arch Intern Med* 157:951–9, 1997.

Panel on Antiretroviral Guidelines for Adults and Adolescents. Guidelines for the use of antiretroviral agents in HIV-1-infected adults and adolescents. Department of Health and Human Services. March 27, 2013; 1–240. Available at http://www.aidsinfo.nih.gov/contentfiles/lvguidelines/adultandadolescentgl.pdf.

Piliero PJ. Interaction between ritonavir and statins. *Am J Med* 112:510–1, 2002.

Rathbun RC, Rossi DR. Low-dose ritonavir for protease inhibitor pharmacokinetic enhancement. *Ann Pharmacother* 36:702–6, 2002.

Shepp DH, Stevens RC. Ritonavir boosting of HIV protease inhibitors. *Antibiotics for Clinicians* 9:301–11, 2005.

Website: www.TreatHIV.com

Saquinavir (Invirase) SQV

Drug Class: Antiretroviral protease inhibitor

Usual Dose: 1000 mg (PO) BID (see comments) with ritonavir 100 mg (PO) BID, or 400 mg (PO) BID with ritonavir 400 mg (PO) BID

How Supplied: Oral Capsule: 200 mg; Oral Tablet: 500 mg

Pharmacokinetic Parameters:

Peak serum level: 0.07 mcg/mL
Bioavailability: hard-gel (4%)
Excreted unchanged (urine): 13%
Serum half-life (normal/ESRD): 13 hrs/no data
Plasma protein binding: 98%
Volume of distribution (V_d): 10 L/kg

Primary Mode of Elimination: Hepatic

Dosage Adjustments*

CrCl 50–80 mL/min	No change
CrCl 10–50 mL/min	No change

"Usual dose" assumes normal renal/hepatic function. * For renal insufficiency, give usual dose × 1 followed by maintenance dose per CrCl. For dialysis patients, dose the same as for CrCl < 10 mL/min and give supplemental (post-HD/PD dose) immediately after dialysis. CrCl = creatinine clearance; CVVH = continuous veno-venous hemo-filtration; HD/PD = hemodialysis/peritoneal dialysis. See pp. 214–216 for explanations, pp. xi–xii for abbreviations.

CrCl < 10 mL/min	No change
Post-HD dose	None
Post-PD dose	None
CVVH dose	No change
Moderate hepatic insufficiency	No change
Severe hepatic insufficiency	Use caution

Antiretroviral Dosage Adjustments

Darunavir	Avoid
Delavirdine	No Information
Efavirenz	(SQV 1,000 mg + RTV 100 mg) BID
Indinavir	No information
Lopinavir/ritonavir 3 capsules BID	Saquinavir 500 mg BID
Nelfinavir	Saquinavir 1 gm BID or 1200 mg BID
Nevirapine	(SQV 1,000 mg + RTV 100 mg) BID
Ritonavir	Ritonavir 100 mg BID + saquinavir 1 gm BID
Rifampin	Contraindicated
Rifabutin	Avoid
Etravirine	(SQV 1,000 mg + RTV 100 mg) BID
Maraviroc	300 mg BID
Raltegravir	No data

Drug Interactions: Antiretrovirals, rifabutin, rifampin (see dose adjustment grid, above); astemizole, terfenadine, benzodiazepines, cisapride, ergotamine, statins, St. John's wort (avoid if possible); carbamazepine, phenytoin, phenobarbital, dexamethasone, prednisone (↓ saquinavir levels, ↑ interacting drug levels; monitor anticonvulsant levels); clarithromycin, erythromycin, telithromycin (↑ saquinavir and macrolide levels); grapefruit juice, itraconazole, voriconazole, ketoconazole (↑ saquinavir levels); sildenafil (do not give > 25 mg/48 hrs); tadalafil (max. 10 mg/72 hrs), vardenafil (max. 2.5 mg/72 hrs); rivaroxaban (↑ rivaroxaban); Warfarin (↑ warafrin, monitor INR).

Adverse Effects: Anorexia, headache, anemia, leukopenia, hyperglycemia (including worsening diabetes, new-onset diabetes, DKA), ↑ cholesterol/triglycerides (evaluate risk for coronary disease/pancreatitis), ↑ SGOT/SGPT, hyperuricemia, fat redistribution, possible increased bleeding in hemophilia. May cause QT interval prolongation when combined with ritonavir.

Allergic Potential: Low

Safety in Pregnancy: B

Comments: Take with food. Avoid garlic supplements, which ↓ saquinavir levels ~ 50%. Boosted dose: 1 gm saquinavir/100 mg ritonavir (PO) BID. Preferred formulation is 500 mg hard-gel capsule (Invirase 500). Soft-gel capsules (Fortovase) no longer available.

Cerebrospinal Fluid Penetration: < 1%

REFERENCES:

Borck C. Garlic supplements and saquinavir. *Clin Infect Dis* 35:343, 2002.

Cameron DW, Japour AJ, Xu Y, et al. Ritonavir and saquinavir combination therapy for the treatment of HIV infection. *AIDS* 13:213–24, 1999.

Cardiello PF, van Heeswijk RP, Hassink EA, et al. Simplifying protease inhibitor therapy with once-daily dosing of saquinavir soft-gelatin capsules/ritonavir

---

"Usual dose" assumes normal renal/hepatic function. * For renal insufficiency, give usual dose × 1 followed by maintenance dose per CrCl. For dialysis patients, dose the same as for CrCl < 10 mL/min and give supplemental (post-HD/PD dose) immediately after dialysis. CrCl = creatinine clearance; CVVH = continuous veno-venous hemo-filtration; HD/PD = hemodialysis/peritoneal dialysis. See pp. 214–216 for explanations, pp. xi–xii for abbreviations.

(1600/100 mg): HIVNAT 001.3 study. *J Acquir Immune Defic Syndr* 29:464–70, 2002.

Hsu A, Granneman GR, Cao G, et al. Pharmacokinetic interactions between two human immunodeficiency virus protease inhibitors, ritonavir and saquinavir. *Clin Pharmacol Ther* 63:453–64, 1998.

Murphy RL, Brun S, Hicks C, et al. ABT-378/ritonavir plus stavudine and lamivudine for the treatment of antiretroviral-naïve adults with HIV-1 infection: 48-week results. *AIDS* 15:F1–9, 2001.

Noble S, Faulds D. Saquinavir: a review of its pharmacology and clinical potential in the management of HIV infection. *Drugs* 52:93–112, 1996.

Panel on Antiretroviral Guidelines for Adults and Adolescents. Guidelines for the use of antiretroviral agents in HIV-1-infected adults and adolescents. Department of Health and Human Services. March 27, 2013; 1–240. Available at **http://www.aidsinfo.nih.gov/contentfiles/lvguidelines/adultandadolescentgl.pdf**.

Perry CM, Noble S. Saquinavir soft-gel capsule formation: a review of its use in patients with HIV infection. *Drugs* 55:461–86, 1998.

Vella S, Floridia M. Saquinavir: Clinical pharmacology and efficacy. *Clin Pharmacokinet* 34:189–201, 1998. http://www.fda.gov/Safety/MedWatch/Safety Information/SafetyAlertsforHumanMedicalProducts/ucm201563.htm

Website: www.fortovase.com

Simeprevir (Olysio)

Drug Class: Anti-hepatitis C agent (NS3/4A protease inhibitor)
Usual Dose: 150 mg once daily with food.
How supplied: Oral capsule, 150 mg
Treatment duration: 12 weeks in combination with a 24- or 48-week course of peg-interferon and ribavirin.

Table 9.2. Duration of Treatment with simeprevir, Peginterferon Alfa and Ribavirin

	Treatment with simeprevir, Peginterferon alfa and Ribavirin	Treatment with Peginterferon alfa and Ribavirin*	Total Treatment Duration*
Treatment-naïve and prior relapser patients[†] including those with cirrhosis	First 12 weeks	Additional 12 weeks	24 weeks
Prior non-responder patients[‡] (including partial and null responders) including those with cirrhosis	First 12 weeks	Additional 36 weeks	48 weeks

* Recommended duration of treatment if patient does not meet stopping rule. See next table for details.
† Prior relapser: undetectable HCV RNA at the end of prior interferon-based therapy and detectable HCV RNA during follow-up.
‡ Prior partial responder: prior on-treatment $\geq 2 \log_{10}$ IU/ml reduction in HCV RNA from baseline at Week 12 and detectable HCV RNA at end of prior interferon-based therapy. Prior null responder: prior on-treatment $< 2 \log_{10}$ reduction in HCV RNA from baseline at Week 12 during prior interferon-based therapy.

"Usual dose" assumes normal renal/hepatic function. * For renal insufficiency, give usual dose × 1 followed by maintenance dose per CrCl. For dialysis patients, dose the same as for CrCl < 10 mL/min and give supplemental (post-HD/PD dose) immediately after dialysis. CrCl = creatinine clearance; CVVH = continuous veno-venous hemo-filtration; HD/PD = hemodialysis/peritoneal dialysis. See pp. 214–216 for explanations, pp. xi–xii for abbreviations.

It is unlikely that a patient with inadequate on treatment response will achieve sustained virologic response (SVR), therefore discontinuation of treatment is recommended as shown below:

Table 9.3. Treatment Stopping Rules in Any Patient with Inadequate On-Treatment Virologic Response

HCV RNA	Action
Treatment Week 4: greater than or equal to 25 IU/mL	Discontinue simeprevir, peginterferon alfa and ribavirin
Treatment Week 12: greater than or equal to 25 IU/mL	Discontinue peginterferon alfa and ribavirin (treatment with simeprevir is complete at Week 12)
Treatment Week 24: greater than or equal to 25 IU/mL	Discontinue peginterferon alfa and ribavirin

Studies of peg-interferon, ribavirin, and simeprevir in patients with genotype 1a demonstrated that the presence at baseline of the NS3 Q80K polymorphism reduced treatment response. If this polymorphism is detected on pre-treatment screening, alternate HCV therapies should be considered.

Off-label use for HCV genotype 1: simeprevir 150 mg QD plus sofosbuvir 400 mg QD for 12 weeks (see Chapter 5).

Pharmacokinetic parameters:
Excreted unchanged: 91% (feces)
Serum half-life: 10-13 hours in HCV uninfected; 41 hours in HCV infected
Plasma protein binding: 98.9%
Primary mode of elimination: Hepatic

Dosage Adjustments for Renal and Hepatic Insufficiency

CrCl 50-80 mL/min	No change
CrCl 30-50 mL/min	No change
CrCl < 30 mL/min	No change
Post-HD dose	Not established
Post-PD dose	Not established
Mild hepatic insufficiency	No changee
Moderate-severe hepatic insufficiency	Not established

Drug Interactions:
Simeprevir is primarily metabolized by cytochrome p450 enzyme CYP3A. As such, administration of simeprevir with inhibitors of CYP3A will significantly increase plasma concentrations; while inducers will decrease simeprevir levels. As all HIV non-nucleoside inhibitors, protease inhibitors, and the PK booster cobicistat influence CYP3A, they should not be given with simeprevir.

Other drugs that are not recommended: carbamazepine, oxacarbazepine, phenobarbital, phenytoin, erythromycin, clarithromycin, telithromycin, itraconazole, ketoconazole, posaconazole, fluconazole, voriconazole, rifampin, rifabutin, rifapentine, dexamethasone, cisapride, milk thistle, St John's wort. Numerous other drugs should be used with caution – see prescribing information for details.

"Usual dose" assumes normal renal/hepatic function. * For renal insufficiency, give usual dose × 1 followed by maintenance dose per CrCl. For dialysis patients, dose the same as for CrCl < 10 mL/min and give supplemental (post-HD/PD dose) immediately after dialysis. CrCl = creatinine clearance; CVVH = continuous veno-venous hemo-filtration; HD/PD = hemodialysis/peritoneal dialysis. See pp. 214–216 for explanations, pp. xi–xii for abbreviations.

Adverse effects: Serious photosensitivity reactions have been observed with simeprevir; patients must use sun protection measures and limit sun exposure. Rash, pruritus, and nausea were also reported more commonly in those receiving simeprevir than placebo.

Allergic potential: Moderate

Safety in pregnancy: Category C. Note that ribavirin may cause birth defects and fetal death, and is absolutely contraindicated during pregnancy (Category X).

REFERENCES:

Fried MW, Buti M, Dore GJ, Flisiak R, et al. Once-daily simeprevir (TMC435) with pegylated interferon and ribavirin in treatment-naïve genotype 1 hepatitis C: The randomized PILLAR study. *Hepatology* 58(6):1918–1929, 2013.

Zeuzem S, Berg T, Gane E, Ferenci P, et al. Simeprevir Increases Rate of Sustained Virologic Response Among Treatment-Experienced Patients With HCV Genotype-1 Infection: A Phase IIb Trial. *Gastroenterology* S0016-5085(13)01576, 2013.

Product Information, Olysio (simeprevir) capsules. Janssen Pharmaceuticals, Titusville, New Jersey, 2013.

Sofosbuvir (Sovaldi)

Drug Class: Anti-hepatitis C agent (nucleotide polymerase inhibitor)

Usual Dose: 400 mg once daily with or without food.

How supplied: Oral tablet, 400 mg

Treatment duration: 12 or 24 weeks

HCV Mono-infected and HCV/HIV-1 Co-infected	Treatment	Duration
Genotype 1 or 4	sofosbuvir + peg-interferon alfa + ribavirin	12 weeks
Genotype 2	sofosbuvir + ribavirin	12 weeks
Genotype 3	sofosbuvir + ribavirin	24 weeks

Sofosbuvir in combination with ribavirin for 24 weeks can be considered for patients with genotype 1 who are interferon ineligible.

Pharmacokinetic parameters)

Excreted unchanged: 80% (urine), 14% (feces), 2.5% (air)

Serum half-life of the primary circulating metabolite GS-331007: 27 hours

Plasma protein binding: 61-65% for sofosbuvir, minimal for GS-331007

Primary mode of elimination: Renal

Dosage Adjustments for Renal and Hepatic insufficiency

CrCl 50-80 mL/min	No change
CrCl 30-50 mL/min	No change
CrCl < 30 mL/min	Not established
Post-HD dose	Not established
Post-PD dose	Not established
Mild-moderate hepatic insufficiency	No change
Severe hepatic insufficiency	No change

Dosage Adjustments with antiretroviral agents: None required.

Drug interactions: Sofosbuvir is a substrate of P-gp and breast cancer resistance protein (BCRP), while GS-331007 (the primary circulating metabolite) is not. Drugs that are potent P-gp inducers in the intestine (e.g. rifampin or St John's wort) may decrease

---

"Usual dose" assumes normal renal/hepatic function. * For renal insufficiency, give usual dose × 1 followed by maintenance dose per CrCl. For dialysis patients, dose the same as for CrCl < 10 mL/min and give supplemental (post-HD/PD dose) immediately after dialysis. CrCl = creatinine clearance; CVVH = continuous veno-venous hemo-filtration; HD/PD = hemodialysis/peritoneal dialysis. See pp. 214–216 for explanations, pp. xi–xii for abbreviations.

Concomitant Drug Class: Drug Name	Effect on Concentration[b]	Clinical Comment
Anticonvulsants: carbamazepine phenytoin phenobarbital oxcarbazepine	↓ sofosbuvir ↓ GS-331007	Coadministration of sofosbuvir with carbarnazepine, phenytoin, phenobarbital or oxcarbazepine is expected to decrease the concentration of sofosbuvir, leading to reduced therapeutic effect of sofosbuvir. Coadministration is not recommended.
Antimycobacterials: rifabutin rifampin rifapentine	↓ sofosbuvir ↓ GS-331007	Coadministration of sofosbuvir with rifabutin or rifapentine is expected to decrease the concentration of sofosbuvir, leading to reduced therapeutic effect of sofosbuvir. Coadministration is not recommended. sofosbuvir should not be used with rifampin, a potent intestinal P-gp inducer
Herbal Supplements: St. John's wort (*Hypericum perforatum*)	↓ sofosbuvir ↓ GS-331007	sofosbuvir should not be used with St. John's wort a potent intestinal P-gp inducer
HIV Protease Inhibitors: tipranavir/ritonavir	↓ sofosbuvir ↓ GS-331007	Coadministration of sofosbuvir with tiipranavir/ritonavir is expected to decrease the concentration of sofosbuvir, leading to reduced therapeutic effect of sofosbuvir. Coadministration is not recommended.

a   This table is not all inclusive. See prescribing information for full details.
b   ↓ = decrease

sofosbuvir's plasma concentration and should not be used. See table below for other potentially significant drug-drug interactions.
Adverse effects: The most common adverse events (incidence greater than or equal to 20%, all grades) observed with sofosbuvir in combination with ribavirin were fatigue and headache. The most common adverse events observed with sofosbuvir in combination with peginterferon alfa and ribavirin were fatigue, headache, nausea, insomnia and anemia. These side effects are seen with these agents when not given with sofosbuvir.
Allergic potential: Low
Safety in pregnancy: Category B. Note that ribavirin may cause birth defects and fetal death, and is absolutely contraindicated during pregnancy (Category X).

"Usual dose" assumes normal renal/hepatic function. * For renal insufficiency, give usual dose × 1 followed by maintenance dose per CrCl. For dialysis patients, dose the same as for CrCl < 10 mL/min and give supplemental (post-HD/PD dose) immediately after dialysis. CrCl = creatinine clearance; CVVH = continuous veno-venous hemo-filtration; HD/PD = hemodialysis/peritoneal dialysis. See pp. 214–216 for explanations, pp. xi–xii for abbreviations.

REFERENCES:

Jacobson IM, Gordon SC, Kowdley KV, Yoshida EM, et al. Sofosbuvir for Hepatitis C Genotype 2 or 3 in Patients without Treatment Options. *N Engl J Med* 368:1867–1877, 2013.

Lawitz, E, Mangia A, Wyles, D, Rodriguez-Torres M, et al. Sofosbuvir for Previously Untreated Chronic Hepatitis C Infection. *N Engl J Med* 368:1878–1887, 2013.

Lawitz E, Poordad FF, Pang PS, Hyland RH, et al. Sofosbuvir and ledipasvir fixed-dose combination with and without ribavirin in treatment-naive and previously treated patients with genotype 1 hepatitis C virus infection (LONESTAR): an open-label, randomised, phase 2 trial. The Lancet 13:62121–62122, 2013.

Product Information, SOLVADI (sofosbuvir) tablets. Gilead Sciences, Foster City, CA, 2013.

Stavudine (Zerit) d4t

Drug Class: Antiretroviral NRTI (nucleoside reverse transcriptase inhibitor)

Usual Dose: ≥ 60 kg: 40 mg (PO) BID; < 60 kg: 30 mg (PO) BID

How Supplied:

Generic—Oral Capsule: 15 mg, 20 mg, 30 mg, 40 mg

Zerit—Oral Capsule: 15 mg, 20 mg, 30 mg, 40 mg, Oral Powder for Suspension: 1 mg/mL

Pharmacokinetic Parameters:

Peak serum level: 4.2 mcg/mL
Bioavailability: 86%
Excreted unchanged (urine): 40%
Serum half-life (normal/ESRD): 1.0/5.1 hrs
Plasma protein binding: 0%
Volume of distribution (V_d): 0.5 L/kg

Primary Mode of Elimination: Renal

Dosage Adjustments* ≥ 60 kg/(≤ 60 kg)

| CrCl 50–80 mL/min | 40 mg (PO) BID (30 mg [PO] BID) |
| CrCl 25–50 mL/min | 20 mg (PO) BID (15 mg [PO] BID) |

CrCl ~ 10–25 mL/min	20 mg (PO) QD (15 mg [PO] QD)
Post-HD dose	20 mg (PO) (15 mg [PO])
Post-PD dose	No information
CVVH dose	20 mg (PO) QD (15 mg [PO] QD)
Moderate hepatic insufficiency	No change
Severe hepatic insufficiency	No change

Drug Interactions: Ribavirin (↓ stavudine efficacy, ↑ risk of lactic acidosis); zidovudine (↓ stavudine levels); dapsone, INH, other neurotoxic agents (↑ risk of neuropathy), didanosine (↑ risk of neuropathy, lactic acidosis).

Adverse Effects: Drug fever/rash, nausea, vomiting, GI upset, diarrhea, headache, insomnia, dose dependent peripheral neuropathy, myalgias, pancreatitis, ↑ SGOT/SGPT, ↑ cholesterol, facial fat pad wasting, lipodystrophy, thrombocytopenia, leukopenia, lactic acidosis with hepatic steatosis (rare, but potentially life-threatening toxicity with use of NRTIs).

Allergic Potential: Low

Safety in Pregnancy: C

Comments: Pancreatitis may be severe/fatal. Avoid coadministration with AZT or ddC. Decrease dose in patients with peripheral neuropathy to 20 mg (PO) BID. Pregnant women may be at increased risk for lactic acidosis/liver damage when stavudine is used with didanosine (ddI).

Cerebrospinal Fluid Penetration: 30%

"Usual dose" assumes normal renal/hepatic function. * For renal insufficiency, give usual dose × 1 followed by maintenance dose per CrCl. For dialysis patients, dose the same as for CrCl < 10 mL/min and give supplemental (post-HD/PD dose) immediately after dialysis. CrCl = creatinine clearance; CVVH = continuous veno-venous hemo-filtration; HD/PD = hemodialysis/peritoneal dialysis. See pp. 214–216 for explanations, pp. xi–xii for abbreviations.

REFERENCES:

Berasconi E, Boubaker K, Junghans C, et al Abnormalities of body fat distribution in HIV-infected persons treated with antiretroviral drugs: the Swiss HIV Cohort Study. *J Acquir Immune Defic Syndr* 31:50–5, 2002.

Dudley MN, Graham KK, Kaul S, et al. Pharmacokinetics of stavudine in patients with AIDS and AIDS-related complex. *J Infect Dis* 166:480–5, 1992.

FDA notifications. FDA changes information for stavudine label. *Aids Alert* 17:67, 2002.

Joly V, Flandre P, Meiffredy V, et al. Efficacy of zidovudine compared to stavudine, both in combination with lamivudine and indinavir, in human immunodeficiency virus-infected nucleoside-experienced patients with no prior exposure to lamivudine, stavudine, or protease inhibitors (Novavir trial). *Antimicrob Agents Chemother* 46:1906–13, 2002.

Lea AP, Faulds D. Stavudine: A review of its pharmacodynamic and pharmacokinetic properties and clinical potential in HIV infection. *Drugs* 51: 846–64, 1996.

Miller KD, Cameron M, Wood LV, et al. Lactic acidosis and hepatic steatosis associated with use of stavudine: report of four cases. Ann Intern Med 133:192–96, 2000.

Murphy RL, Brun S, Hicks C, et al. ABT-378/ritonavir plus stavudine and lamivudine for the treatment of antiretroviral-naïve adults with HIV-1 infection: 48-week results. *AIDS* 15:F1–9, 2001.

Panel on Antiretroviral Guidelines for Adults and Adolescents. Guidelines for the use of antiretroviral agents in HIV-1-infected adults and adolescents. Department of Health and Human Services. March 27, 2013; 1–240. Available at **http://www.aidsinfo.nih.gov/contentfiles/lvguidelines/adultandadolescentgl.pdf**.

Website: www.zerit.com

Telaprevir (Incivek®)

Drug Class: Anti-Hepatitis C agent (Protease inhibitor)

Usual Dose: 750 mg (PO) TID with a meal (must be administered with both peginterferon alfa and ribavirin) for chronic hepatitis C virus, genotype 1 infection

How Supplied: Oral Tablet: 375 MG

Pharmacokinetic Parameters:

Peak serum level: 3510 nanograms/mL
Bioavailability: unknown
Excreted unchanged: 31.9% (feces) 1% (urine)
Serum half-life (normal/ESRD): 9–11 hours / no data
Plasma protein binding: 59–76%
Volume of distribution (Vd): 252 L
Primary mode of Elimination: Feces

Dosage Adjustments*

CrCl 50–80 mL/min	No Change
CrCl 30–49 mL/min	No Change
CrCl < 30 mL/min	No Change
ESRD	No Change
Post-HD dose	No Change
Post-PD dose	No Change
CVVH dose	No Change
Mild – moderate hepatic insufficiency	No Change
Severe hepatic insufficiency	Not recommended

Antiretroviral Dosage Adjustments: do not co-administer telaprevir with the following HIV antiretroviral medications: darunavir/ritonavir, fosamprenavir/ritonavir, and lopinavir/ritonavir Coadministration with raltegravir based HAART my be feasible.

Drug Interactions: Telaprevir is a substrate of CYP3A and an inhibitor of CYP3A and P-gp. Telaprevir may affect the plasma concentrations of the following co-administered drugs: ↑ antiarrhythmics, ↑ digoxin, ↑ macrolide antibiotics

---

"Usual dose" assumes normal renal/hepatic function. * For renal insufficiency, give usual dose × 1 followed by maintenance dose per CrCl. For dialysis patients, dose the same as for CrCl < 10 mL/min and give supplemental (post-HD/PD dose) immediately after dialysis. CrCl = creatinine clearance; CVVH = continuous veno-venous hemo-filtration; HD/PD = hemodialysis/peritoneal dialysis. See pp. 214–216 for explanations, pp. xi–xii for abbreviations.

(↓ telaprevir), ↑ or ↓ warfarin, ↑ carbamazepine (↓ telaprevir), ↑ or ↓ Phenobarbital (↓ telaprevir), ↑ or ↓ phenytoin (↓ telaprevir), ↓ escitalopram, ↑ desipramine, ↑ antifungals [trazodone, ketoconazole, itraconazole, posaconazole, voriconazole (↑ telaprevir)], ↑ colchicine, ↑ rifabutin (↓ telaprevir – contraindicated), ↑ rifampin (↓ telaprevir – contraindicated), ↑ alprazolam, ↑ midazolam, ↓ zolpidem, ↑ calcium channel blockers, ↑ prednisone, ↑ methylprednisolone, ↔ dexamethasone (↓ telaprevir), ↑ fluticasone, ↑ budesonide, ↑ bosentan, ↑ atazanavir (↓ telaprevir), ↓ efavirenz (↓ telaprevir), ↑ telaprevir, ↓ ethinyl estradiol, ↑ cyclosporine, ↑ sirolimus, ↑ tacolimus, ↑ salmeterol, ↓ methadone, ↑ PDE5 inhibitors (sildenafil max 25mg q48H, tadalafil max 10mg q72h, vardenafil max 2.5mg q72h)

Adverse Effects: pruritus 47; rash 56%; Stevens-Johnson syndrome <1%; ↑ uric acid level 73%; anorectal adverse events (eg, hemorrhoids, anorectal discomfort, anal pruritus, and rectal burning) 29%; diarrhea 26%; nausea 39%; vomiting 13%; Hematologic adverse effects associated with ribavirin (anemia, ↓ lymphocyte count, ↓ platelet count, ↓ white blood cell count); leukocytosis 12%; ↑ Serum bilirubin 41%; fatigue 56%

Allergic Potential: high

Safety in Pregnancy: B (when taken w/ ribavirin X)

Comments: Must be taken with 7–9 hours apart with a meal that is high in fat. Must not be used as monotherapy for HCV and must only be used in combination with peginterferon alfa and ribavirin. A high proportion of previous null responders (particularly those with cirrhosis) did not achieve sustained virologic response (SVR) and had telaprevir resistance-associated substitutions emerge during treatment.

The safety and efficacy of telaprevir have not been established in patients co-infected with HCV/HIV or HCV/HBV. Rash is a very common side effect and can be severe.

Cerebrospinal Fluid Penetration: no data

Alias: VX-950

REFERENCES:

McHutchison JG, Everson GT, Gordon SC, et al. Telaprevir with peginterferon and ribavirin for chronic HCV genotype 1 infection. N Engl J Med. Apr 30 2009;360(18):1827–1838.

Hezode C, Forestier N, Dusheiko G, et al. Telaprevir and peginterferon with or without ribavirin for chronic HCV infection. N Engl J Med. Apr 30 2009;360(18):1839–1850.

McHutchison JG, Manns MP, Muir AJ, et al. Telaprevir for previously treated chronic HCV infection. N Engl J Med. Apr 8 2010;362(14):1292–1303.

Jacobson IM, McHutchison JG, Dusheiko G, et al. Telaprevir for previously untreated chronic hepatitis C virus infection. N Engl J Med. Jun 23 2011;364(25):2405–2416.

Zeuzem S, Andreone P, Pol S, et al. Telaprevir for retreatment of HCV infection. N Engl J Med. Jun 23 2011;364(25):2417–2428.

C Kasserra, E Hughes, M Treitel, et al. Clinical Pharmacology of BOC: Metabolism, Excretion, and Drug-Drug Interactions. 18th Conference on Retroviruses and Opportunistic Infections (CROI 2011). Boston. February 27–March 2, 2011. Abstract 118.

R van Heeswijk, A Vandevoorde, G Boogaerts, et al. Pharmacokinetic Interactions between ARV Agents and the Investigational HCV Protease Inhibitor TVR in Healthy Volunteers. 18th Conference on Retroviruses and Opportunistic Infections (CROI 2011). Boston. February 27–March 2, 2011. Abstract 119.

Ramanathan S, Mathias AA, German P, Kearney BP. Clinical pharmacokinetic and pharmacodynamic profile of the HIV integrase inhibitor elvitegravir. *Clinical pharmacokinetics.* Apr 2011;50(4): 229–244.

Website: https://www.incivek.com

"Usual dose" assumes normal renal/hepatic function. * For renal insufficiency, give usual dose × 1 followed by maintenance dose per CrCl. For dialysis patients, dose the same as for CrCl < 10 mL/min and give supplemental (post-HD/PD dose) immediately after dialysis. CrCl = creatinine clearance; CVVH = continuous veno-venous hemo-filtration; HD/PD = hemodialysis/peritoneal dialysis. See pp. 214–216 for explanations, pp. xi–xii for abbreviations.

Telbivudine (Tyzeka) LDT

Drug Class: Anti-Hepatitis B agent (nucleoside reverse transcriptase inhibitor)
Usual Dose: 600 mg (PO) QD
How Supplied: Oral Tablet: 600 mg
Pharmacokinetic Parameters:
Peak serum level: 3.69 mcg/mL
Bioavailability: The absolute bioavailability is unknown
Excreted unchanged: 0% (feces), 42% (urine)
Serum half-life (normal/ESRD): 40–49 hrs/ no data
Plasma protein binding: 3.3%
Volume of distribution (V_d): not studied
Primary Mode of Elimination: Renal
Dosage Adjustments*

CrCl 50–80 mL/min	No change
CrCl 30–49 mL/min	600 mg q2d
CrCl < 30 mL/min	600 mg q3d
ESRD	600 mg q4d
Post-HD dose	Give dose after HD
Post-PD dose	Not studied
CVVH dose	Not studied
Mild to moderate hepatic insufficiency	No change
Severe hepatic insufficiency	No change

Antiretroviral Dosage Adjustments: None
Drug Interactions: Telbivudine Use with Peginterferon Alfa-2a: Increased Risk of Peripheral Neuropathy. Telbivudine is not metabolized by the liver and it is not a substrate or inhibitor of the cytochrome P450 enzyme system, and no drug other drug interactions have been established.

Adverse Effects: Boxed Warnings; Lactic acidosis/hepatomegaly, including fatal cases, have been reported with the use of nucleoside analogues alone or in combination with other antiretrovirals. Signs/symptoms of lactic acidosis include; nausea, vomiting, abdominal pain, tachypnea, decreased renal function, or decreased liver function. Severe acute exacerbations of hepatitis B have been reported in patients who have discontinued anti-hepatitis B therapy. Myopathy has also been associated with telbivudine use. Other less serious adverse effects include: abdominal pain, dizziness, headache, nasopharyngitis, malaise, and fatigue.
Allergic Potential: Low
Safety in Pregnancy: B
Comments: May be administered without regard to food. Telbivudine does not exhibit any clinically relevant activity against HIV type 1. The efficacy and safety in patients co-infected with HIV, hepatitis C virus, hepatitis D virus, a history or signs of hepatic decompensation, or a history of alcohol or illicit substance abuse within the preceding 2 years are unknown. Severe, acute exacerbation of hepatitis B may occur upon discontinuation. Monitor liver function several months after stopping treatment; re-initiation of anti-hepatitis B therapy may be required.
Cerebrospinal Fluid Penetration: no data

REFERENCES:
Chan HL, Heathcote EJ, Marcellin P. Treatment of hepatitis B e antigen positive chronic hepatitis with telbivudine or adefovir: a randomized trial. *Ann Intern Med* 147(11):745–54, 2007.
Gane E, Lai CL, Liaw YF, et al. Phase III comparison of telbivudine vs lamivudine in HBeAg-positive patients with chronic hepatitis B: efficacy, safety,

---

"Usual dose" assumes normal renal/hepatic function. * For renal insufficiency, give usual dose × 1 followed by maintenance dose per CrCl. For dialysis patients, dose the same as for CrCl < 10 mL/min and give supplemental (post-HD/PD dose) immediately after dialysis. CrCl = creatinine clearance; CVVH = continuous veno-venous hemo-filtration; HD/PD = hemodialysis/peritoneal dialysis. See pp. 214–216 for explanations, pp. xi–xii for abbreviations.

and predictors of response at 1 year. *J Hepatol* 44 (suppl 2):S183–S184, 2006.

Lai CL, Gane E, Liaw YF, et al. Maximal early HBV suppression is predictive of optimal virologic and clinical efficacy in nucleoside-treated hepatitis B patients: scientific observations from a large multinational trial (the GLOBE study). *Hepatology* 42(S1):232A–3A, 2005.

Lai CL, Gane E, Liaw YF, et al. Telbivudine (LdT) vs. lamivudine for chronic hepatitis B: first-year results from the international phase III GLOBE trial. *Hepatology* 42(Supp 1):748A, 2005.

Lai CL, Gane E, Liaw YF, et al. Telbivudine versus lamivudine in patients with chronic hepatitis B. *N Engl J Med* 357(25):2576–88, 2007.

Lai CL, Leung N, Teo EK, et al. A 1-year trial of telbivudine, lamivudine, and the combination in patients with hepatitis B e antigen-positive chronic hepatitis B. *Gastroenterology* 129(2):528–36, 2005.

Product Information: TYZEKA(TM) oral tablets, telbivudine oral tablets. Novartis Pharmaceuticals Corporation, East Hanover, NJ, 2006.

Zhou X, Marbury TC, Alcorn HW, et al. Pharmacokinetics of telbivudine in subjects with various degrees of hepatic impairment. *Antimicrob Agents Chemother* 50(5):1721–26, 2006.

Zhou XJ, Lloyd DM, Chao GC, et al. Absence of food effect on the pharmacokinetics of telbivudine following oral administration in healthy subjects. *J Clin Pharmacol* 46(3):275–81, 2006.

Zhou XJ, Myers M, Chao G, et al. Clinical pharmacokinetics of telbivudine, a potent antiviral for hepatitis B, in subjects with impaired hepatic or renal function. *J Hepatol* 40(Suppl 1):452, 2004.

Website: www.tyzeka.com

Tenofovir disoproxil fumarate (Viread) TDF

Drug Class: Antiretroviral (nucleotide analogue) (HIV) (HBV)

Usual Dose: 300 mg (PO) QD (HIV); 300 mg (PO) QD (HBV)

How Supplied: Oral Tablet: 300 mg

Pharmacokinetic Parameters:

Peak serum level: 0.29 mcg/mL
Bioavailability: 25%/39%
(fasting/high-fat meal)
Excreted unchanged (urine): 32%
Serum half-life (normal/ESRD): 17 hrs/no data
Plasma protein binding: 0.7–7.2%
Volume of distribution (V_d): 1.3 L/kg

Primary Mode of Elimination: Renal

Dosage Adjustments*

CrCl ≥ 50 mL/min	No change
CrCl 30–49 mL/min	300 mg (PO) q2d
CrCl 10–29 mL/min	300 mg (PO) 2x/week
CrCl < 10 mL/min	No information
Post-HD dose	300 mg q7d or after 12 hours on HD
Post-PD dose	No information
CVVH dose	No information
Moderate hepatic insufficiency	No change
Severe hepatic insufficiency	No change

Drug Interactions: Didanosine (if possible, avoid concomitant didanosine due to impaired CD4 response and increased risk of virologic failure); valganciclovir (↑ tenofovir levels); atazanavir, lopinavir/ritonavir (↑ tenofovir levels)(↓ atazanavir levels; use atazanavir 300 mg/ritonavir 100 mg with tenofovir); no clinically significant interactions with lamivudine, efavirenz, methadone, oral contraceptives. Not a substrate/inhibitor of cytochrome P-450 enzymes.

"Usual dose" assumes normal renal/hepatic function. * For renal insufficiency, give usual dose × 1 followed by maintenance dose per CrCl. For dialysis patients, dose the same as for CrCl < 10 mL/min and give supplemental (post-HD/PD dose) immediately after dialysis. CrCl = creatinine clearance; CVVH = continuous veno-venous hemo-filtration; HD/PD = hemodialysis/peritoneal dialysis. See pp. 214–216 for explanations, pp. xi–xii for abbreviations.

Adverse Effects: Mild nausea, vomiting, GI upset, asthenia, headache, diarrhea, lactic acidosis with hepatic steatosis (rare, but potentially life-threatening with NRTIs), renal tubular acidosis, acute renal failure, and Fanconi syndrome have been reported, ↓ bone density (clinical significance unknown).

Allergic Potential: Low

Safety in Pregnancy: B

Comments: Eliminated by glomerular filtration/tubular secretion. May be taken with or without food. If possible, avoid concomitant didanosine (see drug interactions).

Cerebrospinal Fluid Penetration: No data

REFERENCES:

Gallant JE, DeJesus D, Arribas JR, et al. Tenofovir DF, emtricitabine, and efavirenz vs. zidovudine, lamivudine, and efavirenz for HIV. *N Engl J Med* 354:251–60, 2006.

Gallant JE. Efficacy and safety of tenofovir DF vs. stavudine in combination therapy in antiretroviral-naïve patients: a 3-year randomized trial. *JAMA* 292: 191–201, 2004.

Gallant JE, Deresinski S. Tenofovir disoproxil fumarate. *Clin Infect Dis* 37:944–50, 2003.

Jullien V, Treluye JM, Rey E, et al. Population pharmacokinetics of tenofovir in human immunodeficiency virus-infected patients taking highly active antiretroviral therapy. *Antimicrobial Agents and Chemotherapy* 49:3361–66, 2005.

Marcellin P, Heathcote EJ, Buti M, et al: Tenofovir disoproxil fumarate versus adefovir dipivoxil for chronic hepatitis B. *N Engl J Med* 2008; 359(23):2442–2455.

Nelson M, Portsmouth S, Stebbing J, et al: An open-label study of tenofovir in HIV-1 and hepatitis B virus co-infected individuals. *AIDS* 17(1): F7–F10, 2003.

Nunez M, Perez-Olmeda M, Diaz B, et al: Activity of tenofovir on hepatitis B virus replication in HIV-co-infected patients failing or partially responding to lamivudine. *AIDS* 16(17):2352–54, 2002.

Panel on Antiretroviral Guidelines for Adults and Adolescents. Guidelines for the use of antiretroviral agents in HIV-1-infected adults and adolescents. Department of Health and Human Services. March 27, 2013; 1–240. Available at **http://www. aidsinfo.nih.gov/contentfiles/lvguidelines/ adultandadolescentgl.pdf**.

Terrault NA. Treatment of recurrent hepatitis B infection in liver transplant recipients. *Liver Transpl* 8(suppl 1): S74–81, 2002.

Thomson CA. Prodrug of tenofovir diphosphate approved for combination HIV therapy. *Am J Health Syst Pharm* 59:18, 2002.

Website: www.viread.com

Tipranavir (Aptivus) TPV

Drug Class: Protease inhibitor

Usual Dose: 500 mg (PO) with ritonavir 200 mg (PO) BID

How Supplied: Oral Capsule, Liquid Filled: 250 mg, Oral Solution: 100 mg/mL

Pharmacokinetic Parameters:

Peak serum level: 77–94 mcg/mL

Bioavailability: No data

Excreted unchanged (urine): 44%

Serum half-life (normal/ESRD): 5.5–6 hrs/ no data

Plasma protein binding: 99.9%

Volume of distribution (V_d): 7–10 L/kg

Primary Mode of Elimination: Hepatic

Dosage Adjustments*

CrCl 50–80 mL/min	No change
CrCl 10–50 mL/min	No change
CrCl < 10 mL/min	No change

"Usual dose" assumes normal renal/hepatic function. * For renal insufficiency, give usual dose × 1 followed by maintenance dose per CrCl. For dialysis patients, dose the same as for CrCl < 10 mL/min and give supplemental (post-HD/PD dose) immediately after dialysis. CrCl = creatinine clearance; CVVH = continuous veno-venous hemo-filtration; HD/PD = hemodialysis/peritoneal dialysis. See pp. 214–216 for explanations, pp. xi–xii for abbreviations.

Post-HD dose	No change
Post-PD dose	No change
CVVH dose	No change
Mild hepatic insufficiency	No change
Moderate or severe hepatic insufficiency	Avoid

Drug Interactions: Rifabutin (↑ levels), clarithromycin (↑ levels), loperamide (↓ levels), statins (↑ risk of myopathy); abacavir, saquinavir, tenofovir, zidovudine, amprenavir/RTV, lopinavir/RTV (↓ levels). Aluminum/magnesium antacids (↓ absorption 25–30%). Ritonavir (↑ risk of hepatitis). St. John's wort (↓ tipranavir levels). Keep refrigerated 2–8°C. Metabolized via CYP 3A4. Maraciroc - dose at 300 mg BID. Rivaroxaban (↑ rivaroxaban), Warfarin (↑ warfrin, monitor INR)

Adverse Effects: Contraindicated in moderate/severe hepatic insufficiency. ↑ risk of hepatotoxicity in HIV patients co-infected with HBV/HCV. Case reports of intracerebral hemorrhage—use with caution in patients with coagulopathies.

Allergic Potential: High. Tipranavir is a sulfonamide; use with caution in patients with sulfonamide allergies

Safety in Pregnancy: C

Comments: Should be taken with food. Increased bioavailability when taken with meals. Must be coadministered with 200 mg ritonavir. Tipranavir contains a sulfonamide moiety (as do darunavir and fosamprenavir).

Cerebrospinal Fluid Penetration: No data

REFERENCES:

Barbaro G, Scozzafava A, Mastrolorenzo A, et al. Highly active antiretroviral therapy: current state of the art, new agents and their pharmacological interactions useful for improving therapeutic outcome. Curr Pharm Des 11:1805–43, 2005.

Clotet B. Strategies for overcoming resistance in HIV-1 infected patients receiving HAART. AIDS Rev 6:123–30, 2004.

Croom KF, Keam SJ. Tipranavir: a ritonavir-boosted protease inhibitor. Drugs 65:1669–79, 2005.

de Mendoza C, Soriano V. Resistance to HIV protease inhibitors: mechanisms and clinical consequences. Curr Drug Metab 5:321–8, 2004.

Gulick RM. New antiretroviral drugs. Clin Microbiol Infect 9:186–93, 2003.

Hicks CB, Cahn P, Cooper DA, et al. Durable efficacy of tipranavir-ritonavir in combination with an optimised background regimen of antiretroviral drugs for treatment-experienced HIV-1-infected patients at 48 weeks in the Randomized Evaluation of Strategic Intervention in multi-drug resistant patients with Tipranavir (RESIST) studies: an analysis of combined data from two randomized open-label trials. Lancet 368:466–75, 2006.

Kandula VR, Khanlou H, Farthing C. Tipranavir: a novel second-generation nonpeptidic protease inhibitor. Expert Rev Anti Infect Ther 3:9–21, 2005.

Kashuba AD. Drug-drug interactions and the pharmacotherapy of HIV infection. Top HIV Med 13:64–9, 2005.

Panel on Antiretroviral Guidelines for Adults and Adolescents. Guidelines for the use of antiretroviral agents in HIV-1-infected adults and adolescents. Department of Health and Human Services. March 27, 2013; 1–240. Available at http://www.aidsinfo.nih.gov/contentfiles/lvguidelines/adultandadolescentgl.pdf.

Plosker GL, Figgitt DP. Tipranavir. Drugs 63:1611–8, 2003.

Turner D, Schapiro JM,Brenner BG, Wainberg MA. The influence of protease inhibitor profiles on selection of HIV therapy in treatment-naïve patients. Antivir Ther 9:301–14, 2004.

Yeni P. Tipranovir: a protease inhibitor from a new class with distinct antiviral activity. J Acquir Immune Defic Syndr 34 (Suppl 1):S91–4, 2003.

Website: www.aptivus.com

Zidovudine (Retrovir) ZDV

Drug Class: Antiretroviral NRTI (nucleoside reverse transcriptase inhibitor)
Usual Dose: 300 mg (PO) BID (see comments).
IV solution 10 mg/mL (dose 1 mg/kg 5–6 x/day)
How Supplied:
Generic—
Oral Capsule: 100 mg
Oral Syrup: 50 mg/5 mL
Oral Tablet: 300 mg
Retrovir—
Intravenous Solution: 10 mg/mL
Oral Capsule: 100 mg
Oral Syrup: 50 mg/5 mL
Oral Tablet: 300 mg
Pharmacokinetic Parameters:
Peak serum level: 1.2 mcg/mL
Bioavailability: 64%
Excreted unchanged (urine): 16%
Serum half-life (normal/ESRD): 1.1/1.4 hrs
Plasma protein binding: < 38%
Volume of distribution (V_d): 1.6 L/kg
Primary Mode of Elimination: Hepatic
Dosage Adjustments*

CrCl 50–80 mL/min	No change
CrCl 10–50 mL/min	No change
CrCl < 10 mL/min	300 mg (PO) QD
HD/PD	100 mg (PO) q6–8h
Post-HD/PD dose	None
CVVH dose	300 mg (PO) QD
Moderate or severe hepatic insufficiency	No information

Drug Interactions: Acetaminophen, atovaquone, fluconazole, methadone, probenecid, valproic acid (↑ zidovudine levels); clarithromycin, nelfinavir, rifampin, rifabutin (↓ zidovudine levels); dapsone, flucytosine, ganciclovir, interferon alpha, bone marrow suppressive/cytotoxic agents (↑ risk of hematologic toxicity); indomethacin (↑ levels of zidovudine toxic metabolite); phenytoin (↑ zidovudine levels, ↑ or ↓ phenytoin levels); ribavirin (↓ zidovudine effect; avoid).
Adverse Effects: Nausea, vomiting, GI upset, diarrhea, malaise, anorexia, leukopenia, severe anemia, macrocytosis, thrombocytopenia, headaches, ↑ SGOT/SGPT, hepatotoxicity, myalgias, myositis, symptomatic myopathy, insomnia, blue/black nail discoloration, asthenia, lactic acidosis with hepatic steatosis (rare, but potentially life-threatening toxicity with use of NRTIs).
Allergic Potential: Low
Safety in Pregnancy: C
Comments: Antagonized by ganciclovir or ribavirin. Also a component of Combivir and Trizivir. Patients on IV therapy should be switched to PO as soon as able to take oral medication. For IV administration, dilute in D5W to a concentration no greater than 4 mg/mL and infuse over 1 hour.
Cerebrospinal Fluid Penetration: 60%

REFERENCES:
Barry M, Mulcahy F, Merry C, et al. Pharmacokinetics and potential interactions amongst antiretroviral agents used to treat patients with HIV infection. *Clin Pharmacol* 36:289–304, 1999.
Been-Tiktak AM, Boucher CA, Brun-Vezinet F, et al. Efficacy and safety of combination therapy with delavirdine and zidovudine: a European/Australian phase II trial. *Intern J Antimcrob Agents* 11: 13–21, 1999.

"Usual dose" assumes normal renal/hepatic function. * For renal insufficiency, give usual dose × 1 followed by maintenance dose per CrCl. For dialysis patients, dose the same as for CrCl < 10 mL/min and give supplemental (post-HD/PD dose) immediately after dialysis. CrCl = creatinine clearance; CVVH = continuous veno-venous hemo-filtration; HD/PD = hemodialysis/peritoneal dialysis. See pp. 214–216 for explanations, pp. xi–xii for abbreviations.

McDowell JA, Lou Y, Symonds WS, et al. Multiple-dose pharmacokinetics and pharmacodynamics of abacavir alone and in combination with zidovudine in human immunodeficiency virus-infected adults. *Antimicrob Agents Chemother* 44:2061–7, 2000.

Montaner JS, Reiss P, Cooper D, et al. A randomized, double-blind trial comparing combinations of nevirapine, didanosine, and zidovudine for HIV-infected patients: The INCAS trial. Italy, the Netherlands, Canada and Australia Study. *J Am Med Assoc* 279:930–7, 1998.

Panel on Antiretroviral Guidelines for Adults and Adolescents. Guidelines for the use of antiretroviral agents in HIV-1-infected adults and adolescents. Department of Health and Human Services. March 27, 2013; 1–240. Available at **http://www.aidsinfo.nih.gov/contentfiles/lvguidelines/adultandadolescentgl.pdf**.

Piscitelli SC, Gallicano KD. Interactions among drugs for HIV and opportunistic infections. *N Engl J Med* 344:984–996, 2001.

Simpson DM. Human immunodeficiency virus-associated dementia: A review of pathogenesis, prophylaxis, and treatment studies of zidovudine therapy. *Clin Infect Dis* 29:19–34, 1999.

"Usual dose" assumes normal renal/hepatic function. * For renal insufficiency, give usual dose × 1 followed by maintenance dose per CrCl. For dialysis patients, dose the same as for CrCl < 10 mL/min and give supplemental (post-HD/PD dose) immediately after dialysis. CrCl = creatinine clearance; CVVH = continuous veno-venous hemo-filtration; HD/PD = hemodialysis/peritoneal dialysis. See pp. 214–216 for explanations, pp. xi–xii for abbreviations.

Appendix 1[*]

* Reprinted with permission from the IAS-USA. Johnson VA, Calvez V, Günthard HF, Paredes R, Pillay D, Shafer RW, Wensing AM, and Richman DD. Update of the drug resistance mutations in HIV-1: March 2013. *Topics in Antiviral Medicine*. 2013;21(1): 6–14. ©2013 IAS–USA. Updated information and User Notes are available at www.iasusa.org.

MUTATIONS IN THE REVERSE TRANSCRIPTASE GENE ASSOCIATED WITH RESISTANCE TO REVERSE TRANSCRIPTASE INHIBITORS

Nucleoside and Nucleotide Analogue Reverse Transcriptase Inhibitors (nRTIs)[a]

Multi-nRTI Resistance: 69 Insertion Complex[b] (affects all nRTIs currently approved by the US FDA)

M	A	▼ K			L	T	K
41	62	69	70		210	215	219
L	V	Insert	R		W	Y	Q
						F	E

Multi-nRTI Resistance: 151 Complex[c] (affects all nRTIs currently approved by the US FDA except tenofovir)

A	V	F	F	Q	
62	75	77	116	151	
V	I	L	Y	M	

Multi-nRTI Resistance: Thymidine Analogue-Associated Mutations[d,e] (TAMs; affect all nRTIs currently approved by the US FDA)

M	D	K		L	T	K
41	67	70		210	215	219
L	N	R		W	Y	Q
					F	E

Abacavir[f,g]

K	L	Y	M
65	74	115	184
R	V	F	V

Didanosine[g,h]

K	L
65	74
R	V

Emtricitabine

K	M
65	184
R	V
	I

Lamivudine

K	M
65	184
R	V
	I

Stavudine[d,e,g,i,j,k]

41	65	67	70	210	215	219
M	K	D	K	L	T	K
L	R	N	R	W	Y / F	Q / E

Tenofovir[l]

65	70
K	K
R	E

Zidovudine[d,e,j,k]

41	67	70	210	215	219
M	D	K	L	T	K
L	N	R	W	Y / F	Q / E

Nonnucleoside Analogue Reverse Transcriptase Inhibitors (NNRTIs)[a,m]

Efavirenz

100	101	103	106	108	181	188	190	225	230
L	K	K	V	V	Y	Y	G	P	M
I	P	N / S	M	I	C	L	S / A	H	L

Etravirine[n]

90	98	100	101	106	138	179	181	188	190	230
V	A	L	K	V	E	V	Y	Y	G	L
I	G	I*	E / H / P*	I	A / G / K / Q	D / F / T	C* / I* / V*	L	S / A	L

Nevirapine

100	101	103	106	108	181	188	190	230
L	K	K	V	V	Y	Y	G	M
I	P	N / S	A / M	I	C / I	C / L / H	A	L

Rilpivirine[o]

101	138	179	181	188	221	227	230
K	E	V	Y	Y	H	F	M
E / P	A / G / K / Q / R	L	C / I / V	L	Y	C	I / L

MUTATIONS IN THE PROTEASE GENE ASSOCIATED WITH RESISTANCE TO PROTEASE INHIBITORS[p,q,r]

Drug	L10	V11	G16	K20	L24	V32	L33	E34	M36	M46	I47	G48	I50	F53	I54	D60	I62	L63	I64	A71	G73	T74	L76	V77	V82	I84	I85	N88	L89	L90	I93
Atazanavir +/– ritonavir[s]	I/F/V/C		E	R/M/T/V	I		I/F/V	Q	I/L/V			V	L	L/Y	L/V/M/T/A	E	V		L/M/V	V/I/T/L	C/S/T/A				A/T/F/I	V	V	S		M	L/M
Darunavir/ ritonavir[t]		I				I	F				V		V		L/M							P	V			V			V		
Fosamprenavir/ ritonavir[u]	F/I/R/V					I				I/L	V		V		L/V/M						S		V		A/F/S/T	V				M	
Indinavir/ ritonavir[u]	I/R/V			M/R	I	I			I	I/L					V					V/T	S/A		V	I	A/F/T	V				M	
Lopinavir/ ritonavir[v]	F/I/R/V			M/R	I	I	F			I/L	V/A		V	L	V/L/A/M/T/S			P		V/T	S		V		A/F/T/S	V				M	

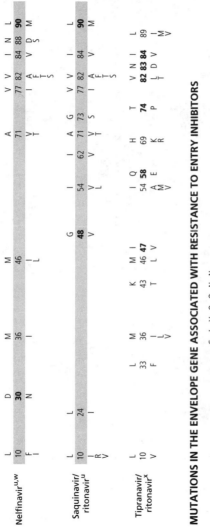

Nelfinavir[u,w]

Saquinavir/ritonavir[u]

Tipranavir/ritonavir[x]

MUTATIONS IN THE ENVELOPE GENE ASSOCIATED WITH RESISTANCE TO ENTRY INHIBITORS

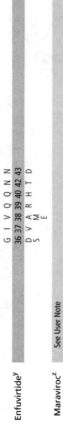

Enfuvirtide[y]

Maraviroc[z]   See User Note

MUTATIONS IN THE INTEGRASE GENE ASSOCIATED WITH RESISTANCE TO INTEGRASE INHIBITORS

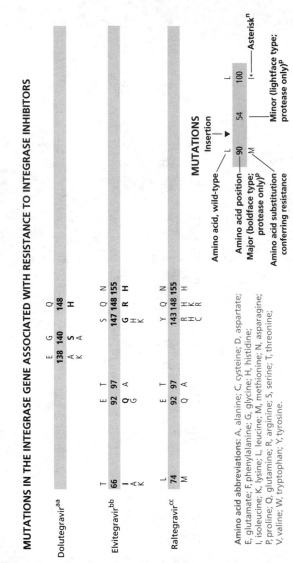

Dolutegravir[aa]

	E	G	Q
	138	140	148
	A	S	H
	K	A	

Elvitegravir[bb]

T	E	T	S	Q	N
66	92	97	147	148	155
I	Q	A	G	R	H
A	G		H		
K			K		

Raltegravir[cc]

L	E	T	Y	Q	N
74	92	97	143	148	155
M	Q	A	R	H	H
			H	K	R
			C	R	

MUTATIONS

Insertion ▶

Amino acid, wild-type ————— L ————— L

Amino acid position ————— 90 54 100 (boldface type; protease only)[p]

Major (boldface type; protease only)[p]

Amino acid substitution conferring resistance ————— M

Minor (lightface type; protease only)[p]

Asterisk[n] ————— I*

Amino acid abbreviations: A, alanine; C, cysteine; D, aspartate; E, glutamate; F, phenylalanine; G, glycine; H, histidine; I, isoleucine; K, lysine; L, leucine; M, methionine; N, asparagine; P, proline; Q, glutamine; R, arginine; S, serine; T, threonine; V, valine; W, tryptophan; Y, tyrosine.

IAS–USA DRUG RESISTANCE MUTATIONS IN HIV-1: March 2013

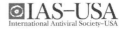

The IAS–USA Drug Resistance Mutations Group reviews new data on HIV-1 drug resistance that have been published or presented at scientific conferences to maintain a current list of mutations associated with antiretroviral drug resistance. The compilation includes mutations that may contribute to a reduced virologic response to a drug. It should not be assumed that the list presented here is exhaustive. Drugs that have been approved by the US Food and Drug Administration (FDA) as well as any drugs available in expanded access programs are included and listed in alphabetic order within each drug class.

The mutations listed have been identified by 1 or more of the following criteria: (1) in vitro passage experiments or validation of contribution to resistance by using site-directed mutagenesis; (2) susceptibility testing of laboratory or clinical isolates; (3) nucleotide sequencing of viruses from patients in whom the drug is failing; (4) correlation studies between genotype at baseline and virologic response in patients exposed to a drug. The availability of recently approved drugs that cannot be tested as monotherapy precludes assessment of the impact of resistance on antiretroviral activity that is not seriously confounded by activity of other drug components in the background regimen. Readers are encouraged to consult the literature and experts in the field for clarification or more information about specific mutations and their clinical impact. Polymorphisms associated with impaired treatment responses that occur in wild-type viruses should not be used

in epidemiologic analyses to identify transmitted HIV-1 drug resistance. For more in-depth reading and an extensive reference list, see the 2008 IAS–USA panel recommendations for resistance testing (Hirsch MS, Günthard HF, Schapiro JM, et al, Clin Infect Dis, 2008;47:266–285).

> **Updates and reference list are posted at www.iasusa.org**

USER NOTES

a. Some nucleoside (or nucleotide) analogue reverse transcriptase inhibitor (nRTI) mutations, like T215Y and H208Y,[1] may lead to viral hypersusceptibility to the nonnucleoside analogue reverse transcriptase inhibitors (NNRTIs), including etravirine,[2] in nRTI-treated individuals. The presence of these mutations may improve subsequent virologic response to NNRTI-containing regimens (nevirapine or efavirenz) in NNRTI-naive individuals,[3-7] although no clinical data exist for improved response to etravirine in NNRTI-experienced individuals. Mutations at the C-terminal reverse transcriptase domains (amino acids 293–560) outside of regions depicted on the figure bars may prove to be important for nRTI and NNRTI HIV-1 drug resistance. The clinical relevance of these connection domain mutations arises mostly in conjunction with thymidine analogue-associated mutations (TAMs) and M184V and have not been associated with increased rates of virologic failure of etravirine or rilpivirine in clinical trials.[8-10]

b. The 69 insertion complex consists of a substitution at codon 69 (typically T69S) and an insertion of 2 or more amino acids

(S-S, S-A, S-G, or others). The 69 insertion complex is associated with resistance to all nRTIs currently approved by the US FDA when present with 1 or more thymidine analogue–associated mutations (TAMs) at codons 41, 210, or 215.[11] Some other amino acid changes from the wild-type T at codon 69 without the insertion may be associated with broad nRTI resistance.

c. Tenofovir retains activity against the Q151M complex of mutations.[11] Q151M is the most important mutation in the complex (i.e., the other mutations in the complex [A62V, V75I, F77L, and F116Y] in isolation may not reflect multidrug resistance).

d. Mutations known to be selected by thymidine analogues (M41L, D67N, K70R, L210M, T215Y/F, and K219Q/E, termed TAMs) also confer reduced susceptibility to all approved nRTIs.[12] The degree to which cross-resistance is observed depends on the specific mutations and number of mutations involved.[13–16]

e. Although reverse transcriptase changes associated with the E44D and V118I mutations may have an accessory role in increased resistance to nRTIs in the presence of TAMs, their clinical relevance is very limited.[17–19]

f. The M184V mutation alone does not appear to be associated with a reduced virologic response to abacavir in vivo. When associated with TAMs, M184V increases abacavir resistance.[20,21]

g. As with tenofovir, the K65R mutation may be selected by didanosine, abacavir, or stavudine (particularly in patients with nonsubtype-B clades) and is associated with decreased viral susceptibility to these drugs.[20,22,23] Data are lacking on the potential negative impact of K65R on clinical response to didanosine.

h. The presence of 3 of the following mutations—M41L, D67N, L210W, T215Y/F, K219Q/E—is associated with resistance to didanosine.[24] The presence of K70R or M184V alone does not decrease virologic response to didanosine.[25]

i. K65R is selected frequently (4%–11%) in patients with nonsubtype-B clades for whom stavudine-containing regimens are failing in the absence of tenofovir.[26,27]

j. The presence of M184V appears to delay or prevent emergence of TAMs.[28] This effect may be overcome by an accumulation of TAMs or other mutations.

k. The T215A/C/D/E/G/H/I/L/N/S/V substitutions are revertant mutations at codon 215 that confer increased risk of virologic failure of zidovudine or stavudine in antiretroviral-naive patients.[29,30] The T215Y mutant may emerge quickly from 1 of these mutations in the presence of zidovudine or stavudine.[31]

l. The presence of K65R is associated with a reduced virologic response to tenofovir.[11] A reduced response also occurs in the presence of 3 or more TAMs inclusive of either M41L or L210W.[11] The presence of TAMs or combined treatment with zidovudine prevents the emergence of K65R in the presence of tenofovir.[32–34]

m. The sequential use of nevirapine and efavirenz (in either order) is not recommended because of cross-resistance between these drugs.[35]

n. Resistance to etravirine has been extensively studied only in the context of coadministration with darunavir/ritonavir. In this context, mutations associated with virologic outcome have been assessed and their relative weights (or magnitudes of impact) assigned. In addition, phenotypic cutoff values have been calculated, and assessment of genotype-phenotype correlations from a large clinical database have determined relative importance of the various mutations. These 2 approaches are in agreement for many, but not all, mutations and weights.[36–38] The single mutations Y181C*/I*/V*, K101P*, and L100I* reduce clinical utility. The presence of K103N alone does not affect etravirine response.[40] Accumulation of several mutations results in greater reductions in susceptibility and virologic response than do single mutations.[41–43]

o. Fifteen mutations have been associated with decreased rilpivirine susceptibility (K101E/P, E138A/G/K/Q/R, V179L, Y181C/I/V, H221Y, F227C, and M230I/L).[44–46] A 16th mutation, Y188L, reduces rilpivirine susceptibility 6 fold.[47] K101P and Y181I/V reduce rilpivirine susceptibility approximately 50 fold and 15 fold, respectively, but are uncommonly observed in patients receiving rilpivirine.[48–50] K101E, E138K, and Y181C, each of which reduces rilpivirine susceptibility 2.5 fold to 3 fold, occur commonly in patients receiving rilpivirine. E138K, and to a lesser extent K101E, usually occur in combination with the nRTI resistance mutation M184I, which alone does not reduce rilpivirine susceptibility. When M184I is combined with E138K or K101E, rilpivirine susceptibility is reduced approximately 7 fold and 4.5 fold, respectively.[50–53]

p. Often, numerous mutations are necessary to substantially impact virologic response to a ritonavir-boosted protease inhibitor (PI).[54] In some specific circumstances, atazanavir might be used unboosted. In such cases, the mutations that are selected are the same as with ritonavir-boosted atazanavir, but the relative frequency of mutations may differ.

q. Resistance mutations in the protease gene are classified as "major" or "minor."

Major mutations in the protease gene (positions in **bold** type) are defined as those selected first in the presence of the drug or those substantially reducing drug susceptibility. These mutations tend to be the primary contact residues for drug binding.

Minor mutations generally emerge later than major mutations and by themselves do not have a substantial effect on phenotype. They may improve replication of viruses containing major mutations. Some minor mutations are present as common polymorphic changes in HIV-1 nonsubtype-B clades.

r. Ritonavir is not listed separately, as it is currently used only at low dose as a pharmacologic booster of other PIs.

s. Many mutations are associated with atazanavir resistance. Their impacts differ, with I50L, I84V, and N88S having the greatest effect. Higher atazanavir levels obtained with ritonavir boosting increase the number of mutations required for loss of activity. The presence of M46I plus L76V might increase susceptibility to atazanavir when no other related mutations are present.[55]

t. HIV-1 RNA response to ritonavir-boosted darunavir correlates with baseline susceptibility and the presence of several specific PI mutations. Reductions in response are associated with increasing numbers of the mutations indicated in the figure bar. The negative impact of the protease mutations I47V, I54M, T74P, and I84V and the positive impact of the protease mutation V82A on virologic response to darunavir/ritonavir were shown in 2 data sets independently.[56,57] Some of these mutations appear to have a greater effect on susceptibility than others (e.g., I50V vs V11I). A median darunavir phenotypic fold-change greater than 10 (low clinical cutoff) occurs with 3 or more of the 2007 IAS–USA mutations listed for darunavir[58] and is associated with a diminished virologic response.[59]

u. The mutations depicted on the figure bar cannot be considered comprehensive because little relevant research has been reported in recent years to update the resistance and cross-resistance patterns for this drug.

v. In PI-experienced patients, the accumulation of 6 or more of the mutations indicated on the figure bar is associated with a reduced virologic response to lopinavir/ritonavir.[60,61] The product information states that accumulation of 7 or 8 mutations confers resistance to the drug.[62] However, there is emerging evidence that specific mutations, most notably I47A (and possibly I47V) and V32I, are associated with high-level resistance.[63–65]

The addition of L76V to 3 PI resistance–associated mutations substantially increases resistance to lopinavir/ritonavir.[55]

w. In some nonsubtype-B HIV-1, D30N is selected less frequently than are other PI mutations.[66]

x. Clinical correlates of resistance to tipranavir are limited by the paucity of clinical trials and observational studies of the drug. The available genotypic scores have not been validated on large, diverse patient populations. The presence of mutations L24I, I50L/V, F53Y/L/W, I54L, and L76V have been associated with improved virologic response to tipranavir in some studies.[67–69]

y. Resistance to enfuvirtide is associated primarily with mutations in the first heptad repeat (HR1) region of the gp41 envelope gene. However, mutations or polymorphisms in other regions of the envelope (eg, the HR2 region or those yet to be identified) as well as coreceptor usage and density may affect susceptibility to enfuvirtide.[70–72]

z. The activity of CC chemokine receptor 5 (CCR5) antagonists is limited to patients with virus that uses only CCR5 for entry (R5 virus). Viruses that use both CCR5 and CXC chemokine receptor 4 (CXCR4; termed dual/mixed [D/M] virus) or only CXCR4 (X4 virus) do not respond to treatment with CCR5 antagonists. Virologic failure of these drugs frequently is associated with outgrowth of D/M or X4 virus from a preexisting minority population present at levels below the limit of assay detection. Mutations in HIV-1 gp120 that allow the virus to bind to the drug-bound form of CCR5 have been described in viruses from some patients whose virus remained R5 after virologic failure of a CCR5 antagonist. Most of these mutations are found in the V3 loop, the major determinant of viral tropism. There is as yet no consensus on specific signature mutations for CCR5 antagonist resistance, so they are not depicted in the figure. Some CCR5 antagonist-resistant viruses selected in vitro have shown mutations in gp41 without mutations in V3;[73] the clinical significance of such mutations is not yet known.

aa. Cross-resistance studies with raltegravir- and elvitegravir-resistant viruses in vitro indicate that Q148H and G140S in combination with mutations L74I/M, E92Q, T97A, E138A/K, G140A, or N155H are associated with 5-fold to 20-fold reduced dolutegravir susceptibility[74] and reduced virologic suppression in patients.[75–81] Results of the phase III dolutegravir study in antiretroviral treatment-naive patients are expected to provide additional resistance information.

bb. Six elvitegravir codon mutations have been observed in integrase strand transfer inhibitor treatment-naive and -experienced patients in whom therapy is failing.[82–88] T97A results in only a 2-fold change in elvitegravir susceptibility and may require additional mutations for resistance.[85,86] The sequential use of elvitegravir and raltegravir (in either order) is not recommended because of cross-resistance between these drugs.[85]

cc. Raltegravir failure is associated with integrase mutations in at least 3 distinct genetic pathways defined by 2 or more mutations including (1) a signature (major) mutation at Q148H/K/R, N155H, or Y143R/H/C; and (2) 1 or more additional minor mutations. Minor mutations described in the Q148H/K/R pathway include L74M plus E138A, E138K, or G140S. The most common mutational pattern in this pathway is Q148H plus G140S, which also confers the greatest loss of drug susceptibility. Mutations described in the N155H pathway include this major mutation plus either L74M, E92Q, T97A, E92Q plus T97A, Y143H, G163K/R, V151I, or D232N.[89] The Y143R/H/C mutation is uncommon.[90–94] E92Q alone reduces susceptibility to elvitegravir more than 20-fold and causes limited (< 5 fold) cross resistance to raltegravir.[84,95–97] N155H mutants tend to predominate early in the course of raltegravir failure but are gradually replaced by viruses with higher resistance, often bearing mutations G140S plus Q148H/R/K, with continuing raltegravir treatment.[90]

These updated figures and additional information about the IAS–USA Drug Resistance Mutations Group are also available on the IAS–USA Web site (www.iasusa.org). To purchase copies of this card, call (415) 544-9400, e-mail the request to info2013@iasusa.org, or write to IAS–USA, 425 California Street, Suite 1450, San Francisco, CA 94104-2120. For permission to reprint or adapt the figures, please contact the IAS–USA.

Reprinted with permission from the IAS–USA. Johnson VA, Calvez V, Günthard HF, Paredes R, Pillay D, Shafer RW, Wensing AM, and Richman DD. Update of the drug resistance mutations in HIV-1: March 2013 *Topics in Antiviral Medicine*. 2013;21(1): 6–14. ©2013 IAS–USA. Updated information and User Notes are available at www.iasusa.org.

Appendix 2

SELECTED KEY INTERNET RESOURCES

- AIDSinfo—A Service of the Department of Health and Human Services (www.aidsinfo.nih.gov)
- Chronic Hepatitis C: Current Disease Management (http://digestive.niddk.nih.gov/ddiseases/pubs/chronichepc/)
- Clinical Care Options (www.clinicaloptions.com/HIV.aspx)
- Comprehensive HIV/AIDS Resource (www.thebody.com)
- Hep C Connection (www.hepc-connection.org)
- HIV Drug Interactions: www.HIV-druginteractions.org
- HIV Hepatitis Resources (www.mpaetc.org/hep)
- HIV and Hepatitis.com (www.hivandhepatitis.com)
- HIV and Observations (blogs.jwatch.org/hiv-id-observations/)
- International AIDS Society—USA (www.iasusa.org)
- Johns Hopkins Hepatitis C and HIV Coinfection Information (www.hopkins hivguide.org/diagnosis/opportunistic_infections/viral/full_hepatitis_c.html)
- Journal Watch: AIDS Clinical Care (aids-clinical-care.jwatch.org)
- Medscape HIV/AIDS (www.medscape.com/hiv)
- National AIDS Treatment Advocacy Project (www.natap.org)
- National Clinicians' Post-exposure Prophylaxis Hotline (www.ucsf.edu/hivcntr/Hotlines/PEPline.html)
- National HIV/AIDS Clinicians' Consultation Center (www.nccc.ucsf.edu/)
- National Institute of Allergy and Infectious Diseases (www3.niaid.nih.gov/)
- National Library of Medicine—AIDS Portal (sis.nlm.nih.gov/hiv.html)
- National Library of Medicine—MedlinePlus AIDS page (www.nlm.nih.gov/medlineplus/)

REFERENCE

1. Krakower D, Kwan CK, Yassa DS, Colvin RA. iAIDS: HIV-Related Internet Resources for the Practicing Clinician <http://www.ncbi.nlm.nih.gov/pubmed/20738185>. Clin Infect Dis 2010, Aug 25.

INDEX